THE ENCYCLOPEDIA OF

# THE DIGESTIVE SYSTEM
# AND
# DIGESTIVE DISORDERS

THE ENCYCLOPEDIA OF

# THE DIGESTIVE SYSTEM
# AND
# DIGESTIVE DISORDERS

Anil Minocha, M.D.
Christine Adamec

☑®
Facts On File, Inc.

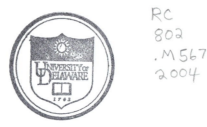

## The Encyclopedia of the Digestive System and Digestive Disorders

Facts On File, Inc.
132 West 31st Street
New York NY 10001

### Library of Congress Cataloging-in-Publication Data

Minocha, Anil.
The encyclopedia of the digestive system and digestive disorders / Anil Minocha, Christine Adamec.
p. cm.
ISBN 0-8160-4993-9 (alk. paper)
1. Gastrointestinal system—Encyclopedias. 2. Digestive organs—Encyclopedias. 3. Gastrointestinal system—Diseases—Encyclopedias. 4. Digestive organs—Diseases—Encyclopedias.
[DNLM: 1. Digestive System—Encyclopedias. 2. Digestive System Diseases—Encyclopedias. WI 13 M666e 2004] I. Adamec, Christine A., 1949- II. Title.
RC802.M567 2004
616.3'003—dc222003021432

Facts On File books are available at special discounts when purchased in bulk quantities for businesses, associations, institutions, or sales promotions. Please call our Special Sales Department in New York at (212) 967-8800 or (800) 322-8755.

You can find Facts On File on the World Wide Web at http://www.factsonfile.com

Text and cover design by Cathy Rincon

Printed in the United States of America

VB FOF 10 9 8 7 6 5 4 3 2 1

This book is printed on acid-free paper.

Dr. Minocha would like to dedicate this book to his loving parents, Ram S. Minocha and Kamla Devi Minocha, and to his daughter, Geeta P. Minocha.

Christine Adamec would like to dedicate this book to her husband, John Adamec, in grateful appreciation of his continued support throughout this project.

# CONTENTS

# FOREWORD

I am both a practicing gastroenterologist and a medical school professor, as well as an author of medical journal articles and self-help books for the general public, such as *How to Stop Heartburn* and *Natural Stomach Care.* My different roles dovetail to provide me with a broad and current overview of both common and rare diseases and disorders of the digestive system. From these perspectives, I perceive the present as a very exciting time of major advances. In fact, a broad array of amazing diagnostic and therapeutic breakthroughs has occurred over the course of my career, and I have also seen the development of many exciting new techniques and treatments that help patients with digestive diseases and disorders.

Let me illustrate with just a few examples to show readers how far medical science has advanced in the field of digestive health in a relatively short period. In the not-so-distant past (in the 1980s and the early 1990s), many physicians worldwide believed that peptic ulcers (painful sores of the stomach and of the duodenum, which is the upper part of the small intestine) were solely caused by severe stress and/or diets high in fatty or spicy foods. Now doctors know that the majority of ulcers are caused by bacteria called *Helicobacter pylori* and that most of the remaining ulcers are caused by medications, primarily nonsteroidal anti-inflammatory drugs (NSAIDs) that are taken for other illnesses such as arthritis.

This knowledge has effectively enabled physicians to prevent the recurrence of ulcers by treating them with antibiotics (if the cause is bacterial) or by recommendation of the avoidance of ulcer-inducing medications, if the cause is an NSAID medication. If NSAIDs must be used, an additional medication to protect against the ulcerogenic effect can be taken along with the NSAID. We physicians also offer newer medications with high-tech names like *proton pump inhibitors* that decrease the level of stomach acidity and give the stomach a chance to recover from the ulcer.

Even more exciting than this breakthrough in peptic ulcer disease is the fact that medical researchers have made dramatic advances in diagnosing and treating cancer, which have the potential to extend the lives of patients for years. Colorectal cancer, the second most prominent form of cancer in the United States, can be readily screened with tests, not just the fecal occult blood test (FOBT) or the colonoscopy, a procedure that enables physicians to look inside the colon and small intestine and check for disease, but also a virtual colonoscopy! Tests that are now available can check the stool for genetically altered cells that are shed by a colonic tumor.

Wireless endoscopy has arrived, allowing physicians a noninvasive means to visualize regions of the small bowel that are not easily within the reach of standard endoscopy, thus increasing the likelihood of pinpointing the causes of obscure gastrointestinal bleeding and other digestive problems.

Medical science has also identified risk factors for colorectal cancer as well as many other forms of cancer and other digestive diseases and disorders; thus, provided with a complete medical history, doctors know the illnesses for which they should especially screen their patients. If the colonoscopy identifies polyps that may be precancerous, they can be removed, averting the risk of damage and death from colon cancer.

More good news is that improvements in sanitation save lives of people worldwide as individuals are educated globally about the importance of identifying and avoiding contaminated food and water. (Sadly, however, this is not always possible for all individuals.)

We have known about the effects of bacteria for more than a hundred years, but despite this knowledge, many patients worldwide have died of illnesses such as bacterial and parasitic infections that were transmitted through contaminated food and water. As recently as the 20th century, many babies died in infancy because of severe diarrhea, which was often caused by a bacterial or viral infection. Simple awareness of the need to wash hands frequently and to clean meats and vegetables has enabled many infants and children to live normal lives. However, many people still suffer from a variety of different infectious diseases including parasitic infections that are primarily caused by poor sanitation. So not everyone is aware of the importance of cleanliness.

Many digestive enigmas have not been resolved yet. There remains much to learn, and important research continues. For example, many forms of cancer are still rapid killers, such as pancreatic cancer or esophageal cancer, which frequently cause no symptoms or signs until the disease is far advanced. Other diseases and disorders, although they usually do not kill patients, may cause them misery for years or even for decades, such as Crohn's disease or irritable bowel syndrome. However, because of medical advances, instead of wearing an osteomy bag after the removal of the colon for ulcerative colitis, patients now have the option of having newer surgeries that allow continent bowel function through the anal canal. Future scientific findings should improve the digestive health of many more citizens of the world.

Sometimes even prosperity causes a worsening of some digestive diseases. One unfortunate "side effect" of the general well-being of many people that is seen in the United States and other developed countries has been an increase in obesity, which itself leads to an increased risk of many other digestive diseases and disorders, such as gallstones, stomach and liver cancer, high cholesterol level, and diabetes.

In fact, more than half of all Americans and Canadians are overweight, and many people in Europe and on other continents are also excessively heavy. This is a problem, because obesity itself increases the risk for development of many health problems, such as heart disease, high blood pressure, diabetes, stroke, and other diseases and disorders. A 2003 study published in the *New England Journal of Medicine* found a direct correlation between body weight and the development of many forms of cancer, including major digestive cancers such as colorectal cancer and stomach cancer. These topics are covered in this book.

There are other health problems that can directly or indirectly lead to digestive diseases or disorders. Alcoholism leads to numerous digestive diseases, including heart disease, pancreatitis, vitamin and mineral deficiencies, and, for some people, damage and destruction of the liver (liver cirrhosis), for which the only cure may be a liver transplantation.

Another questionable habit of about a quarter of all Americans is cigarette smoking, which contributes to many digestive diseases and makes others worse. Patients who have Crohn's disease worsen with continued smoking, as do individuals who have gastroparesis (slow stomach emptying). Paradoxically, smoking is protective against ulcerative colitis.

In this volume, I provide a comprehensive overview of the major as well as the less well-known digestive diseases and disorders, including a definition and a description of the disease and what is known about what causes it (if anything). I also provide information on the epidemiological characteristics of the disease or disorder, which identify the people for whom the condition is most likely to be contracted or developed.

My coauthor and I also explain how most doctors diagnose digestive diseases and disorders, discussing the laboratory tests and diagnostic tests that are used to determine whether the disease is present and to rule out other diseases. In addition, we provide information on treatments for diseases—if there are any available treatments. (Sadly, sometimes there is no known treatment or cure for a digestive disease or disorder.) In many cases, there are actions that patients can take to improve their condition: changing their diet, losing weight, avoiding certain activities, requesting specific laboratory tests, and so forth. Even something as seemingly minor as raising the level of the head end of the bed or using a reflux wedge can provide significant pain relief to many patients with chronic heartburn.

My personal goals with *The Encyclopedia of the Digestive System and Digestive Disorders* are to provide a basic overview of digestive illnesses to nonphysician readers so that they can be better educated and they can also be aware of key questions to ask their physicians. Knowing that I could not describe all of the information on every digestive disease that can possibly be contracted or developed, I have selected the major illnesses that may occur as well as an assortment of rare diseases. I hope that readers find this encyclopedia to be helpful and informative.

—Anil Minocha, M.D.

# ACKNOWLEDGMENTS

The authors would like to thank Marie Mercer, reference librarian at the DeGroodt Public Library in Palm Bay, Florida, for her assistance in locating very hard-to-find journal articles on many different digestive diseases and conditions. In addition, they would like to thank Mary Jordan, interlibrary loan librarian at the Central Library Facility in Cocoa, Florida, for her research assistance.

# INTRODUCTION AND HISTORY OF DIGESTIVE DISEASES AND DISORDERS

The digestion of food is necessary to allow life to continue. This fact is as true today, in the 21st century of high technology and a dazzling array of medications and therapeutic medical devices, as it was when humans actively hunted or farmed for the food that they needed to survive. Modern computerized equipment and even the most remarkable discoveries and improvements in medicine that have occurred since the dawn of humankind cannot change one unalterable fact: everyone needs to eat and to digest food in order to stay alive; the only other option is feeding through tubes or intravenously, both of which are prone to complications.

The Wall Street genius, the street child, and the retired person in a nursing home all share the common need to feed, along with every other human who is alive on the planet, although the components of their diet and even the way they eat may vary quite considerably. The gourmet delicacies that may be taken for granted by the wealthy are very different from the garbage scraps that a street child must subsist on, and both of these types of food are also very different from the nutrition that is directly placed into the feeding tube or the intravenous line of the severely ill nursing home or hospital patient. But to the digestive system, whether it is oysters and elegant chocolate that are consumed by a person or leftover fast food from the trash can, or material that is inserted into a feeding tube, it is all basically the same thing: food that must be broken down, processed, used up, and its waste material eliminated, for the primary purpose of keeping the individual alive. (Note that the food that is placed into the body intravenously is already processed or digested and need only be assimilated into the body for its use.)

The need for nutrition occurs even before birth. The fetus is nourished in the mother's womb through the umbilical cord. After the baby is born, whether the child is fed with mother's breast milk or with baby formula, the infant's digestive system actively works to extract everything needed for its continued life as well to propel the child forward on a course of active growth and development. This need for food and the necessity to digest the food continue on until death.

Of course, sometimes the digestive system malfunctions and does not properly digest the food that is ingested. A broad array of problems can also occur with the digestive system, ranging from transient and easily correctable illnesses to chronic and/or severe problems that must be treated by physicians. In most cases, doctors can provide efficacious medications, procedures, and treatments to improve the broad array of digestive diseases and disorders that many people experience. In other cases, serious diseases, such as colorectal cancer, can be detected in time with procedures such as colonoscopies, and often patients with early stages of colorectal cancer can be cured. Sometimes, as with some forms of advanced cancers of the esophagus or pancreas, physicians can only keep patients as pain-free as possible while the illness implacably progresses to destroy the organs and the patient's life.

It is very easy to take the digestive system for granted, and most people do so until a peptic ulcer, gastroesophageal reflux disease, or another digestive ailment develops.

# A Marvel of Cooperation: The Digestive System

Digestion is an amazingly complicated process. The digestive system manages a marvelous process that no machine could possibly duplicate in its thousands or perhaps millions of interactive tasks, both with other organs and with the blood, the bones and nerves, and other systems of the body.

The food that is so necessary to sustain life must be completely broken down with special enzymes and digestive juices and then absorbed and assimilated by the body, in a complex symphony of cooperation among many different organs. In the digestive system—which includes the oral cavity, the esophagus (the food tube that connects to the stomach), the stomach, the pancreas, the liver, the gallbladder, the small intestine, and the colon— several organs play critically important roles in managing the very complex process of digestion and absorption. The process begins when a person takes the very first bite of food, and it continues on until there is no further use for what is left, and that in turn is excreted from the body, transformed into fecal matter.

Actually, however, rather than a start–stop type of operation, the digestive system is nearly a "24–7" operation that rarely shuts down altogether. Often while breakfast and a midmorning snack are being processed and assimilated, a person may be eating lunch, and, thus, the stomach, the small intestine, and the colon are all involved in various processes of breaking down and absorbing the nutrients from food, and ultimately in excreting what is left over and not needed in the fecal mate-

rial. No factory on Earth could sustain such a continuous operation for 70 or more years of life, and it is not surprising that in the digestive system minor and major problems develop in the course of an individual's life.

*When the Digestive System Goes Awry* Sometimes problems with digestion arise from factors that may stem from within or from outside a person's body. At some point in their life most people's digestive system will malfunction in a minor and usually a self-correcting way, such as when a person has stomachache and heartburn caused by eating too much of a heavy holiday meal that did not "agree" with the body in some minor way, causing stomach pain or diarrhea. In most cases, the body successfully and eventually rids itself of the excessive or disagreeable food or illness, and the signs and symptoms of disease go away too.

At other times an individual's digestive system malfunctions in a far more serious way, and cancerous growths, inflammatory diseases, or other severe and possibly life-threatening chronic medical problems, such as pancreatitis (an inflammation of the pancreas), cirrhosis (dangerous scarring) of the liver, or other very serious digestive diseases and disorders, develop. In other cases, problems develop but may not manifest immediately, such as gallstones that increase in number and that may in some but not all cases cause pain and/or infection or pancreatitis that requires an individual to have surgery.

*Considering Food-Borne and Waterborne Illnesses* Digestive problems can also be caused by influences impinging from outside the body. Nearly all individuals have been affected by a food-borne illness, whether they realize it or not. Often illness is caused by ingesting bacteria transmitted in some contaminated food prepared by someone who fails to wash the hands *after* using the toilet and before preparing food. Sometimes bacteria are passed on in contaminated water.

People who think that they have never had a digestive ailment that was caused by contaminated food or water may be right; however, most people who are affected by contaminated food or water experience relatively mild symptoms such as diarrhea, nausea, and a mild fever at some point in time, and they or their physicians often assume that their problem was caused by an unknown virus that is said to be "going around." Only if the individual's stools were actually analyzed and checked by a laboratory, a process that is not routinely performed in every case, could anyone know whether a digestive illness was or was not caused by food- or waterborne bacteria, parasites, or viruses. Even after exhaustive testing, sometimes an offending pathogen may not be identified.

Many people in the United States, Canada, and other developed countries assume that because their sanitation is usually significantly better in these countries when compared to general conditions that are found in developing countries, then infectious diseases causing digestive ailments just do not occur in their country. Although it is true that there are fewer per capita cases of diseases spread by contaminated food and water in developed countries, and certainly fewer fatalities, cases of food and water contamination clearly still happen. A study that was jointly conducted by the American Gastroenterological Association and TAP Pharmaceuticals revealed that an astounding estimated 135 million cases of food-borne digestive diseases occurred in the United States in 2000.

Sometimes large numbers of people are affected by digestive problems en masse, and in such cases, the cause is usually contaminated food. Although no one died in 1994 in a national outbreak of *Salmonella* poisoning, experts estimated that 224,000 people (nearly a quarter of a million individuals) became very ill as a result of eating contaminated ice cream. According to an article describing the case and the discovery of the probable cause in a 1996 issue of the *New England Journal of Medicine,* the experts believed that because pasteurized premixed ice cream, made in Minnesota and distributed nationwide, was transported in tanker trucks that had previously carried unpasteurized eggs, contamination by those eggs led to the infection with *Salmonella* organisms that made so many people extremely sick.

In some cases, an infection affecting the digestive system is spread in unclean water, as in Milwaukee, Wisconsin, in 1993, when more than 400,000 people became sick from *Cryptosporidium* bacteria that were ingested from contaminated water.

### Medications Can Cause Digestive Diseases

There are also many other causes of digestive illnesses beyond contaminated food and water; for example, medications can cause many short- or long-term digestive problems. Nonsteroidal antiinflammatory drugs (NSAIDs) that are taken to alleviate the severe and chronic pain of arthritis or other illnesses can also be harmful to the stomach, and their use has led to the development of peptic ulcers in thousands of patients. The use of acetaminophen (Tylenol) in high doses can also harm the liver, especially among individuals with alcoholism. Many other medications that are prescribed for a broad array of illnesses may cause the side effects of nausea, vomiting, diarrhea or constipation, heartburn, and other distressing side effects.

Sometimes narcotics that are prescribed to treat chronic and severe pain can lead to digestive problems, such as severe constipation, narcotic bowel syndrome, and even fecal impaction. Whenever possible, patients need to work with their doctors to taper off the narcotic gradually, as well as to take laxatives and consume plenty of fluids and fiber to keep their bowels working well.

### A Combination of Causes May Exist

The body can be affected by *both* internal and external influences. For example, the excessive consumption of alcohol can lead to disease of the liver and the pancreas. The ailing and weakened liver or pancreas may then cause the individual to become more prone to development of cancerous tumors or other internal problems.

Often it is a combination of causes that results in digestive diseases; for example, when people who have a diet that is heavy in caffeine, fatty foods, and alcohol, along with an innate genetic propensity for development of the disease, diseases such as gastroesophageal reflux disease (GERD) as well as other digestive disorders, can result. In other cases, nontreatment of an existing disease such as GERD can result in a precancerous condition such as Barrett's esophagus, which eventually may lead to esophageal cancer, a very difficult form of cancer to treat.

It is also true that some medical problems are associated with a risk of development of a digestive disease; for example, hepatitis C, when it leads to liver cirrhosis, can increase the risk of the development of liver cancer. Patients with diabetes are often at risk for development of gastroparesis, or slow stomach emptying. Many illnesses are correlated with other illnesses. They are not inevitably linked, but the probability is greater when a patient has one disease that he may also suffer from other specific diseases. It is important to remember, however, that medicine is an art as well as a science, and statistics may not apply to an individual.

### Severe Symptoms Do Not Always Indicate the Presence of Severe Diseases   It is also interesting to note that the presence of pain is not always an indicator of a severe digestive problem, just as the absence of pain does not mean a disorder is a minor one. Some relatively minor and correctable digestive diseases, such as the early stages of chronic acid reflux (gastroesophageal reflux disease), may cause far more discomfort than is seen in some cases of cancerous tumors of the digestive system. For this reason, recurrent digestive problems should be discussed with physicians, and individuals should also have regular physical examinations to help detect any underlying medical problems.

### Many People Experience Digestive Diseases and Disorders   Digestive diseases are very common, and according to the Centers for Disease Control and Prevention (CDC), in the National Ambulatory Medical Care Survey, released in 2002, patients in the United States made nearly 38 million office visits to physicians for symptoms that were related to the digestive system in 2000. About 12.5 million office visits to doctors were specifically due to the complaints of stomach pain, cramps, and spasms. In addition, doctors diagnosed a digestive disease in 29.4 million patients in 2000.

Many patients feel so ill that they do not wait to see a doctor in an office but instead go to the nearest emergency room. There were about 13.4 million visits to emergency rooms in 2000 by people

with symptoms that were related to the digestive system, according to the CDC.

Among the 108 million visits to the emergency room for all purposes in 2000, about 6.8 million visits were for stomach and abdominal pain, cramps, and spasms.

### Differences among People Who Have Digestive Diseases and Disorders   Digestive diseases are not randomly dispersed by gender, age, and ethnicity; for example, men are more likely to be diagnosed with cancer of the esophagus than women. In the United States, men have a greater risk of development of cirrhosis of the liver, liver cancer, and stomach cancer, as well as alcoholic pancreatitis and hemochromatosis than women. On the other hand, women in the United States face a higher risk than men for development of gallstones, gallbladder cancer, and irritable bowel syndrome.

In looking at ulcer disease only, according to data provided by the National Center for Health Statistics, about 2 million females of all ages suffer from ulcers, compared to 1.7 million men. Men are more likely to suffer from frequent indigestion. About 1.9 million males younger than age 45 have frequent indigestion, compared to 1.3 million females. Children may also suffer from many different digestive diseases; nearly 2 million children younger than age five have a digestive disorder.

The overall incidence of digestive diseases may also vary by age. Often, middle-aged and older people are more likely to have digestive diseases; however, in some cases, younger people are more likely to be diagnosed with diseases. For example, most people who are diagnosed with Crohn's disease, a severe inflammatory disease of the colon and/or the small intestine, are between the ages of 10 and 30 years. Middle-aged and older people are more likely to suffer from most cancers.

Sometimes there are racial and ethnic differences among people suffering from one digestive disease or another; for example, blacks are more than three times more likely than whites to have sarcoidosis, a systemic disease that can harm the digestive system, just as they are much more likely to be diagnosed with hepatocellular carcinoma, a form of severe liver cancer. In addition, blacks are more likely to suffer from adverse consequences of an infection with hepatitis C, whereas whites are more likely to suffer from Barrett's esophagus and its related esophageal cancer (adenocarcinoma).

Combined risk factors may increase the odds of development of a digestive disease or disorder; for example, in considering gender and age, women between the ages of 20 and 60 years have double to triple the risk of development of gallstones of men of the same age. In considering race and gender, black women have a higher risk than others of development of type 2 diabetes.

*Considering Possible Genetic Links*   Many diseases also have a genetic basis, and if a parent or sibling is diagnosed with a digestive disorder, such as polyps in the colon or cancer, this often indicates that the health risk of development of the illness is increased for other family members. This is true of hemochromatosis, celiac sprue, diabetes, most forms of cancer, and many other digestive diseases and disorders. Of course, diagnosis of an illness in a relative does not mean that everyone in the family is doomed to development of the disease as well. It means, however, that often the risk is increased for development of the disease, and, thus, it is important for patients to report such a family history to physicians.

*Taking into Account the Value of Lifestyle Changes*   When a digestive disease or disorder is diagnosed by a physician, patients need to know what, if anything, they can do about their illness. In many cases, lifestyle changes, such as giving up smoking and drinking, losing weight, and sleeping properly, can improve chronic digestive disorders. However, in many cases, patients also need to have medications and other treatments.

## Looking at the Gastrointestinal System

To understand digestive diseases and disorders, it is important to have a basic understanding of the gastrointestinal system and the organs that it comprises and an understanding of the digestive process itself. Digestion actually begins at the mouth, where individuals produce the saliva that helps to break down the food even before it enters the esophagus and begins its passage down the gastrointestinal system.

The gastrointestinal system is primarily composed of a series of connecting hollow and looping tubes. This system processes and moves food along it, breaking down the food for fuel. The digestive system starts with the mouth and throat, proceeding on to the gut, which begins with the esophagus (the food tube) and continues on through the stomach and small intestine, where the absorption of most nutrients occurs. It ends at the colon, also known as the large intestine, where the unused excrement is eliminated via the rectum and through the anus.

Of course, there are other important organs that are actively involved in digestion as well. The gallbladder, the pancreas, and the liver are all intimately involved in providing special secretions of the enzymes and substances that are essential in order to break down and absorb the food that individuals consume into usable energy to fuel the body for yet another day.

The gallbladder, pancreas, and liver can also malfunction—become infected, inflamed, or cancerous—as well as experience other medical problems. For example, the person's body may store too much iron (hemochromatosis), causing damage to the liver, the pancreas, and the heart, or too much copper (Wilson's disease), causing an overload of metal that can become dangerous or toxic to the liver and the brain. Occasionally, the first manifestation of Wilson's disease may be a life-threatening fulminant hepatic failure, which necessitates an urgent liver transplantation.

*When Problems Develop in the Digestive System*   Most of the time, the digestive system works very well for most individuals. However, millions of people of all ages, from infancy to their retirement years, suffer from an array of acute or chronic digestive ailments in their lifetime. Such disorders are so prevalent in society that virtually every family, at some point in time, can name family members who are touched by a significant digestive illness, whether it is gastroenteritis, colorectal cancer, a peptic ulcer, or another disease or disorder. Billions of dollars are spent each year in treating these diseases with medications, hospitalizations, and outpatient visits to physicians.

There are also indirect economic costs of digestive diseases; for example, according to the National Center for Health Statistics, Americans lose nearly 14 million workdays per year because of digestive problems. Days are also lost from school or from family events because the person is simply too ill to participate in these activities.

In 2001, the American Gastroenterological Association (AGA), with TAP Pharmaceuticals, released the results of an extensive survey of digestive disorders. The results surprised even the participating gastroenterologists in the study. Said Mark Donowitz, a member of the AGA's study advisory board and a professor of medicine at Johns Hopkins University, "We expected the study to reveal a high burden, but we had no idea how titanic that burden would be, and because this study only includes 17 out of 300 digestive disorders, even these results do not fully reflect the burden."

Some of these results, which Dr. Donowitz said are actually conservative in their estimates, are summarized in the table.

**MAJOR CHRONIC DIGESTIVE DISEASES AND NUMBER OF SUFFERERS IN THE UNITED STATES, 2000***

| Disease | Number of Sufferers (in Millions) |
| --- | --- |
| Gallbladder disease | 20.5 |
| Gastroesophageal reflux disease | 18.6 |
| Irritable bowel syndrome | 15.4 |
| Peptic ulcer disease | 6.7 |
| Total | 61.2 |

*Data provided by a study conducted by the American Gastroenterological Association and TAP Pharmaceutical Products, released in May 2001. The total does not include cancers and other major chronic or acute diseases, digestive diseases and disorders.

**INCIDENTS OF GASTROENTERITIS IN 2000***

| | |
| --- | --- |
| **Food-borne** | 135 million cases |
| **Nonfood-borne** | 76 million cases |

*Data provided by a study conducted by the American Gastroenterological Association and TAP Pharmaceutical Products, released in May 2001.

**Costs of Gastrointestinal Diseases**   In their analysis of the numbers of incidents and the costs of gastrointestinal diseases, the American Gastroenterological Association and TAP Pharmaceuticals found that the costs of five digestive diseases

totaled nearly $28 billion in the United States in 2000. The costs in 2003 were at least that high and probably significantly greater.

| Disease | Estimated Cost (in Billions of Dollars)* |
| --- | --- |
| Gastroesophageal reflux disease | 10.0 |
| Gallbladder disease | 6.5 |
| Colorectal cancer | 5.3 |
| Peptic ulcer disease | 3.4 |
| Diverticular disease | 2.6 |
| Total Cost of Five Diseases | 27.8 |

*Data provided by a study conducted by the American Gastroenterological Association and TAP Pharmaceutical Products, released in May 2001.

**Considering the Statistics**   The statistics provided in these tables are not all-inclusive: they do not even include most digestive diseases because they do not include all of the cancers of the gastrointestinal system, such as cancer of the liver, the stomach, the pancreas, the gallbladder, or the esophagus. For example, 24,000 people are diagnosed with stomach cancer each year in the United States.

It is also very important to note that the statistics from this study can provide only a snapshot of the estimated annual numbers of incidents of key digestive diseases; however, the pervasiveness and pain of gastrointestinal diseases are actually much greater. For example, according to the Centers for Disease Control and Prevention (CDC), one in every 10 Americans suffers from peptic ulcer disease in his or her lifetime. When all digestive diseases, in addition to ulcers, cancers, and the many other ailments that may occur, are considered together, the problem is clearly an enormous one.

**Ignorance May be Harmful or Even Deadly**
Many people are ignorant of the basics of digestive diseases; for example, most people have no idea that at least 50 to 90 percent of all peptic (stomach and duodenal) ulcers are caused by bacteria known as *Helicobacter pylori.* Most of the rest of ulcers are caused by nonsteroidal anti-inflammatory drugs (NSAIDs). A few of the non–*H. pylori,* non-NSAID ulcers may be caused by newly discovered bacteria called *Helicobacter heilmaniis.*

Most people continue to believe mistakenly that if they alleviate stress in their life as much as possible and eat right, then they will feel better. The reality is that only antibiotics can cure an ulcer that was caused by bacteria and prevent it from recurring. Acid blocking medications temporarily heal an ulcer, but an ulcer due to *H. pylori* infection is likely to return unless the patient takes antibiotics. Similarly, patients with history of or at risk for NSAID-induced ulcers need preventative treatment with cyclooxygenase-2 (COX-2) inhibitors and/or NSAID prophylaxis with another medication to combat the ulcerogenic effect of the NSAID. Untreated ulcer disease can further accelerate, causing blood loss, anemia, and other medical complications, including perforation of the stomach or the small intestine, resulting in life-threatening illness.

Knowledge of digestive diseases can help patients and their physicians counteract the impact of the disease. Information and education cannot eradicate all digestive diseases, but they can help people to obtain diagnoses in the early stages of disease, when they are usually easier to treat, and to avoid behavior that worsens the digestive system, such as smoking, overeating, failing to exercise, and drinking to excess.

## A Global Look at Digestive Diseases and Disorders

Some digestive diseases that are unknown or very rare in the United States, Canada, and other developed countries are very common in the poorer countries of the world. It is unthinkable to most individuals that more than a few people could actually die of diarrhea or dehydration, and yet that is what happens every day to many people living in some countries in Africa and Asia, primarily because of contaminated food and water, and also because of the extreme overcrowding of the population, combined with poor or nonexistent medical care.

According to the World Health Organization (WHO), 1.7 million people die each year worldwide primarily as a result of infectious diarrhea that is spread by contaminated water and poor sanitation. In fact, diarrheal diseases represent the

third leading infectious cause of death in the world. Ninety percent of those who die are children.

Cholera is one of the diseases that cause diarrhea, and in 2000, a team at the National Institute of Allergy and Infectious Diseases (NIAID) broke the code on the deoxyribonucleic acid (DNA) sequence of *Vibrio cholerae*. The scientists discovered that many of the genes that constitute *Vibrio cholerae*, the bacterium that causes cholera, are similar to those found in *Escherichia coli*. Further study should provide extremely helpful information for combating cholera.

Acquired immunodeficiency syndrome (AIDS), caused by the human immunodeficiency virus (HIV), is one of the most deadly infectious diseases in the world. According to the National Institute of Allergy and Infectious Diseases, there were 36.1 million people worldwide in 2000 who had HIV/AIDS, including 1.4 million children below the age of 15 years. The overwhelming majority of AIDS cases (95 percent) occur in developing countries, and 70 percent of the patients live in sub-Saharan Africa. An estimated 600,000 children were newly infected with HIV in 2000.

HIV infection and AIDS increase the risk of development of many digestive infections and diseases, because of the compromised immune system that results from the disease. People with AIDS are more likely than others to have anal cancer, anemia, anal warts, rectal fissures, esophagitis, pernicious anemia, Kaposi's sarcoma, non-Hodgkin's lymphoma and, pancreatitis. Because of the high prevalence of AIDS and HIV in developing countries, such digestive problems are common.

Malnutrition and undereating are major digestive problems today, and many people in the world are severely malnourished and underweight. According to *The World Health Report 2002*, there were 170 million underweight children living in poor countries in 2002, and 3 million children die of underweight each year in countries in Asia and Africa. Most of the underweight children are younger than five years old. According to the World Health Organization in their 2003 report on chronic diseases worldwide, 60 percent of the 10.9 million deaths of children below the age of five years were either caused by or associated with malnutrition.

It seems highly ironic that at the other extreme from malnutrition lies the problem of overeating that causes obesity, which is also an increasing health problem in both developed and many developing countries. Obesity often leads to the development of type 2 diabetes and of nonalcoholic fatty liver disease (NAFLD) and many other digestive diseases and health problems. According to the World Health Organization, more than 500,000 people in North America and Europe died of obesity-related illnesses in 2000, including 220,000 people in the United States and Canada and 320,000 people in the 20 countries of Western Europe. WHO estimates that there are about 150 million people worldwide with type 2 diabetes, and this number is expected to double by 2025, primarily because of projected increases in China and India. Diabetes, of course, predisposes one to many digestive illnesses.

Parasitic diseases causing diarrhea and other digestive ailments are also very common in poor countries, where children and adults are more likely to be exposed to protozoa, worms, and other parasites that cause infections. In some cases, these infections not only damage the digestive organs, but also may cause medical problems outside the gut, such as in the lungs, the heart, and the brain. Parasitic infections weaken infected individuals, making them more susceptible to the ravages of bacterial and viral infections transmitted in contaminated food and water, as well as airborne pathogens.

Another major problem throughout the world is the presence of severe vitamin and mineral deficiencies. According to the WHO, iron deficiency is a highly prevalent problem. WHO estimates that *two billion* people worldwide may have an iron deficiency, which causes nearly a million deaths each year.

Children and their mothers are at the greatest risk for suffering from iron deficiencies, because of the high need for iron during growth and pregnancy. Vitamin A deficiency is another serious problem, and it is a key cause of acquired blindness among children. Other severe deficiencies globally include iodine deficiencies, which can cause thyroid damage, and zinc deficiencies, which may result in a variety of disorders, such as dermatitis, short stature, and impaired immune function, and also leads to an increase of diarrhea, malaria, and

respiratory infections. There are also still many children and adults in the world who suffer from deficiencies of vitamin C and vitamin D, as well as of many other vitamins.

## Considering Modern Threats to Digestive Health

A new fearsome threat emerged with the attack on the World Trade Center on September 11, 2001, when Americans and people in many other countries realized the fragility of life and the potential power of terrorism. Key people in federal, state, and municipal governments immediately began to rethink scenarios in which bacterial and viral strains could theoretically cause severe digestive diseases and other types of diseases leading to permanent harm or even fatalities. For example, anthrax causes not only respiratory illness but also causes a predominantly digestive illness leading to death. It is beyond the scope of this book to describe how to resolve such problems; however, it is clear that an awareness of them is both chilling and necessary at this time.

On the plus side, it appears that the governments in the United States and other countries have developed effective systems to maintain far greater vigilance since September 11 to deal with potential terrorist threats and possible biological warfare that could lead to widespread disease and death. Scientists at NIAID and in other organizations in the United States, such as the Defense Advanced Research Products Agency, have accelerated their research on biological agents that may represent one element of the "weapons of mass destruction." Clearly, this is an issue of paramount importance to the United States, which invaded Iraq in 2003 because of the concern that Iraq was developing and possessed weapons of mass destruction, including biological agents. As of this writing, the occupying coalition forces have not found any weapons of mass destruction in Iraq.

In 2002, NIAID released their agenda on biological agents, including their key concerns about pathogens: botulism, anthrax, and plague agents. Said the investigators in their 2002 report, "Deciphering Pathogens: Blueprints for New Medical Tools,"

Scientists continue to decipher the genetic secrets of infectious microbes and the organisms that transmit them to people. By understanding the underlying genes that make those microbes tick, researchers will continue to make advances in the diagnosis, prevention, and treatment of infectious diseases.

Another issue to consider with regard to the transmission of digestive diseases, and particularly pathogens such as *E. coli,* is that many people travel extensively worldwide, and thus, diseases may be transmitted far more readily than in past years, when most people were far less mobile. In part because of globalization, some diseases that are not commonly found in the United States and Canada, for example, mad cow disease, may be transmitted. In addition, *E. coli* 0157:H7 is a relatively new and very virulent strain of *E. coli* bacteria, which causes hemolytic uremic syndrome in 10 to 15 percent of those who are infected by it. This is a very serious complication that can lead to kidney failure and death. Children and elderly individuals, as well as others who are immunocompromised (such as cancer patients, transplantation patients, or patients with AIDS) are especially at risk.

## Looking Back in Time

People have had digestive diseases throughout recorded time, and certainly they also had digestive illnesses well before written records were ever kept. The hunters and gatherers of the ancient past primarily faced death from other animals as well as from bacterial diseases such as tuberculosis and cholera and from some parasitic diseases (which still exist today) such as hookworm and trichinosis. The Pilgrims favored regular enemas as a key to a healthy digestive system. In the 18th and 19th centuries, antimony, arsenic, and mercury were remedies that were administered for ulcerlike symptoms.

Remedies to treat the common diseases of the time as well as the more exotic ailments of the esophagus, stomach, small intestine, colon, liver, and other digestive organs ranged from providing patients with medications that were copiously laced with opium or alcohol to giving treatments such as "bleeding" them or purging them with antiemetics that caused vomiting.

In considering food products alone, we have come a long way from past years, when dairy products were not pure because Louis Pasteur had not yet developed pasteurization. There was no Food and Drug Administration (FDA) in the United States, and consequently there was no regulation of foods or drugs. There were abuses in the meat industry, which first came very prominently to light in one chapter of Upton Sinclair's popular novel *The Jungle,* which caused such an intense furor that Congress passed a law regulating the meatpacking industry in 1938. In that same year, a law regulating foods and drugs was also passed.

In addition, many medications to treat diseases, such as penicillin, were not yet discovered. It was not until 1921 that the Canadian physicians Banting and Best discovered that insulin could be used to treat type 1 diabetes patients. Before their discovery, everyone who had that form of diabetes died, usually a slow and agonizing death.

### *Past Remedies for Digestive Complaints*
Treatments for digestive ailments through the ages have ranged from the possibly efficacious to the ridiculous and also to the dangerous. Doctors in past years did not have a basic knowledge of microbiology, the importance of sanitation, or the basic anatomy of the internal organs and did not know about many other aspects of medicine that are taken for granted today. In addition, many doctors in previous centuries received little or no training, other than an apprenticeship to an existing physician. Knowledge (and ignorance) about medicine was passed on from generation to generation. Some remedies that were actually useful in the past, such as use of senna (an ingredient in some modern laxatives) for constipation, ipecac (to treat some poisoning cases), and opium (narcotics that are still used in many painkilling drugs and anesthetics), are still used today.

In early America, Dover's powder, invented by Thomas Dover in 1740, was a popular medication for digestive disorders such as dyspepsia or dysentery. This concoction comprised 10 percent ipecac, 10 percent opium, and 80 percent potassium sulfate. Of course, such a concoction could not kill the bacteria or viruses that undoubtedly infected many people; however, some people eventually felt better, probably because their immune system destroyed the infection. However, they may have mistakenly attributed their improved health to the drug.

Some remedies for digestive ailments were quite bizarre; for example, the fifth-century Greek physician Anthimus considered bacon a cure for intestinal parasites and partridge flesh cooked in goat's milk a good remedy for dysentery.

Some ancient physicians did have a basic understanding of some diseases but did not have access to the medications and treatments of the 21st century. For example, the great physician Hippocrates believed that patients suffering from tuberculosis (also called "consumption" for many years and later the "white plague" because of the customary pallor it caused in patients) should leave the city for the country, rest, and eat nutritious foods. The famed physician Galen also recommended that patients with tuberculosis go to warmer climates and rest. He also noted the infectious nature of tuberculosis, in that people who slept in the same bed and shared clothes with an infected person often contracted tuberculosis.

From ancient times and until the early 20th century, digestive diseases were treated with narcotics and/or alcoholic drinks. In the Russia of the Middle Ages, scurvy (a vitamin C deficiency) was treated with gold in the form of gold leaf on bread. It was not until the 18th century that doctors and the general public finally realized that in the case of scurvy, lime juice is actually more effective than precious metals such as gold.

Some remedies for illnesses were truly startling. For example, according to Christine El Mahdy in her book *Mummies, Myth and Magic in Ancient Egypt,* from the 14th to the 16th century, wealthy Europeans believed that Egyptian mummies had amazing healing properties and that drinking a concoction that was composed of ground-up mummy dust would help to resolve many medical problems.

This remedy failed to work at all, and in fact, it reportedly (and not surprisingly) made the consumers who actually tried this concoction feel much worse. But for a while, this remedy was so popular that Egyptian mummy dust sellers ran out of old mummies, and the demand for the mummy dust created what amounted to almost a production line of mummies to satisfy the intense European demand for the alleged mummy dust cure.

Said the French surgeon Ambroise Pare, in decrying the mummy dust remedy as a treatment, "It causes great pain in their stomachs, gives them evil smelling breath and brings about serious vomiting."

Another popular remedy for a wide variety of diseases in England, and one that many people fervently believed in, was that the laying on of hands by particular people was curative. It was considered particularly beneficial to be touched by a king. According to Benjamin Lee Gordon in his book *Medieval and Renaissance Medicine,* in one instance, so many people surged forward to receive the "king's touch" from Charles II that seven people were trampled to death. King Charles's touch apparently had little therapeutic properties, and many people nevertheless died of scrofula, then a prevalent form of tuberculosis. Says Gordon, "It is of interest to note that more people died of scrofula during the time of Charles II than at any other period in English history."

For centuries, medical knowledge of the digestive system was lacking and/or mostly wrong. Physicians believed that "tickling" a patient's abdomen with the application of leeches would somehow take out the "bad blood." Bloodletting was also used to treat indigestion, constipation, and many other ailments.

Not all past medical recommendations were nonsensical. The 18th-century inventor, author, and political leader Benjamin Franklin, although he was not a physician, had some recommendations that doctors today would consider valid. According to Kirsner in *The Early Days of American Gastroenterology,* "Franklin's rules of health included a vegetarian diet, exercise, and the avoidance of tobacco."

Many digestive remedies available in the late 19th and early 20th centuries were concoctions that were liberally laced with alcohol, opium, or cocaine. These drugs were sold directly to consumers, who often had no idea which ingredients they included, since there were no labeling laws at the time and no Food and Drug Administration in the United States.

In the past, sometimes even the fashion of the day actually caused digestive ailments; for example, very tight corsets that constricted the stomach and abdomen could make smooth functioning of the digestive system difficult in some people (usually they were women who wore such garments). However, people who sneer at such fashions of the past should consider their own modern fashions; for example, some people in the 21st century favor wearing very tight-fitting jeans, which essentially have the same effect on the abdomen as did the Victorian corset.

### Medical Breakthroughs of the Nineteenth and Twentieth Centuries

A variety of medical discoveries made in the 19th and 20th centuries, now accepted as commonplace, have become invaluable to physicians and to patients with digestive diseases as well as other disorders; for example, Manuel Garcia invented the laryngoscope (the precursor to the endoscope) in 1855, and X rays were discovered by W. K. Roentgen in 1895. Joseph Lister first wrote about the effect of bacteria on wounds in 1867; unfortunately, it was years before his work demonstrating the necessity for sterile conditions was actually heeded by surgeons and other physicians.

It was also in the 19th century that Koch discovered both the tuberculosis and the anthrax bacteria and when August Gärtner in Germany first isolated *Salmonella* bacteria in a case of food poisoning. Then in 1928, Sir Alexander Fleming discovered penicillin, which was not used as a drug to treat humans with bacterial infections until it was first tried on soldiers in 1940. In 1944, Selman Waksman at Rutgers University discovered streptomycin and physicians began using the drug as an antibiotic. After this point, doctors began using antibiotics on a large scale in the United States and in other countries.

Surgery was an agonizing procedure in past centuries, and it was rarely done because it was so often fatal. The only available anesthetic drug for surgical patients was opium before Sir Humphry Davy discovered nitrous oxide in 1798 and J. C. Warren and then W. Morton developed ether in 1846. Since then, many anesthetics that allow virtually pain-free surgery have been developed by researchers.

Breakthroughs in medical procedures occurred as well in the 18th and 19th centuries; for example, the first cholecystectomy (removal of the gallbladder) in the United States was performed in 1867. However, at that time (and in many cases, for years afterward), many people with digestive disorders requiring surgery did not have the surgery and either recovered from their illness or died.

Medical devices and therapeutic techniques were developed and improved in the 20th century; for example, the semiflexible gastroscope, a device invented by Rudolf Schindler in 1932, preceded the flexible endoscope that was later developed by Basil Hirschowitz in 1957. Endoscopic ultrasonography, an ultrasound method of imaging the internal organs through an endoscope placed into the gut lumen, was first developed in the 1980s.

The development of ultrasound technology further advanced the ability of physicians to diagnose many different digestive diseases and disorders; for example, studies have shown that the use of ultrasound imaging of the appendix can provide physicians with an accurate diagnosis of appendicitis in the majority of cases.

Better tests were created for diagnosing disease, such as the Schilling test developed in 1953 to detect the presence of both pernicious anemia and vitamin $B_{12}$ malabsorption and breath tests created in the late 20th century to detect the presence of the *Helicobacter pylori* bacteria that cause the majority of peptic ulcers. Breath tests are also used to detect lactose intolerance.

Physicians also discovered illnesses that had previously not been identified and diagnosed, such as irritable bowel syndrome. Researchers and doctors have increasingly recognized and treated this common gastroenterological problem.

The formation of the American Gastroenterological Association in 1897 and of subsequent organizations such as the American College of Gastroenterology and the American Society for Gastrointestinal Endoscopy has further advanced the state of knowledge of digestive diseases and disorders. However, gastroenterology as a medical specialty did not actually "take off" until the 1950s and the 1960s, according to the medical historian Joseph B. Kirsner.

Other medical advances, including some truly amazing developments, occurred in the 20th century, such as the ability to perform liver transplantation. The first liver transplantations, performed in 1967 as heroic lifesaving measures, kept the patients alive briefly; for example, a one-and-a-half-year-old child lived for 400 days after a liver transplantation. Then in 1979, the antirejection drug cyclosporine came on the market. According to the physician Thomas E. Starzl in his chapter in *The Growth of Gastroenterologic Knowledge during the Twentieth Century,* "Of our first 12 liver recipients treated with cyclosporine and prednisone in the first 8 months of 1980, 11 lived for more than a year and 7 are still alive more than 12 years later."

Since Starzl's success with liver transplantations, some medical facilities have been successful with partial liver donations from living liver donors, usually for family members and friends.

### The Era of Health and Safety Regulations: The 19th Century to Today

In the United States and other developed countries, it is generally taken for granted that meat to be sold to the public will first be inspected for parasites and bacteria. It is also taken for granted that drug companies must perform massive clinical studies of new medications before physicians are allowed to prescribe these new drugs. Few people think about the existing government-dictated processes that sanitize the water or that sterilize dairy products in order to minimize the risk of harboring harmful pathogens that could be passed on to consumers. Most people do not thank an unknown government entity every time that they flush a toilet and the waste material goes somewhere far away from their home environment.

Health and sanitation requirements that are assumed to be the norm today were completely unknown in past centuries, when thousands of people died of diseases caused by infections spread through contaminated food or water. It is still true that in developing nations, the major cause of death among infants is diarrhea, which is usually caused by poor sanitation and a lack of medical treatment such as simple drugs taken for granted by people in developed countries.

In 1906 President Theodore Roosevelt signed into law the Food and Drugs Act, which banned the interstate commerce of misbranded and adulterated foods and drinks. On the same day in 1906 the Meat Inspection Act, based on the revelations of extremely unsanitary conditions that had led to diseases, was also passed. In 1938 the Federal Food, Drug and Cosmetic Act was passed, initiating the regulation of drugs. This law also required factory inspections and a variety of other procedures created for the public safety.

According to the Food and Drug Administration (FDA), its origin occurred in 1862, when President Lincoln appointed the chemist Charles M. Wetherill to the newly created Department of Agriculture. The Bureau of Chemistry later developed into the Food and Drug Administration. In 1883 Dr. Harvey W. Wiley, the "Father of the Pure Food and Drugs Act," expanded the bureau's work on food adulteration.

In 1927 the Bureau of Chemistry was subdivided into the Food, Drug, and Insecticide Administration of the Bureau of Chemistry and Soils. Then in 1930 the name was shortened to the Food and Drug Administration.

In 1962 on the heels of thousands of birth defects caused by thalidomide, introduced as a sleep remedy and for the nausea and vomiting of pregnancy, the Kefauver-Harris Drug Amendments were passed. They required pharmaceutical companies to prove to the FDA that their products were safe before they were allowed to sell them. In 1973 the U.S. Supreme Court upheld the court-challenged 1962 law.

In response to deaths caused by adulterated Tylenol, in 1983 Congress passed the Tamper-Resistant Packaging regulations, making it a crime to tamper with packaged consumer products. In 1990 Congress passed the Nutrition Labeling and Education Act, requiring all packaged foods to provide nutritional information and standardizing such terms as *low-fat* and *light.*

Because of the intense consumer interest in vitamin and mineral supplements, in 1994 Congress passed the Dietary Supplement Health and Education Act, which classifies dietary supplements as foods rather than drugs and does not require manufacturers to prove their products are safe or effective. Instead, the FDA can remove products from the market only if it finds that they were unsafe.

## Looking to the Future

Many exciting advances lie ahead in the near-future for patients with digestive diseases and disorders and the physicians who treat them; for example, in wireless capsule endoscopy, patients swallow a tiny camera that is about the size of a capsule, which then transmits imaging information to the cordless receiver that is worn by the patient. The data on the receiver set can then be downloaded to a computer so that the doctor can view the capsule in the gut lumen as it travels down the patient's gastrointestinal system. If problems are detected, further diagnostic and therapeutic procedures and a "regular" endoscopy can then be performed on the patient. As of this writing, there are several limitations to the wireless camera (also known as a pill or capsule camera), such as that it is primarily used for visualization of the areas hard to reach through endoscopy such as the small intestines.

The virtual colonoscopy is also in use in a few medical centers, where radiologic imaging enables physicians to image the colon to determine whether polyps or other potential medical problems are present. In addition, modern advances may allow patients to forgo bowel purging when they have a virtual colonoscopy, purging that is still a requirement for the standard colonoscopy. If problems are noted in the virtual colonoscopy, then patients will have a standard colonoscopy so that their physicians can remove any existing polyps, as well as take biopsy specimens or perform any other actions that are needed when disease is present. The virtual colonoscopy has been investigated for its effectiveness in colorectal cancer screening and it may be as good as real-time colonoscopy; however, therapeutics cannot be done, and if a lesion is found, the patient has to have a full colonoscopy.

Research actively continues on the genetic causes of diseases, and this information has the potential to be extremely helpful to doctors and patients. If doctors know that a patient has a family history of a disease that is largely or even partly hereditary, they can then test the patient for those diseases and therefore may be able to provide treatment early on in the course of the illness, before any long-term ill effects will have occurred. Such testing is already commonly done for families with a medical history of familial adenomatous polyposis and hemochromatosis.

Researchers are also studying methods of treating serious illnesses such as inflammatory bowel disease, rheumatoid arthritis, cancer, and other diseases with immunotherapy, to enable the body to fight off disease.

Colon cancer diagnostic breakthroughs are on the horizon; for example, first-generation stool tests to check for several genetic mutations in the tumor cells shed in stool are already available, and advanced stool testing for an expanded number of genetic mutations is being developed and should be available to the general public within several months to years of this writing. In addition, researchers are finding a potentially increased role for chemoprophylaxis to treat both Barrett's esophagus and prevent recurrence of colon polyps.

## Conclusion

Major and minor digestive diseases and disorders play a role in the lives of many people worldwide. Gone are the days when patients with digestive diseases were largely treated with opium, bloodletting, or enemas, and today many patients are fortunate to have their life extended by the major advances in diagnosis and treatment based on research that was performed in the past and that continues in the present. The future looks even brighter. At the same time, doctors cannot do everything for patients, and it is increasingly clear that, just as Benjamin Franklin believed in the 18th century, patients who desire good digestive health need to eat vegetables, and to exercise and to maintain (or to adopt) healthy lifestyle habits.

Ackerknecht, Erwin H., M.D. *A Short History of Medicine.* Rev. ed. Baltimore: Johns Hopkins University Press, 1982.

American Gastroenterological Association. "AGA Announces Results of Landmark Study: More than 283 Million Cases of Gastrointestinal Disease Cost at Least $42 Billion Dollars Annually." News release, May 21, 2001.

Blackwell, D. L., J. G. Collins, and R. Coles. "Summary Health Statistics for U.S. Adults: National Health Interview Survey, 1997." National Center for Health Statistics. *Vital Health Statistics* 10, no. 205 (2002).

Cherry, Donald K., and David A. Woodwell. Division of Health Care Statistics. "National Ambulatory Medical Care Survey: 2000 Summary." *Advance Data* no. 328 (June 5, 2002).

El Mahdy, Christine. *Mummies, Myth and Magic in Ancient Egypt.* New York: Thames & Hudson, 1989.

Food and Drug Administration. "The Story of the Laws behind the Labels. Part 1. 1906 Food and Drugs Act." *FDA Consumer,* June 1981.

Gordon, Benjamin Lee, M.D. *Medieval and Renaissance Medicine.* New York: Philosophical Library, 1959.

Hennessy, Thomas W., M.D., et al. "A National Outbreak of *Salmonella enteritidis* Infections from Ice Cream." *New England Journal of Medicine* 334, no. 20 (May 16, 1996): 1,281–1,286.

Joint World Health Organization and Food and Agriculture Organization of the United Nations. "Diet, Nutrition and the Prevention of Chronic Diseases: Report of a Joint WHO/FAO Expert Consultation." *WHO Technical Report,* Series 916. Geneva, Switzerland, 2003.

Kirsner, Joseph B. *The Early Days of American Gastroenterology.* Cedar Knolls, N.J.: Lippincott-Raven Healthcare, 1996.

Kirsner, Joseph B., M.D. *The Growth of Gastroenterologic Knowledge during the Twentieth Century.* Philadelphia: Lea & Febiger, 1994.

National Institute of Allergy and Infectious Diseases. "Deciphering Pathogens: Blueprints for New Medical Tools." National Institutes of Health, NIH Publication no. 02-4987, September 2002.

National Institute of Allergy and Infectious Diseases. "Microbes: In Sickness and in Health." National Institutes of Health, NIH Publication no. 01-4914, September 2001.

National Institute of Allergy and Infectious Diseases. "NIAID Global Health Research Plan for HIV/AIDS, Malaria, and Tuberculosis." Undated.

Petit, William A., Jr., M.D., and Christine Adamec. *The Encyclopedia of Diabetes.* New York: Facts On File, 2002.

Porter, Roy, ed. *Cambridge Illustrated History of Medicine.* Cambridge: Cambridge University Press, 1996.

Satin, Morton. *Food Alert! The Ultimate Sourcebook for Food Safety.* New York: Facts On File, 1999.

Schoenborn, Charlotte A., Patricia F. Adams, and Patricia M. Barnes. "Body Weight Status of Adults: United States, 1997–1998," *Advance Data from Vital and Health Statistics,* no. 330 (September 6, 2002).

Starzl, Thomas E. "The Contribution of Transplantation to Gastroenterologic Knowledge." In *The Growth of Gastroenterologic Knowledge during the Twentieth Century.* Philadelphia: Lea & Febiger, 1994.

World Health Organization. "The World Health Report 2002: Reducing Risks, Promoting Healthy Life." Geneva, Switzerland, 2002.

# ENTRIES A–Z

**abdominal pain**   Mild to severe discomfort that occurs in the midsection of the body. Abdominal pain may be caused by a variety of conditions, such as ULCERS, PANCREATITIS, CHOLECYSTITIS, biliary colic, CONSTIPATION, gastroenteritis, FOOD-BORNE ILLNESSES, infections, inflammation, menstrual cramps, or a reaction to a medication. The pain may be a temporary condition that lasts a few minutes to hours to a few days, or it may be chronic, lasting months to years. It may also be acute pain that is caused by APPENDICITIS or by other severe and acute life-threatening ailments that require medical or surgical treatment.

Sometimes abdominal pain is referred pain: the patient experiences pain at a site away from its actual source; for example, the pain of a gallbladder attack may be felt in the shoulder blade. Similarly the pain of a heart attack may be felt in the abdomen.

See also PAIN.

**achalasia**   An uncommon digestive disorder of the esophagus, in which the lower esophageal sphincter (the opening that allows food to move from the esophagus into the stomach) does not relax. In addition, peristalsis, which is the wavelike muscle movement that helps to propel the food downward, does not occur in the esophagus. Achalasia is due to the degeneration of the nerve cells of the myenteric plexus in the esophagus. The cause of this disorder is unknown, but it is speculated to be an autoimmune disorder.

### Risk Factors

Achalasia occurs in about one in 100,000 people, and men and women are affected equally. The disorder usually occurs in adulthood, in individuals who are between 25 and 60 years old.

### Signs and Symptoms

The major indicator of achalasia is dysphagia (trouble with swallowing). Most patients have difficulty swallowing liquids and solids. In addition, the majority of patients have difficulty with belching, although most patients must be specifically asked about this by their doctors, since it does not occur to them that having difficulty belching is a symptom of disease.

Other symptoms that may occur are as follows:

- Chest pain
- Heartburn
- Unintended weight loss
- Regurgitation of the food, undigested food ingested several hours or a day earlier, from the esophagus.

### Diagnosis and Treatment

Many patients have achalasia almost five years or more before they are diagnosed. Often they are treated for gastroesophageal reflux disease or other digestive disorders before achalasia is diagnosed.

Diagnostic tests for achalasia include the barium swallow test, which is nearly 95 percent accurate in diagnosing this condition. To confirm the presence of achalasia, doctors also usually order MANOMETRY to measure esophageal pressures. In addition, an ENDOSCOPY can be useful in diagnosis, especially to exclude any other diseases, such as cancer mimicking achalasia.

Achalasia cannot be cured, but it can be improved. Medications in the calcium channel blocker class and nitrates can help to relax the lower esophageal sphincter, although they may be effective over the short term only. Patients take these drugs sublingually (under the tongue) 10 to 15 minutes before eating meals.

Other treatments for achalasia include botulinum toxin (Botox) injections to relax the lower esophageal sphincter (LES) and pneumatic balloon dilation. Botulinum injections have been highly effective in some patients; however, the effect usually lasts only a few months and is reserved for patients who have other severe illnesses that preclude surgery as an option. Usually either a dilation of the LES via an endoscopy or a surgical myotomy is performed to improve achalasia. Since myotomy predisposes to increased acid reflux, some surgeons perform an antireflux procedure along with the myotomy.

**acid blocking agents**  Prescribed or over-the-counter medications that prevent acid formation in the stomach. Prescribed medications are generally but not always stronger and of longer duration than are over-the-counter medications. Both kinds of medications may be taken by people with chronic heartburn, which is also known as GASTROE-SOPHAGEAL REFLUX DISEASE. These medications also heal peptic ulcers.

See also ACID REFLUX; HEARTBURN; HISTAMINE-2 BLOCKERS; PROTON PUMP INHIBITORS.

**acid reflux**  A backward flow, in an upward direction, of acidified food (up from the stomach toward the mouth, rather than downward and toward the intestines). Some degree of acid reflux is normal in relation to meals. When acid reflux becomes excessive, and it causes symptoms or complications, it is then called GASTROESOPHAGEAL REFLUX DISEASE (GERD). Acid reflux is also sometimes referred to as heartburn. In addition to heartburn, chronic acid reflux may cause chest pain, asthma, hoarseness, loss of dental enamel, and bad breath. Long-standing acid reflux can cause a precancerous condition of the esophagus that is known as BARRETT'S ESOPHAGUS.

Excessive acid reflux or GERD can be treated with medications, such as over-the-counter (OTC) medications and prescribed ACID BLOCKING AGENTS, including ranitidine (Zantac), cimetidine (Tagamet), famotidine (Pepcid), omeprazole (Prilosec), lansoprazole (Prevacid), pantoprazole (Protonix), rabeprazole (Aciphex), and esomeprazole (Nexium).

GERD may also be treated with lifestyle recommendations, such as patients' avoiding eating heavy meals at night and sleeping with the head of the bed tilted upward. Patients who have chronic acid reflux should be evaluated by physicians if they have heartburn more than once a week, before their condition worsens further. Long-term acid reflux can lead to complications, including cancer.

See also HISTAMINE-2 BLOCKERS; PROTON PUMP INHIBITORS; ULCERS, PEPTIC.

Minocha, Anil, M.D., and Christine Adamec. *How to Stop Heartburn: Simple Ways to Heal Heartburn and Acid Reflux.* New York: John Wiley & Sons, 2001.

**acquired immunodeficiency syndrome**  AIDS, the disease that is caused by the human immunodeficiency virus (HIV) can create severe digestive problems, such as painful swallowing, abdominal pain, and DIARRHEA.

See also CACHEXIA; CANCER, ANAL; *CRYPTOSPORIDIUM*; CYTOMEGALOVIRUS; HUMAN IMMUNODEFICIENCY VIRUS; KAPOSI'S SARCOMA; FISSURE; FUNGI; PANCREATITIS; TROPICAL SPRUE; TUBERCULOSIS; WHIPPLE'S DISEASE.

**activated charcoal**  A remedy for a drug overdose. The charcoal is highly refined into very small particles to give it a very large surface area to which the poison or drug can attach, thus preventing the poison from becoming absorbed from the digestive tract and into the bloodstream. Use of activated charcoal has also been advocated for excessive gas, although its efficacy is controversial.

See also POISONS.

**acute abdomen**  A condition of sudden and severe abdominal pain. The condition is sometimes accompanied by nausea, vomiting, abdominal distention, failure of passage of the stools, or loose stools. Physicians take into account the location and severity of the pain as well as the patient's medical history and other symptoms and signs in order to make a diagnosis and determine the treatment that is needed. Some patients do not present with typical signs and symptoms, especially the elderly and the immune compromised, such as those who have DIABETES MELLITUS and acquired immunodeficiency syndrome (AIDS).

There are many different possible causes for acute abdomen, including an inflammation or rupture of the appendix, an obstruction such as a gallstone that is blocking the cystic duct and causing inflammation of the gallbladder (acute CHOLECYSTITIS), a stone in the ureter (ureteric colic), or an inflammation that is caused by either PANCREATITIS or DIVERTICULITIS. The medical problem may also be a systemic one, stemming from a Herpes zoster infection, a heart attack, or heavy metal poisoning. These are only a few of the many possibilities that physicians must consider when determining the cause of acute abdomen.

### Diagnosing Acute Abdomen

In addition to taking a medical history from the patient (or from others, if the patient is unable to provide sufficient details), the doctor performs a physical examination to ascertain where the pain is most severe and what its effects are on the adjacent structures and the rest of the body. Gentle pressure may reveal that an organ is enlarged or that a mass is present. A gentle tapping of the abdomen may reveal to the physician that there is a source of inflammation in the abdomen.

Physicians usually also order laboratory tests, such as a complete blood count. In cases of acute abdomen, whatever the cause, the white blood cell count is often higher than normal, especially when the cause is an infection or an inflammation. An elevation of the serum amylase level usually indicates the presence of PANCREATITIS, but an elevation may also occur with intestinal perforation.

An elevated level of serum bilirubin may indicate an overproduction of bilirubin due to a breakdown of red blood cells. This overproduction of bilirubin is seen with conditions such as a sickle cell crisis, a blockage of flow of bile through the bile ducts, with gallstones causing pancreatitis, or with liver disease.

A plain X ray of the abdomen is done to look for any intestinal obstruction or perforation. A computed tomography (CT) scan may reveal some evidence of the source of the pain, showing existing conditions such as pancreatitis, cholecystitis, and appendicitis. A CT scan may also indicate further complications, such as an abscess.

For patients who have ASCITES (fluid-filled abdomen), physicians may perform a diagnostic PARACENTESIS, in which fluid is withdrawn for laboratory analysis.

### Treatment

The treatment for acute abdomen is directly linked to the diagnosis. In some cases, exploratory surgery may be indicated, such as in an emergency or when APPENDICITIS is suspected; in other cases, the patients may be observed to see whether the condition improves or worsens. If the condition does not improve over the course of 24 to 48 hours, the physician may decide that exploratory surgery cannot be avoided.

See also ABDOMINAL PAIN.


**adhesions**    Scar tissue that occurs between different organs in the abdomen and between the loops of bowel, usually as a result of recent or long past surgery. Abdominal adhesions may cause abdominal discomfort or pain, even to the extent of causing an intestinal obstruction that may require surgery to break the adhesions and to relieve the obstruction.

See also ABDOMINAL PAIN; SURGERY.


**adolescents and digestive diseases**    Minor or major digestive upsets that occur to children who are in or who have already completed puberty (generally children between the ages of 12 and 18 years old). Adolescents may suffer from many of the same digestive diseases that affect adults, such as GASTROESOPHAGEAL REFLUX DISEASE, DIARRHEA, and CONSTIPATION. Some adolescents have EATING DISORDERS, such as ANOREXIA NERVOSA (self-starvation) or BULIMIA NERVOSA (self-induced vomiting, usually after bingeing on a large meal), which are problems that are more prevalent among adolescents (particularly female adolescents) than adults.

Many adolescents also suffer from OBESITY, which is a matter of deep concern to health officials and educators, because adolescents who are obese find it particularly difficult to attain a normal weight in adulthood, when most are considerably less physically active than they are in their teenage years.

**albumin**    A protein that is synthesized by the liver and that circulates in the blood. Albumin performs many important functions in the body, such as maintenance of the plasma oncotic pressure. This pressure holds water inside the blood vessels. If the albumin level is low, water then leaks out of the vessels, causing edema. Albumin also helps to transport numerous substances in the body.

If the liver is damaged, the albumin levels in the blood are decreased. Sometimes albumin is found in the urine, and that presence may be an indicator of kidney disease. In some kidney diseases, the loss of protein in the urine is so severe that blood levels are low. Low serum albumin level may also be a sign of MALNUTRITION.

**alcohol abuse and dependence/alcoholism**
Severe problem drinking, a disorder that may also cause serious heart as well as digestive diseases, such as cirrhosis of the liver, liver failure, and death. It also increases the risk for development of HEPATITIS. This form of hepatitis is usually caused by heavy drinking rather than by an infectious illness. Severe alcoholic hepatitis may be fatal.

The difference between alcohol abuse and alcohol dependence is a matter of degree and depends on whether or not physical dependency is present. Both forms of excessive alcohol consumption are injurious to health; chronic alcohol dependence is the worse of the two types.

Alcohol abuse is the chronic use of alcohol based on a strong psychological need. Conversely, alcoholism includes both a psychological and a physical dependency, and it is an even more serious problem than is chronic alcohol abuse. The Substance Abuse and Mental Health Services Administration (SAMSA) reports that about 7 to 10 percent of people in the United States have an alcohol problem. As a result, about 14 to 20 million people have serious problems with alcohol, and they also have risks of development of a variety of digestive diseases as well as other health problems.

Many people who are heavy drinkers are also heavy smokers, and the combination of the two types of behavior can worsen any existing digestive problems or create new health problems; for example, people who drink and smoke are more prone to development of various forms of CANCER such as esophageal cancer than are people who do not drink or smoke.

### Causes of Alcohol Abuse and Alcoholism
Experts disagree on the cause of alcoholism. It may be caused by a genetic factor or by biochemical abnormalities that predispose some individuals to the inability to limit their alcohol consumption. Social pressure may play some role in alcohol abuse, although few cultures condone chronic alcohol abuse or alcoholism.

### Alcohol and Digestive Problems
Both alcohol abuse and alcoholism can severely and permanently affect the digestive system (particularly the liver); although the effect on alcoholics is more profound, to the point that alcoholism may cause the patient's death from cirrhosis of the liver or from other digestive diseases. Alcoholism is also linked to an increased risk of development of STOMACH CANCER, ESOPHAGEAL CANCER, and COLORECTAL CANCER. It may cause ANEMIA, particularly among alcoholics who are eating very little food and who are obtaining most or all of their caloric intake from alcohol. Alcohol has poor nutritional value, although it has many calories.

Many alcoholics have vitamin deficiencies, which may be extremely severe. They may be particularly deficient in thiamine (vitamin $B_1$), and this deficiency may seriously damage the brain and may also cause memory and other intellectual problems.

Chronic heavy drinking can lead to alcoholic pancreatitis, an illness that causes severe abdominal pain and vomiting. Alcoholic men in their 40s have the greatest risk of development of alcoholic pancreatitis. This disease can cause death if it becomes severe. In general, the person with an attack of alcoholic pancreatitis may need to be hospitalized and given intravenous painkillers. He or she must subsequently give up alcohol completely, to increase the interval between attacks.

The alcoholic may also suffer from MALLORY–WEISS SYNDROME, a digestive disorder that is experienced by many alcoholics. This medical problem results in mild to heavy internal bleeding due to a tear in the area where the esophagus joins the stomach. It is usually caused by vomiting and retching, which are common actions among many people with severe alcohol problems.

Pregnant women who are heavy drinkers or alcoholics may cause their infant to suffer from fetal alcohol syndrome, a condition that is characterized by physical and intellectual deficits and birth defects.

### Risk Factors and General Information on Alcoholics in the United States

Males are more typically problem drinkers or alcoholics than females, although women can experience these problems as well. Women who are alcoholics are more likely to deny and/or to minimize their alcohol problem. In considering heavy chronic drinking, men are about four times as likely to fit an alcoholic pattern as women. Even among younger people, such as teenagers, it is usually adolescent boys who are heavy drinkers rather than teenage girls.

In looking at race alone, Hispanics and whites in the United States are the heaviest drinkers. Many Native Americans also have severe problems with alcohol abuse and alcoholism; for example, a 1995 study of car crash deaths caused by alcohol revealed that Native Americans and Alaska Natives had a rate of 19.2 crashes per 100,000, which was about three times the car crash death rate for African Americans (6.4) and whites (6.0).

### Indicators/Symptoms of Alcohol Abuse and Alcoholism

According to the National Institute on Alcohol Abuse and Alcoholism (NIAAA) in the United States, alcohol abusers meet at least one of the following criteria due to excessive drinking:

- They fail to fulfill their responsibilities at work, school, or home.
- They drive or operate dangerous equipment when under the influence of alcohol.

- They have been arrested for a problem related to alcohol, such as driving under the influence of alcohol or attacking someone when drunk.
- They drink despite family and relationship problems that are either caused or worsened by their excessive drinking.

Alcohol dependence is characterized by alcohol use that is associated with three or more of the following indicators:

- Tolerance
- Withdrawal symptoms
- Use of a substance in a larger quantity than is intended
- Persistent desire to cut down or control use of alcohol
- Significant time spent obtaining, using, or recovering from the substance
- Neglect of social, occupational, or recreational tasks
- Continued use despite physical and psychological problems

### Diagnosis of Alcoholism

A screening test may be used to screen whether alcohol is a problem for a person: the CAGE questionnaire. It asks the following questions:

- Have you ever felt the need to Cut down on your drinking? (C)
- Have you ever felt Annoyed by criticism of your drinking? (A)
- Have you ever had Guilty feelings about your drinking? (G)
- Have you ever taken a morning Eye opener? (E)

Even one positive response to the CAGE questions suggests the need for further evaluation. Giving two positive answers constitutes an 85 to 90 percent accurate indication of the diagnosis of alcohol abuse and/or alcohol dependency. One drawback is that this test may not differentiate between present and past alcohol abuse.

Physicians diagnose chronic alcohol abuse or alcoholism on the basis of behavior, information provided by family members, and laboratory tests of the blood and liver. Severe alcoholics may exhibit clearly visible symptoms of alcohol use, such as tremors (chronic shaking), bloodshot eyes, and difficulty in thinking. LIVER ENZYME/FUNCTION TESTS may be abnormal and an imaging scan of the liver may show an enlarged, inflamed, or damaged liver.

If the individual is going through acute alcohol withdrawal, which in its severest form is also known as delirium tremens, he or she is clearly ill and may exhibit hallucinations, confusion, hyperactivity, and seizures. The patient may also be severely dehydrated. Withdrawal symptoms are precipitated by the complete lack of alcohol in an alcoholic person, and usually they commence about 12 to 48 hours after the last drink was taken. Delirium tremens generally occur 48 to 72 hours after withdrawal from alcohol, but they may also occur as late as seven days after the last drink. People in this condition require inpatient treatment in a hospital.

### Treating Alcoholism

Residential treatment at a clinic is commonly used for long-term alcoholics, and there are many residential facilities in the United States, Canada, and other countries.

Some experts also treat patients with medications. In the past, disulfuram (Antabuse) was the drug most commonly used to treat alcoholism. An alcoholic person who took Antabuse and later consumed even a small amount of alcohol became violently nauseous and sick. More recently, experts have claimed some success with naltrexone (ReVia), a drug that blocks the pleasure centers of the brain, prevents the "high" from drug abuse and reduces the craving for alcohol. If the alcoholic normally obtains a feeling of euphoria and well-being from drinking, such feelings do not occur with drinking while naltrexone is in the system.

Persuading alcoholics to take any antidrinking medication is not easy, and they can be very resistant to this therapy. Often another person must administer the drug and must actually watch the person taking it to ensure that it is really taken.

Some alcoholics find success with antialcohol organizations such as Alcoholics Anonymous (AA), which require complete abstinence from alcohol and offer considerable support in helping the alcoholic achieve that goal. Alcoholics Anonymous, an international organization that has more than one million members in the United States in about 50,000 groups nationwide and an additional 770,000 members worldwide, was founded in 1935. AA does not charge dues, and the only membership requirement is a sincere commitment to drinking no alcohol (abstinence).

For further information, contact the following organizations:

Alcoholics Anonymous
Grand Central Station
P.O. Box 459
New York, NY 10163
http://www.alcoholics-anonymous.org

National Institute on Alcohol Abuse and
    Alcoholism (NIAAA)
6000 Executive Boulevard, Wilco Building
Bethesda, MD 20892
http://www.niaaa.nih.gov

See also ANEMIA; CANCER, COLORECTAL; CANCER, ESOPHAGEAL; CANCER, LIVER; CIRRHOSIS; HEPATOCELLULAR CARCINOMA; LIVER; LIVER FAILURE; LIVER TRANSPLANTATION; PANCREAS; PANCREATITIS; VITAMIN DEFICIENCIES; WERNICKE'S ENCEPHALOPATHY.

Bagnardi, Vincenzo, et al. "Alcohol Consumption and the Risk of Cancer." *Alcohol Research & Health* 25, no. 4 (2001): 263–269.
Minocha, Anil, et al. "Impairment of Cognitive and Psychomotor Function by Ethanol in Social Drinkers." *Veterinary and Human Toxicology* 27 (1985): 533–536.

**alcoholic pancreatitis**   See ALCOHOL ABUSE AND DEPENDENCE/ALCOHOLISM.

**allergies, food**   An immune response of the body to certain foods that causes the body to release protective chemicals that may lead to reactions that may sometimes be severe and even life-threatening.

Some food allergies are extreme and may be fatal, such as a severe allergic reaction to eating peanuts. Some individuals are extremely allergic to common substances such as wheat. In other cases, the allergy may be a mild one.

Infants may be allergic to either cow's milk or soy milk. Children may be allergic to shellfish, cow's milk, peanuts, soy, wheat, eggs, tree nuts (walnuts, hazelnuts, and so forth), and fish. Adults with food allergies are most likely to be allergic to peanuts, tree nuts, fish, and shellfish.

Sometimes people may believe that they have become ill from a food allergy when, in fact, the food that they ate may have been contaminated with bacteria or other pathogens. Before assuming that a food allergy is present and fastidiously avoiding a food, patients should first consult their physician.

Digestive diseases may also be misdiagnosed as food allergies by patients. Persistent nausea and vomiting or chronic heartburn may be an indicator of another serious disease rather than a reaction to food, and patients should consult physicians for diagnosis and treatment. Untreated diseases such as gastroesophageal reflux disease or duodenal or gastric ulcers can become worse over time, when untreated.

### Food Allergies versus Food Intolerances

A food allergy is not the same as a food intolerance. A food intolerance may cause an adverse reaction, but it is not a reaction that is immunological in nature; for example, a lactase deficiency in a person causes lactose intolerance. The person is not allergic to milk or milk products; instead, he or she is unable to digest them because of an innate lactase deficiency. Another type of food intolerance is a reaction to food colorings or to some chemical additives, such as monosodium glutamate (MSG). The individual does not respond with an allergic reaction but instead may feel ill after consuming foods to which he or she is intolerant.

### Risk Factors

Patients who have shown allergic reactions to food in the past are at risk for other food allergies. Some gastrointestinal disorders and symptoms may be caused by food allergies, such as eosinophilic gastroenteritis. Food allergies also appear to "run" in families, and if a parent or sibling is highly allergic to a food, other family members may need to be tested for the allergy as well.

People who are allergic to one food are often allergic to other similar foods. This phenomenon is called cross-allergy. For example, if a person is allergic to shrimp, he or she may also need to avoid all shellfish, including lobster, crab, and crayfish.

### Symptoms and Signs

There are a variety of symptoms and signs of food allergies, ranging from a skin reaction to asthma and all the way to the most severe reaction, which is anaphylaxis, a medical emergency in which the allergic reaction usually occurs within a few minutes and can be rapidly fatal. The patient experiences nausea and vomiting, and the patient's tongue swells up. In addition, the patient's throat and the air passages start to close, and the patient experiences low blood pressure and then shock. If a person has a true anaphylactic reaction to a certain food, then the individual should respond rapidly to the administration of epinephrine (adrenaline). Additionally, steroids and antihistamines may be used, depending on the severity of the allergic reaction.

### Diagnosis and Treatment

If a patient has been treated and any crisis has passed, the physician attempts to work with the individual to analyze what foods were eaten in relation to when the reaction occurred. For example, a food eaten a week before a reaction is unlikely to have caused the reaction, since it would have been digested and excreted days before.

Doctors may recommend an elimination diet, in which specific foods, such as eggs or nuts or other suspected foods, are avoided. The patient observes whether he or she feels better when not consuming these foods. In some cases, physicians use scratch tests, in which a small amount of the suspected food extract is scratched on the skin, to determine whether there is any allergic reaction. Physicians may also use blood tests to check for food allergies, such as the radioallergosorbent test (RAST) and the enzyme-linked immunosorbent assay (ELISA). These tests determine whether there is a food-specific reaction in the blood.

Once the physician determines that there is a food allergy, and, if there is, the food or foods to which the patient is allergic, the patient is then instructed to avoid these foods. Sometimes this can be difficult: for example, peanuts and peanut oil are added to many foods; consequently, patients must carefully read the labels on food products. In addition, when eating out, it is important to advise the waiter that the patient is highly allergic to whatever the food is and that the waiter should check with the chef to make sure the problem food is not included in the meal. When dining with friends or others, it is very important to share the information about the food allergy.

### Food Allergies in Children

Food allergies in children can be particularly difficult for parents who cannot be with their children constantly to watch them, particularly as the children get older; in addition, children may be resistant to refusing foods to which they are allergic, simply because they want to avoid embarrassment. Parents must make it clear to children that it will be far more embarrassing to have a severe allergic reaction requiring hospitalization than to tell people about their food allergy and/or to refuse a food or fluid to which they are allergic.

### Anaphylaxis: It Can Be Fatal

As mentioned, the most severe allergic reaction to food is anaphylaxis. If untreated, the patient dies. The patient becomes rapidly sick and sicker and requires emergency medical attention. Patients who know that they are allergic to foods should self-inject with epinephrine if it is available. In the United States, the 911 emergency phone number should also be called immediately for an ambulance to treat patients with a reaction to a life-threatening food allergy.

In a study on anaphylaxis in children, reported in a 1997 issue of *Pediatrics,* researchers studied the causes of nonfatal anaphylaxis in 50 patients who were ages one to 19 years old. The researchers found that food was the cause of the anaphylaxis in 25 percent of the cases. (An allergic reaction to latex was even more common: 27 percent of the cases were attributed to that reaction.) Other common causes of anaphylaxis included reactions to

drugs (16 percent) and venoms (15 percent). Small percentages were severely allergic to radiocontrast dye given in diagnostic tests and to reactions to poison ivy. The cause could not be determined in 13 percent of the cases.

Most of the sick children presented with either respiratory or skin symptoms, such as swelling of the lips or face and urticaria. For some children, difficulty in breathing was the first symptom. Few of the children had gastrointestinal symptoms, and 93 percent had skin and/or respiratory symptoms.

The foods most commonly found to cause anaphylaxis in this group of children were nuts, peanuts, and seafood.

### Preventive Actions

Children and adults who have known severe food allergies should wear medical bracelets that state the allergies, their doctors' names, and other emergency information. They should also carry a syringe of epinephrine (adrenaline) to self-inject in the event of an emergency. Parents of minor children should be certain to alert school authorities and make sure that epinephrine is readily available for emergency use. Many schools have a no-drug policy, so children may be prevented from carrying their own syringe, even with a prescription. For this reason, it is imperative that other individuals are trained and alerted to treat the child, if necessary.

For further information, contact the following organizations:

American Academy of Allergy, Asthma and
 Immunology
611 East Wells Street
Milwaukee, WI 53202
(414) 272-6071
(800) 822-2762 (toll-free)
http://www.aaaai.org

Food Allergy & Anaphylaxis Network
10400 Eaton Place
Suite 107
Fairfax, VA 22030
(800) 929-4040 (toll-free)
http://www.foodallergy.org

See also CELIAC SPRUE; LACTOSE INTOLERANCE; TROPICAL SPRUE.

American Gastroenterological Association. "American Gastroenterological Association Medical Position Statement: Guidelines for the Evaluation of Food Allergies." *Gastroenterology* 120 (2001): 1,023–1,025.

Dibs, Susan D., M.D., and M. Douglas Baker, M.D. "Anaphylaxis in Children: A 5-Year Experience." *Pediatrics* 99, no. 1 (January 1997): E7.

O'Leary, Paula, M.D., and Fergus Shanahan, M.D. "Food Allergies." *Current Gastroenterology Reports* 4 (2002): 373–382.

**alternative medicine**  Nontraditional remedies and treatments, also known as complementary medicine. The use of alternative medicines including herbal medicines is based on belief and tradition that are passed on through the generations.

Alternative/complementary medicine includes taking vitamins and nutritional supplements as well as using treatments that are not considered mainstream: acupuncture, acupressure, hypnotherapy, relaxation therapy, yoga, tai chi, and many other treatments. Some patients are turning to the ancient Indian system of medicine known as Ayurveda, which relies upon herbal medications to treat and reorganize the "constitutional imbalances" that have led to disease in people. Many of these alternative remedies or treatments are oriented to people suffering from digestive diseases.

Some patients also use homeopathic remedies. The theory behind homeopathy is that a tiny amount of a substance that would normally be harmful (such as nux vomica, or poison nut) may be beneficial in resolving problems such as chronic heartburn. The amount of the drug is so heavily diluted that it is frequently undetectable.

Aromatherapy is another form of alternative medicine, which uses essential oils and their aromas to ease stress and improve health. Because many people who have digestive problems are under a great deal of stress (whether caused by their own personal problems, anxiety about their digestive disorders, or both), aromatherapy may be beneficial for some.

The alternative remedy market is a multibillion-dollar one in the United States and other countries, and in a study of 508 patients at the Veterans Administration Health Care System in Tucson, Arizona, most patients (50 percent) stated that they use some form of complementary medicine to treat their medical problems. In the United States, one key reason for this huge market was the passage of the Dietary Supplement Health and Education Act of 1994, explained in the next section. The other key reason for the use of alternative medicine is that many patients with chronic and serious illnesses are frustrated by traditional medicine's inability to provide disease and pain relief.

Alternative remedies may be extremely helpful to many people; however, some drugs that are considered natural may be dangerous, particularly if they purport to cure diseases such as diabetes, CANCER, and other serious ailments. In fact, some alternative remedies claim to cure many different diseases, in the same way as did remedies that were sold more than a hundred years ago, which were also useless. These panacea (cure-all) drugs especially should be avoided because they are rarely helpful and may be harmful.

### Dietary Supplement Health and Education Act of 1994

On the basis of this legislation, herbal remedies and vitamin supplements were thereafter regulated differently than both over-the-counter (OTC) and prescribed medications were. Prescribed medications and OTC drugs are regulated much more strictly. However, most consumers do not realize this, and they instead assume that the same government protections established for prescribed and OTC drugs apply to herbs and supplements.

### Problems with Alternative Medicine That Many People Are Unaware Of

One problem with alternative medicine is that many patients assume that if a drug is natural, such as virtually any herbal remedy or mineral supplement that they buy in a health food store or in a pharmacy, it must be completely safe. This is an erroneous belief, because some herbal remedies or supplements, just as with other medications, can be harmful to some individuals. For example, the herb *Ginkgo biloba* is a blood thinner, and if the patient is already taking a blood-thinning medication such as warfarin (Coumadin), the addition of the *Ginkgo biloba* could contribute to internal bleeding and, in rare instances, even to death.

For this reason, it is crucially important that patients who are taking herbal remedies or supplements (or even thinking about taking them) check with their doctor first to make sure that the herb or supplement will not be harmful to them and will not interact with any other medications they are taking. At the least, the drug should not be harmful. It would also be helpful if the drug provided the relief patients seek, although the federal law does not require scientific confirmation that the remedy is efficacious.

Most patients also do not realize that herbal remedies and supplements are only loosely controlled by the Food and Drug Administration (FDA), which can only order the removal of herbs or supplements if they are proved to be harmful. This is a different standard from the one the FDA follows for all prescribed drugs and over-the-counter (OTC) medications, which may not be sold until testing proves that they are effective. No such proof is required with alternative medicine. It is also easier for the FDA to remove prescribed drugs or OTC drugs if they are proved harmful.

The use of alternative medicines, including herbal medicines, is sometimes based on traditional beliefs and anecdotal records. As a result, if the herbal remedy or supplement does not appear to be dangerous, the FDA cannot pull it off the market. Although manufacturers of alternative remedies are supposed to limit the promises they make for their products, it appears that because of the sheer volume of thousands of products on the market, there may be little or no confirmation that they observe this rule.

### Benefits of Alternative Remedies

Despite the problems with alternative remedies, there are also many benefits that people may gain from their use. Some herbal remedies can improve digestion, constipation, and other digestive and health problems (although patients with chronic medical problems should be sure to see their physician to make sure that there are no serious medical risks).

### Popular Herbal Remedies for Digestion

Ginger may be very helpful for chronic digestive problems. According to Elke Langner, Ph.D., and her colleagues in their 1998 article in *Advances in Therapy,* "The active constituents of the [ginger] plant stimulate digestion and absorption but also exert a calming effect on the digestive tract. Ginger relieves constipation, cramps, and flatulence by gently increasing muscular activity in the digestive tract. Regular consumption has been proved to prevent gastritis."

Ginger is also commonly prescribed for the nausea and vomiting that are associated with pregnancy, even by mainstream physicians.

In addition to ginger, other herbs that are used to help people with digestive problems include chamomile, meadowsweet, and ginseng.

For further information, contact the following organizations:

National Center for Complementary and
  Alternative Medicine Clearinghouse
P.O. Box 8281
Silver Spring, MD 20907
(888) 644-6226 (toll-free)
http://nccam.nih.gov

Office of Dietary Supplements
National Institutes of Health
6100 Executive Boulevard
Room 3B01, MSC 7517
Bethesda, MD 20892
(301) 435-2920
http://dietary-supplements.info.nih.gov

See also FISH OIL; IRON; SELENIUM; VITAMINS DEFICIENCIES/EXCESSES.

Baldwin, Carol, M. R. N., et al. "A Profile of Military Veterans in the Southwestern United States Who Use Complementary and Alternative Medicine." *Archives of Internal Medicine* 162, no. 15 (August 12, 2002): 1,697–1,704.

Langner, Elke, Stefan Greifenberg, and Joeg Gruenwald. "Ginger: History and Use." *Advances in Therapy* 15, no. 1 (January/February 1998): 25–44.

Minocha, Anil, M.D., with David Carroll. *Natural Stomach Care.* New York: Penguin Putnam, 2003.

Minocha, Anil, M.D., and Christine Adamec. *How to Stop Heartburn: Simple Ways to Heal Heartburn and Acid Reflux.* New York: John Wiley & Sons, 2001.

**amebiasis** An infection of the intestine or liver that is caused by a parasite that can be found in the human intestinal tract or human feces: *Entamoeba histolytica*. About 40 to 50 million people worldwide experience amebiasis each year, and the disease accounts for an estimated 40,000 deaths per year. The infection is more common in poor countries, although outbreaks can occur in developed countries, such as when water is contaminated.

### Transmission of Amebiasis

Amebiasis is most commonly transmitted through contaminated food or water or contamination that results when people have failed to wash their hands after having a bowel movement and then prepare contaminated food to be consumed by others. The parasite in its cyst form is then transmitted in the food, which is swallowed by the new host. The person's digestive juices break down the cyst, and the parasite is then able to invade the body and grow, unless or until it is diagnosed and treated. The parasite can also be spread during anal intercourse. Usually, only the large intestines of the affected person are involved; however, the liver, lungs, heart, and even brain may also become infected.

### Symptoms

The majority of patients remain asymptomatic. Children, pregnant women, elderly individuals, and patients with cancer, alcoholism, human immunodeficiency virus (HIV), and immunodeficiency are more likely to have symptoms.

The infected person who experiences symptoms may not do so for one to three weeks or longer. When they occur, symptoms include ABDOMINAL PAIN, JAUNDICE, DIARRHEA, DYSENTERY, ANOREXIA, fatigue, and weight loss. If untreated, the PARASITIC INFECTION can cause ulcers in the colon and intestinal blockages, and it can also cause death if the parasite invades organs such as the liver or the brain.

### Diagnosis and Treatment

Physicians may suspect an amebiasis infection because of a patient's symptoms, but cannot be sure until a stool specimen is analyzed and yields a positive result. Blood tests for amebiasis are also used.

The physician may order a lower gastrointestinal study, such as a sigmoidoscopy or a colonoscopy. A liver abscess may be identified by ultrasound or by a computed tomography (CT) scan.

Medications such as metronidazole (Flagyl) are prescribed to destroy the parasite. Chlorine alone is not adequate to kill the amebic cysts when they are found in contaminated water; the water must be boiled. Disinfection with iodine is also effective. It is best to avoid sexual practices that lead to feco-oral contact.

See also CONTAMINATED FOOD OR WATER; PARASITIC INFECTIONS.

**American College of Gastroenterology** A professional organization that was formed in 1932 for physicians involved in the study and treatment of gastrointestinal disorders. The American College of Gastroenterology had about 7,000 members worldwide in 2003.

For further information, contact:

American College of Gastroenterology
4900 B South 31st Street
Arlington, VA 22206
(703) 820-7400
http://www.acgi.gi.org

Related organizations include the following:

American Gastroenterological Association
4930 Del Ray Avenue
Bethesda, MD 20814
(301) 654-2055
http://www.gastro.org

American Society for Gastrointestinal Endoscopy (ASGE)
1520 Kensington Road
Suite 202
Oak Brook, IL 60523
(630) 573-0600
http://www.asge.org

See also Appendix I.

**American Gastroenterological Association (AGA)** Founded in 1897, the American Gastroenterological Association is a nonprofit specialty organization of about 12,000 gastroenterologic physicians and researchers around the world. The AGA is a partner in hosting Digestive Diseases Week, an annual meeting of physicians and researchers interested in digestive diseases.

The AGA publishes *Gastroenterology,* a twice-monthly scientific medical journal. It also publishes guidelines on the diagnosis and treatment of numerous digestive disease and disorders.

For further information, contact the AGA:

American Gastroenterological Association
4930 Del Ray Avenue
Bethesda, MD 20814
(301) 654-2055
http://www.gastro.org


## American Society for Gastrointestinal Endoscopy

An organization that was founded in 1941 as a forum for physicians who perform endoscopies to diagnose and treat diseases of the digestive tract.

For further information, contact the organization:

American Society for Gastrointestinal Endoscopy
1520 Kensington Road
Suite 202
Oak Brook, IL 60523
(630) 573-0600
http://www.asge.org


**amylase**    An enzyme that is produced by the body to break down the carbohydrates in food. Saliva includes amylase in the first phase of digestion when food is first eaten. Most of the amylase that is seen in the blood is secreted by the pancreas so that the final digestion of carbohydrates can be completed in the intestine. Blood levels of amylase are elevated among patients with PANCREATITIS.


**amyloidosis**    A rare disease that is characterized by deposits of amyloid in the organs and tissues. Amyloid is composed of fibrils made up of small subunits of a variety of proteins, many of which may be seen circulating in the blood. The protein fragments may be deposited in the gastrointestinal system, the heart, the kidneys, the brain, the nerves, and the hand. When found in the gastrointestinal system, amyloidosis may cause slow gut motility, and cause GASTROPARESIS and MALABSORPTION syndrome. An estimated one in 100,000 people in the United States carries the genetic mutations for this disease.

There are two forms of amyloidosis: primary amyloidosis and secondary amyloidosis. Primary amyloidosis usually affects the tongue, the gastrointestinal tract, the thyroid gland, the liver, and the spleen. It may also affect the heart and can cause congestive heart failure. Secondary amyloidosis is usually found in conjunction with another disease that is present, such as rheumatoid arthritis or frequent infections. It is more likely to affect the kidneys, liver, and spleen and may also cause skin inflammation. Secondary amyloidosis may cause kidney failure.

### Risk Factors

The risk factors for amyloidosis are unknown, although genetic factors are known to be involved in many cases.

### Symptoms of Amyloidosis

Amyloidosis can cause as well as result from disease of other organs. Symptoms of the disease depend upon the organ where the amyloid is deposited and/or on the underlying condition that led to the amyloidosis. In the digestive system, amyloidosis may cause bleeding due to colitis. It may also produce lazy stomach (GASTROPARESIS) and slow intestinal movements, causing constipation, an overgrowth of bacteria in the small intestine, and intestinal pseudoobstruction. Problems in other systems of the body that can be caused by amyloidosis include heart and kidney failure, irregular heart rhythms, heart attack, weight loss, lightheadedness, shortness of breath, and weakness. The disease eventually kills the patient.

### Diagnosis and Treatment

The diagnosis of amyloidosis can only be made by a biopsy, the removal and examination of tissue. In primary amyloidosis, the organ that is affected is treated. Gastrointestinal amyloidosis usually does not cause death, and the treatment is directed at the problem. For example, patients who have gastroparesis may be helped by taking PROKINETIC medications, and those patients who have a bacterial overgrowth benefit from taking antibiotics. In cases of hepatic amyloidosis, a liver transplantation is needed. In secondary amyloidosis, the treatment involves treating the underlying cause that has led to amyloidosis.

Falk, Rodney H., M.D., Raymond L. Comenzo, M.D., and Martha Skinner, M.D. "The Systemic Amyloidoses." *New England Journal of Medicine* 337, no. 13 (September 25, 1997): 898–909.

Wynbrandt, James, and Mark D. Ludman. "amyloidosis (genetics)." *The Encyclopedia of Genetic Disorders and Birth Defects*. 2d ed. New York: Facts On File, 2000.

**anal cancer** See CANCER, ANAL.

**anal warts** See CONDYLOMA ACUMINATUM.

**anemia** An illness that is characterized by an insufficiency of red blood cells. For practical purposes, it is a reduction in one of the red blood cell measurements, such as hemoglobin, hematocrit, or red blood cell count.

### Causes of Anemia

The most common form of anemia is iron deficiency anemia, which is a medical problem in which the patient has been bleeding or lacks sufficient iron in the body. The other main forms of anemia include sickle cell anemia (which is primarily diagnosed among African Americans) and thalassemia (which is primarily diagnosed among people whose family originated in the Mediterranean area and in tropical areas, as in Africa, Indonesia, and southern China).

Aplastic anemia is a rare condition in which the bone marrow cannot produce red blood cells. It may be induced by exposure to some drugs, chemicals, or heavy metals. Treatment options include bone marrow transplantation and immunosuppressive therapy.

Anemia may be a temporary medical problem that is caused by a debilitating illness or acute bleeding, or it may be a chronic problem that is caused by the slow oozing of blood or by an inherited genetic defect. Sometimes it is caused by a nutritional deficiency. PERNICIOUS ANEMIA is an autoimmune disorder that is characterized by antibodies to intrinsic factor, which is vital for the absorption of vitamin $B_{12}$. This medical problem leads to a deficiency of vitamin $B_{12}$.

Anemia may also be caused by gastrointestinal bleeding or extremely heavy menstrual bleeding. Chronic infections can cause anemia, and for that reason individuals who have the human immunodeficiency virus (HIV) are at high risk for development of anemia, since they have little or no resistance to infections.

Sometimes anemia is caused by medications or treatments, such as chemotherapy that is given to patients in order to treat many forms of cancer. People with chronic alcoholism often have anemia caused by alcohol's suppressing the bone marrow, producing liver dysfunction, as well as leading to poor nutrition. Rarely, if a mild anemia is found in a person who is also a regular runner, the problem may be "runner's anemia," which may be caused by the regular and frequent destruction of blood cells during running when the feet hit the hard ground for a long time and/or when blood is lost from the gut.

### Risk Factors

The risk for development of anemia increases with age and is usually due to the presence of associated diseases rather than aging itself. However, women who have heavy menstrual periods are also at risk for development of anemia.

Race and heredity are other risk factors for anemia: hereditary forms of anemia include sickle cell anemia, found in some blacks, and Fanconi's anemia, found in some Jews of Ashkenazi descent.

The presence of other severe and chronic diseases, such as kidney failure, also increases the risk for development of anemia.

### Symptoms and Signs of Anemia

The key symptoms and signs of anemia are as follows:

- Chronic fatigue
- Weakness
- Headache
- Shortness of breath
- Sore tongue
- Worsening of other illnesses, such as heart disease or cognitive impairment
- Worsening dizziness
- Frequent infections
- PICA (a perverted desire to eat nonfoods, such as dirt or clay, or constantly eat ice [pagophagia]), which results from iron deficiency anemia.

### Considering Types of Forms of Anemia

Various forms of anemia stem from different causes. The major forms of anemia and their causes are covered in this section.

*Iron deficiency anemia*  Iron deficiency anemia is the most common form of anemia that is diagnosed among patients. It may stem from a gastrointestinal blood loss that is caused by peptic ULCERS, tumors, or use of NONSTEROIDAL ANTI-INFLAMMATORY MEDICATIONS (NSAIDs), which are often prescribed to treat many different ailments, such as arthritis, back pain, and other chronic pain disorders. Women and teenage girls who have heavy menstrual periods are also prone to development of iron deficiency anemia, as are pregnant women.

Sometimes an individual's diet can cause iron deficiency anemia, as when a person chooses to eat no meat, poultry, or fish. Vegetarians or others who completely avoid eating meats, poultry, or fish can experience iron deficiency because plants have a lower concentration of iron than is needed by the body. If individuals with this problem improve their diet, in most cases, the deficiency is resolved, although iron supplements may also be required for a brief period. Cooking foods in iron utensils helps to augment their iron content.

Some people are unable to absorb sufficient iron in the food that they eat, and only intravenous iron that is given on a regular basis can resolve their anemia.

Anemia may develop in patients who are undergoing kidney dialysis as a result of a kidney failure. In these cases, many causes may be involved, including a deficiency of the erythropoietin that is produced by the kidneys. (Erythropoietin facilitates red blood cell production.) Patients having dialysis have low levels of iron and may also have deficiencies of folic acid. Other factors leading to anemia for dialysis patients include gastrointestinal blood loss, blood loss that results from having multiple laboratory tests, blood retention in the dialysis machine system, and a shortened red blood cell survival time.

Some good sources of iron are liver, egg yolks, dried fruits, and red meats.

*Inherited forms of anemia*  The best known form of inherited anemia is sickle cell anemia, a hereditary problem that is found among some African Americans. People who have sickle cell anemia are prone to experiencing a high rate of infections, gallstones, and bone damage. Sickle cell anemia patients may require painkilling medications for pain control and may also need transfusions. Bone marrow transplantation offers the only hope for cure of sickle cell anemia as of this writing.

Another inherited form of anemia is thalassemia, which is further subdivided into various forms of the disease. The most prominent forms of thalassemia are thalassemia alpha and beta. Alpha thalassemia is more commonly seen among people from Southeast Asia; beta thalassemia is found among people from the Mediterranean area of the globe. Of the two, thalassemia beta is more severe. It results in an iron overload and skull and facial deformities. Thalassemia beta can also retard growth, can cause heart disease and osteoporosis, and may also lead to other health problems. It is estimated that there are more than 100 different genetic mutations of thalassemia beta; bone marrow transplantation is being increasingly used for the treatment of severe cases.

Fanconi's anemia, named after 20th-century Swiss pediatrician Guido Fanconi, is another inherited disorder of anemia. It causes a form of aplastic anemia. Children who have Fanconi's anemia have low birth weight, poor growth, and short stature.

Children may also have heart defects and deafness. Several different mutations have been identified in the Netherlands as well as among individuals of Ashkenazi Jewish descent.

### Diagnosis and Treatment of Anemia

Anemia is identified with a complete blood count (CBC), a test that determines the number of red blood cells, white blood cells, and platelets. In general, anemia is diagnosed if the patient's hematocrit levels on a blood test are less than 41 percent in adult males and less than 36 percent in adult females. Normal values may vary between laboratories. Anemia is a manifestation of an underlying medical problem; therefore, further testing is needed to determine the specific type of anemia, unless the problem is clearly due to bleeding.

The size of the red blood cell provides clues. Small red blood cell size (microcystic anemia) is seen in iron deficiency, the anemia of chronic disease, and, rarely, copper deficiency. It is also seen with lead poisoning, sideroblastic anemia, thalassemia, and other hemoglobin disorders.

An increase in red blood cell size (macrocystic anemia) occurs with folic acid and vitamin $B_{12}$ deficiency. It is also seen after cancer chemotherapy and with acute leukemias, alcoholism, liver disease, and hypothyroidism (low thyroid level).

The red blood cell size may also be normal in anemia, especially in mild cases or in anemia that is caused by chronic diseases.

The treatment of anemia depends on the cause of the illness. If the physician believes that it is a temporary problem, such as a short-term case of iron deficiency anemia, then use of iron supplements may resolve the anemia. In addition, patients are advised to eat foods that are rich in iron. If the anemia is a long-term, chronic problem, the continued use of supplements may be needed and treatment is targeted at the cause. In some extreme cases of anemia, bone marrow transplantation is the only way to resolve the anemia completely and to prevent further and more severe consequences.

### Use Caution in Taking Iron

Iron supplements should not be taken unless they are recommended by a physician, because an iron overload can become a problem when supplements are not needed. When a doctor recommends iron supplements, avoid enteric-coated iron supplements. Do not take iron with medications such as antacids. In addition, iron should be taken with water or juice on an empty stomach for maximal absorption and effectiveness. People with iron absorption problems should also avoid drinking tea with meals, since it can impair iron absorption.

See also HEMOCHROMATOSIS; IRON; PERNICIOUS ANEMIA; VITAMIN DEFICIENCIES/EXCESSES.

Ammer, Christine. *The New A to Z of Women's Health.* 4th ed. New York: Facts On File, 2000.

Andrews, Nancy C., M.D. "Disorders of Iron Metabolism." *New England Journal of Medicine* 341, no. 26 (December 23, 1999): 1,986–1,995.

Dang, Chi V., M.D. "Runner's Anemia." *Journal of the American Medical Association* 286, no. 6 (August 8, 2001): 714–716.

Izaks, Gerbrand J., M.D., Rudi G. J. Westerndrop, M.D., and Dick L. Knook. "The Definition of Anemia in Older Persons." *Journal of the American Medical Association* 281, no. 18 (May 12, 1999): 1,714–1,717.

Olivieri, Nancy F., M.D. "The ß-Thalassemias." *New England Journal of Medicine* 341, no. 2 (July 8, 1999): 99–109.

**anorexia nervosa**   A very serious EATING DISORDER that is characterized by self-starvation, behavior that, when present, is usually evinced by people (mostly female) who have a distorted body image and who mistakenly believe that they are obese (although the reverse is true). They may also fear that they will become obese should they forgo rigidly controlling their eating. The term *anorexia* indicates a lack of appetite; for example, in some cases, elderly individuals are anorexic because they are too ill to eat much and/or are incapable of preparing their own food or feeding themselves; they do not have anorexia nervosa.

### Risk Factors

Although anorexia nervosa is commonly considered a problem of teenage girls, women, and males of all ages may exhibit its signs. In rare cases, anorexia nervosa may be confused with Addison's disease, which produces similar symptoms of extreme weight loss, nausea and vomiting, and weakness and fatigue.

Sometimes in the early stages of Addison's disease, an endocrine disorder of the adrenal glands, patients have weight loss and lack of appetite and may be misdiagnosed with anorexia nervosa. Patients with anorexia nervosa are more likely to have *high* levels of cortisol in contrast with the hypocortisolism seen in Addison's disease. Anorexia nervosa patients are more likely to be hyperglycemic; patients with Addison's disease are more likely to be hypoglycemic. Last, anorexia nervosa patients often have low potassium blood levels whereas Addison's disease patients are hyperkalemic (have excessively high levels of potassium in the blood).

### Signs and Symptoms

People who have anorexia nervosa may appear extremely thin or may be slender and intent on losing more weight. The absence of menstruation (amenorrhea) for three or more months is one possible sign of anorexia nervosa. A significant weight loss is a possible indicator, particularly if the individual is less than about 85 percent of the normal body weight for his or her height. Patients with anorexia nervosa exhibit a fear of gaining weight. Female athletes, ballet dancers, and models are at elevated risk of development of anorexia nervosa, since very thin body types are admired by their peers. Females (or males) who have type 1 diabetes may appear thin, and diabetes should be ruled out as the cause of a recent weight loss. People who have anorexia nervosa sometimes abuse laxatives in order to keep their weight down.

### Diagnosis and Treatment

Anorexia nervosa may be diagnosed by an internist or a family practitioner, although sometimes it is diagnosed by a psychiatrist and treated in part as an emotional disorder. When medications are prescribed, anorexia nervosa may be treated with antidepressants, such as fluoxetine (Prozac).

Psychological therapy is usually required, to help the individual adjust the distorted body perception to their actual appearance. In extreme cases, individuals with anorexia nervosa may need to be hospitalized, either in a standard hospital or in a rehabilitation facility that specializes in treating people with anorexia nervosa. Inpatient treatment is especially indicated if the patient has the following conditions:

- Hypotension
- A low pulse rate of less than 50 beats per minute or a fast pulse rate greater than 100 beats per minute
- An extremely severe weight loss resulting in body weight that is 25 to 30 percent below normal body weight
- Heart arrhythmias

When a patient's weight increases to within a normal range (about 90 percent of normal body weight), menstruation may resume within about six months.

For further information, contact the following organizations:

Anorexia Nervosa and Related Eating Disorders, Inc.
P.O. Box 5102
Eugene, OR 97405
(503) 334-1144

National Association of Anorexia Nervosa and
   Associated Disorders
P.O. Box 7
Highland Park, IL 60035
(847) 831-3438
http://www.anad.org

See also BULIMIA NERVOSA; LAXATIVE ABUSE; LAXATIVES.

Adams, Robert, M.D., et al. "Prompt Differentiation of Addison's Disease from Anorexia Nervosa during Weight Loss and Vomiting." *Southern Medical Journal* 91, no. 2 (February 1998): 208–211.

Becker, Anne E., M.D., et al. "Eating Disorders." *New England Journal of Medicine* 340, no. 14 (April 8, 1999): 1,092–1,098.

Mehler, Philip S., M.D. "Diagnosis and Care of Patients with Anorexia Nervosa in Primary Care Settings." *Annals of Internal Medicine* 134, no. 11 (June 2001): 1,048–1,059.

**antacids** Over-the-counter medications that significantly neutralize the level of gastric acid in individuals. Antacids are usually used by patients who suffer from acute or chronic indigestion. When antacids are taken infrequently or rarely, they are usually used to treat indigestion or heartburn caused by overeating. However, some individuals take antacids very often and even daily, and such people need medical attention. They may have a peptic ulcer, GASTROESOPHAGEAL REFLUX DISEASE, or a variety of other illnesses that physicians can diagnose and treat. Common antacids contain calcium (Tums), aluminum, and magnesium. Some antacids contain a combination of these elements. Calcium and aluminum cause constipation, whereas magnesium may cause diarrhea.

When treated in the early stages, chronic illnesses that patients sometimes self-treat with antacids may be relatively easy to resolve. However, if patients treat themselves for years with over-the-counter antacids before telling a physician about the problem, the condition may have become very serious over that period. At times, the first-time patient may be seen in the hospital emergency room with a possible bleeding ulcer or a food blockage located in the esophagus (such as a piece of meat) in the case of stricture (narrowing) of the esophagus due to gastroesophageal reflux disease (GERD).

See also ACID REFLUX; HISTAMINE-2 BLOCKERS; PROTON PUMP INHIBITORS.

**antibiotics**  Antibacterial medications that are derived from live organisms and that are given to fight diagnosed or suspected bacterial infections. There are many different types of antibiotics, and many of them may have side effects on the digestive system, causing gastrointestinal upset, diarrhea, or even bleeding. Physicians may advise taking the drug with food or with milk, although some antibiotics may be more effective when taken on an empty stomach.

Patients who know that a particular antibiotic upsets their stomach should advise their physician, who may be able to prescribe a different antibiotic when one is needed. Patients should advise their pharmacist of the problem as well, because pharmacists are aware of medications that are in the same

group and can warn patients and doctors away from some medications, particularly newer drugs.

See also HELICOBACTER PYLORI; LACTOBACILLUS; THRUSH; YEAST.

**antidepressants**  Medications that are given to counteract the effects of clinical depression, a state of extreme and clinical sadness characterized by an inability to find joy in former activities and by constant thoughts of death. However, low doses of antidepressants are also often prescribed for individuals to combat other illnesses, such as IRRITABLE BOWEL SYNDROME (IBS), noncardiac chest pain, and other chronic pain conditions. These doses are too low to combat clinical depression but may be efficacious in other disorders.

**antidiarrheals**  Prescribed or over-the-counter (OTC) drugs that are taken to counteract DIARRHEA. Such drugs may be given in the form of oral medication or liquid suspension. If the drug is an OTC medication, such as loperamide (Imodium), the patient is usually instructed to take it after a bowel movement and then again after any subsequent loose stools that occur. If the medication is a prescribed drug, such as diphenoxylate hydrochloride and atropine sulfate (Lomotil), then similar instructions may be given.

It is important to follow the instructions carefully, because taking too many antidiarrheal drugs can lead to CONSTIPATION, whereas taking too few can be ineffectual. Some patients may also need prescribed ANTIBIOTICS. Patients who have diarrhea that is accompanied by bleeding and weight loss must always consult their physician and not rely on treating themselves with OTC antidiarrheal medications.

See also IRRITABLE BOWEL SYNDROME; LAXATIVE ABUSE; LAXATIVES.

**antiemetics**  Prescribed or over-the-counter drugs that are taken to prevent nausea and vomiting. Commonly used examples are promethazine (Phenergan) and prochlorperazine (Compazine). Newer and more potent antiemetics include ondansetron (Zofran) and granisetron (Kytril). Among alternative medicines, ginger is a popular remedy for the nausea and vomiting of pregnancy.

See also NAUSEA AND VOMITING.

**antigens and antibodies**  Antigens are foreign substances that are perceived by the body as foreign and harmful. In response, the immune system generates the production of antibodies, or chemicals that counteract the effect of antigens. Sometimes the body may erroneously perceive a part of the body or body tissue as a foreign substance, leading to diseases known as autoimmune diseases.

See also ANTIBIOTICS.

**antioxidants**  Substances that dispose of the toxic free radicals that are generated in chemical reactions in the body, thus reducing or preventing damage to body tissues. Antioxidants include vitamins A, C, and E. Many other chemicals, such as selenium, are antioxidants. In addition, vegetables and fruits have antioxidant properties. Antioxidants have been identified as possibly effective in preventing CANCER and are often added to food or taken as supplements. Some foods, such as tomatoes, are high in various vitamins as well as in antioxidants. Researchers performing a variety of clinical studies are seeking to determine the full extent of the effects of antioxidants.

See also CANCER; IRON; SELENIUM; VITAMIN DEFICIENCIES/EXCESSES; ZINC.

**antispasmodics**  Drugs that limit or stop intestinal muscle spasms, such as dicyclomine (Bentyl), hyoscyamine (Levsin), and a combination of atropine, hyoscyamine, scopolamine, and phenobarbital (Donnatal). These and related drugs may be prescribed for patients who have IRRITABLE BOWEL SYNDROME.

**anus**  The end of the digestive tract, which is the opening that leads to the outside of the body. Stools are excreted from the anus.

**appendicitis**  An inflammation of the appendix, an abdominal organ in the lower right side whose purpose is unknown and appears to be vestigial. The appendix is a small pouch or appendage connected to the cecum, which is the beginning of the colon. The appendix can rupture (burst), endangering other organs and even the person's life. Appendicitis is usually but not always very painful and requires an appendectomy, which is the removal of the entire appendix.

The cause of appendicitis is usually a blockage of the appendicial lumen. In young individuals, the blockage occurs as a result of a viral or bacterial infection, causing an increase of the lymph tissue of the appendix and leading to obstruction. In older subjects, the blockage may be due to a hard stool that is impacting the appendix. Appendicitis may also occur among older subjects as a result of cancer, PARASITIC INFECTIONS, or the scarring of the appendix. Untreated appendicitis can lead to gangrene and PERITONITIS, which are both life-threatening conditions.

About 250,000 patients per year are hospitalized for the diagnosis of appendicitis in the United States. Many medical problems can mimic the symptoms of appendicitis, such as bladder infections, severe CONSTIPATION, and acute PANCREATITIS.

Appendicitis is the most common surgical reason for hospitalizing children, and children younger than age 18 have a rate of about four appendectomies per 1,000.

In one study of 524 patients by Anil Minocha, M.D., and colleagues, those who had had a prior appendectomy were compared to a control group of 469 individuals who had no history of appendectomy. The patients with prior appendectomy (the study group) were more likely to have undergone an ENDOSCOPY (33 percent) than the nonappendectomy patients (21 percent). It is unclear what the clinical significance of this finding is, and further study is indicated. In addition, several studies, including one study by Dr. Minocha, have shown that a prior appendectomy may be protective against ulcerative colitis.

### Risk Factors

Appendicitis is slightly more common among males. Most people diagnosed with appendicitis are below age 40, although individuals older than age 40 may experience it. The incidence of appendicitis peaks from the late teens to the early 20s. Younger children may also have appendicitis, but they are usually at least age two when the problem presents itself.

### Symptoms of Appendicitis

The general symptoms of appendicitis are as follows; all symptoms do not occur in all individuals.

- Acute abdominal pain that starts in the midline near the navel and then localizes on the right side of the lower abdomen, usually for less than 72 hours, and is increasingly severe
- Nausea and sometimes vomiting
- Chills and shaking
- Constipation or diarrhea
- Low fever (about 100°F or 37.7°C)
- Lack of appetite
- Severe pain with gentle pressure on the abdomen, especially in the right lower part

### Diagnosis and Treatment

There are no specific blood tests for appendicitis, although an ultrasound and computed tomography (CT) scan can identify the illness with a high degree of accuracy. Appendicitis is diagnosed on the basis of presenting symptoms, and the physician may also order tests such as a complete blood count to check for infection and urinalysis to rule out a bladder infection. The doctor may also order either an ultrasound or a CT scan to determine whether the appendix appears inflamed. Rarely, a laparoscopy is also performed, and if the laparoscopy confirms appendicitis, then the appendix is removed. In general, surgery is performed when patients are suspected to have acute appendicitis. A 15 percent error rate is considered acceptable by experts.

**Medical history is important**   Taking a careful medical history is essential to the diagnosis of appendicitis. The pain of appendicitis usually starts in the navel area and then localizes in the right lower abdomen. If abdominal pains have lasted longer than three to five days, the problem is less likely to be appendicitis, especially in a young patient. On the other hand, diagnosis is often delayed in atypical cases and among elderly subjects; in those cases a high rate of complications and even death results.

The doctor also observes the patient. If the patient is an active child with abdominal pains who is running around while also complaining about abdominal pains, the diagnosis is unlikely to be appendicitis, because patients are typically inactive and clearly in severe pain.

**Using CT scans for diagnosis**   According to the physicians Rao and colleagues in their article on using a CT scan of the appendix in a 1998 issue of the *New England Journal of Medicine,* CT scan is 93 to 98 percent accurate in diagnosing appendicitis. This is important because sometimes doctors misdiagnose appendicitis or diagnosis is delayed, and a delayed diagnosis increases the risk that the appendix may rupture and that postoperative complications may develop.

The researchers performed an appendiceal CT scan on 100 emergency room patients who were hospitalized for suspected appendicitis or who had been diagnosed with appendicitis and were scheduled for surgery. The researchers found that 53 of the 100 patients actually had appendicitis. The CT scan was 98 percent accurate, and the CT results led to treatment changes for more than half (59) of the patients. The researchers concluded that using a CT scan to check for appendicitis resulted in net savings of $447 per patient.

On rare occasions, appendicitis is diagnosed inadvertently during a colonoscopy examination; however, a colonoscopy should not be used for the diagnosis of appendicitis. In some cases, the colonoscopy has been known to induce appendicitis.

Doctors may not prescribe pain medications when they suspect appendicitis because they do not want the pain to mask any symptoms that can help establish a diagnosis.

In cases of appendicitis when the diagnosis is delayed beyond five days and the appendix has ruptured to form an abscess, the illness is initially treated with antibiotics and intravenous fluids, later by surgery.

**Potential dangers**   If the appendix is inflamed and is not removed in a timely manner, it can burst and damage the peritoneum, the sac that covers and protects the abdominal organs. This damage leads to inflammation of the peritoneum, known as peritonitis, and to an abscess in the abdomen that can be life-threatening.

Some patients may have chronic appendicitis, presenting with chronic pain and fever, with evidence of a mass or an abscess that is located in the right lower abdomen. Some of these patients may actually have recurrent acute appendicitis that had improved before the perforation occurred. Other causes of pain must be excluded before the diagnosis of chronic appendicitis is made. Surgery may be considered if no other nonsurgical causes of these symptoms are found.

*The appendectomy* The surgical removal of the appendix (appendectomy) is generally a safe procedure and deaths are rare in the United States (less than 1 percent). Often the appendix is removed through a small incision in the abdomen. The worst surgical risk is that the patient was misdiagnosed and does not actually have appendicitis. In such cases, a 15 percent error rate is considered acceptable.

For further information, contact the following organization:

National Digestive Diseases Information Clearinghouse
2 Information Way
Bethesda, MD 20892
(800) 891-5389 (toll-free)
www.niddk.nih.gov/health/digest/nddic.htm

See also GALLSTONES; LIVER ABSCESS; PAIN.

Minocha, Anil, M.D. "An Endoscopic View of Appendicitis." *New England Journal of Medicine* 339, no. 20 (November 12, 1998): 1,481.

Minocha, Anil, M.D., et al. "Prevalence of Previous Appendectomy among Patients Needing Gastrointestinal Endoscopy." *Southern Medical Journal* 92, no. 1 (January 1994): 41–43.

Quick, Clive R. G., et al. "Appendicitis." In *Essential Surgery: Problems, Diagnosis and Management.* 3d ed. Edinburgh, Scotland: Churchill Livingstone, 2001.

Rao, Patrick M., M.D., et al. "Effect of Computer Tomography of the Appendix on Treatment of Patients and Use of Hospital Resources." *New England Journal of Medicine* 338, no. 3 (January 15, 1998): 141–146.

**appetite**    Normal physical desire and need for food. A normal, healthy appetite enables people to know when they are hungry and when they should eat. Sometimes appetite is impaired by temporary or chronic diseases. A chronic lack of appetite may also stem from an emotional disorder, such as depression, or from a physical disorder, such as cancer. Some people are obese because they ignore their natural appetite and eat to excess beyond the point when they feel satiated. In 2002, the substance GHRELIN, which appears to be a sort of appetite thermostat, was discovered. In some individuals, it malfunctions.

Some individuals lose their appetite because of disorders with the sense of taste or smell. If these problems resolve themselves, the normal appetite usually returns.

See also ANOREXIA NERVOSA; BARIATRIC SURGERY; BULIMIA; DIET PILLS; OBESITY.

**ascites**    An accumulation of excess fluid in the abdomen that frequently causes visible swelling of the abdomen. Ascites may be caused by cancer, cirrhosis of the liver, heart or kidney failure, severe malnutrition, or other medical problems such as blockages in the blood and lymphatic vessels.

### Symptoms of Ascites

Symptoms of ascites include a feeling of pressure and abdominal swelling. The individual may have trouble walking or even breathing. It is essential that the person with ascites receive medical attention, and hospitalization is also required in many cases.

### Diagnosis and Treatment

A physician who knows that an individual has an illness that causes ascites may begin treatment for ascites. Most cases of ascites are related to liver cirrhosis. At least once, all patients with ascites undergo a procedure that is called PARACENTESIS, in which the fluid is removed for diagnostic purposes as well as evaluation for any complications that the patient is experiencing, such as an infection.

In large-volume paracentesis, the fluid is removed to help the patient breathe and feel better. Paracentesis is used when ascites is seen for the first time in a patient, usually at the time of every hospitalization (25 percent of those admitted to the hospital have an infection in the ascitic fluid), and then performed on an as-needed basis afterward. If the physician is unsure of the cause of the ascites, he or she may order blood tests, an ultrasound, or computed tomography (CT) scan and an echocardiogram.

Treatment for ascites is directed to reducing the excessive fluid and treating the underlying condition and exacerbating factors. Diuretics may help rid the body of fluid. Individuals with ascites are also advised to adopt a salt-restricted diet. In some cases, shunts are implanted to help to move the fluid into the bloodstream via a special catheter or stent. Shunts may be placed surgically or in many cases less invasively by radiologists. Shunts placed by radiologists are called transjugular intrahepatic portosystemic shunts (TIPs).

An infection of ascitic fluid (spontaneous bacterial peritonitis) that occurs in patients who have ascites requires antibiotics.

See also BUDD-CHIARI SYNDROME; CANCER, GALLBLADDER; CANCER, LIVER; CIRRHOSIS; EOSINOPHILIC GASTROENTERITIS; HEMOCHROMATOSIS; MALNUTRITION.

Altman, Roberta, and Michael J. Sarg. *The Cancer Dictionary.* Rev. ed. New York: Facts On File, 2001.

**atresia**    Usually the absence of a normal opening or a lumen. When present, atresia may be seen as a blockage of any hollow part, for example, a blockage of any part of the small intestine such as the duodenum, jejunum, or ileum. Biliary atresia, as the name suggests, involves the bile ducts. In rare cases, atresia is found in more than one location. Atresia may also occur in newborns at the site of the esophagus or anus, bile ducts, and other locations, requiring surgery. Atresia is most commonly found in newborn infants, although it may also occur in older children and adults.

Atresia is considered the result of a congenital defect. It occurs in about one in 1,500 newborns. Duodenal atresia is associated with Down syndrome, tracheoesophageal fistula and anorectal malformations.

The symptoms of atresia depend on the site involved; for example, infants with intestinal atresia have abdominal swelling, constipation, and vomiting. Surgery is usually required in such cases. Similarly, esophageal atresia can be surgically corrected, allowing the child subsequently to ingest food.

**back pain**   Pain in the back that may emanate from the digestive organs, such as the pancreas or the colon. Back pain may also be caused by an infection, such as a urinary tract infection or an infection of the prostate gland in a man. Back pain is a very common problem for many people, particularly as they become middle-aged or older. Individuals of all races and both genders suffer from back pain. Diagnosing the cause of the back pain can be challenging for physicians, since there are many different reasons for back pain.

### *Diagnosis and Treatment*

In general, the physician takes a careful medical history from the patient who has back pain and also orders laboratory blood tests to screen for diseases and infections. Urine tests may be ordered to screen for a bladder infection, which is another frequent cause of back pain. A man is also given a rectal examination, including a manual check of the prostate gland for prostatitis (inflammation of the prostate gland). If a specific part of the patient's back hurts, the doctor may order plain X rays or computed tomography (CT), or he or she may order a magnetic resonance imaging (MRI) scan or an ultrasound. A renal ultrasound may be done if kidney problems are suspected.

If the physician does not find any serious illness on the basis of the examination and the results of the laboratory or imaging tests ordered, he or she may treat the patient for pain by prescribing painkillers or muscle relaxants. Massage therapy has also been shown to be of benefit to patients with back pain.

See also PAIN.

**bacteremia**   The presence of bacteria in the blood, indicating an active infection. Bacteremia is

identified by blood cultures. Bacteremia is a severe condition treated aggressively with ANTIBIOTICS. Initially, broad-spectrum antibiotics such as piperacillin/taxobactam (Zosyn), ampicillin/sulbactam (Unasyn), or imipenem/cilastatin (Primaxin) are started, pending the results of the cultures and antibiotic susceptibility testing. Once the antibiotics that are the most likely to be effective have been identified by the laboratory testing, the initial choice of the broad-spectrum antibiotic may be switched to an antibiotic that is specifically targeted at the particular organism.

Sometimes the source of the origin of the bacteremia, for example, cholangitis or abdominal abscesses, can be identified. In such cases, further treatments, such as therapeutic endoscopy or surgery, may be needed in addition to the antibiotics in order to correct the underlying problem.

**balanced diet**   A diet that consists of a variety of different types of nutritious foods containing an optimal balance of carbohydrates, fats, and proteins, as well as minerals and vitamins. What actually constitutes a "balanced diet" is a subject that is constantly debated by nutritionists, physicians, and others.

See also ANTIOXIDANTS; EATING DISORDERS; MALNUTRITION; PICA; VITAMINS.

**balloon distention test**   A test that is usually used in the investigation of the esophagus or rectum. Patients who have IRRITABLE BOWEL SYNDROME, in whom the balloon is inserted rectally, sense the balloon at an earlier stage of inflation than do other patients, probably because of problems with HYPERALGESIA (a higher sensitivity of the colon/rectum to the stimulus and a low tolerance to pain). Similarly, the inflation of a balloon in the esophagus in patients with noncardiac chest pain results in pain at much lower volumes of inflation than in healthy subjects. The rectal balloon distention test is also sometimes used as part of the testing and investigation of a patient's problems with CONSTIPATION and fecal incontinence.

Sometimes patients with constipation are asked to expel the intrarectally inflated balloon in order for the physician to study the defecatory function. This test is known as the balloon expulsion test.

**bariatric surgery** Elective surgery that limits the amount of food that the body can digest and absorb by surgically contracting the capacity of the stomach, with or without a gastric bypass. It is also known as weight reduction surgery. When only the volume of the stomach is restricted, it is known as a gastric restriction procedure. Another form of bariatric surgery is the gastric bypass.

According to the American Society for Bariatric Surgery, at least 63,000 individuals had bariatric surgery in the United States in 2002, and the surgery appears to be increasing in popularity. The female-to-male ratio for the surgery is seven to one, and the average morbidly obese woman who undergoes bariatric surgery is 39 years old and is five feet and three inches tall. In most cases, the surgery is a gastric bypass.

People who are severely obese, those who have a body mass index (BMI) of 40 or greater, who have failed to lose weight on a weight loss diet, may choose to have this particular surgery after other medical weight loss methods have failed them. A BMI of greater than 30 is considered obese.

In some cases, physicians perform the procedure on patients whose BMI is 35 and above, if they have other medical problems that would likely be improved by a significant weight loss: diabetes, hypertension, and other problems.

It may sometimes be very difficult for patients to obtain medical insurance coverage for bariatric surgery, which may be specifically excluded in some insurance policies, because the procedure is considered cosmetic and not medically necessary, despite the patient's physician's opinion. However, sometimes medical insurance does provide such coverage, and obese patients should not assume that coverage is never available for bariatric surgery and should investigate the issue with the help of their physician.

Physicians may limit their patients who have bariatric surgery to those who are older than age 20 and younger than age 60, although some physicians operate on extremely obese adolescents or elderly individuals. Most bariatric surgery patients are female; some males also choose the surgery.

Many physicians require patients who wish to have bariatric surgery to have psychological evaluations to verify that the surgery would be psychologically appropriate and that the patients are not suffering from clinical depression or other emotional disorders. Many physicians require letters of approval for the surgery (preoperative clearance) from the patient's primary care doctor.

All bariatric surgery patients should have a thorough physical examination before the surgery, to rule out any undiagnosed medical problems. Some surgeons also require a presurgical endoscopy as well.

### Types of Surgery

Bariatric surgery may be performed with an abdominal "open" incision or, in some cases, laparoscopically, through small incisions in the belly.

There are several primary ways the surgery is performed, including the malabsorptive surgical bypass procedures and restrictive surgical procedures. The three most common surgeries used currently are biliary-pancreatic diversion (duodenal Switch), Roux-en-Y gastric bypass surgery (RYGB), and laparoscopic adjustable band (Lap-Band), and these can be performed laparoscopically. Malabsorptive procedures limit intestinal absorption by restricting the stomach size and also with bypassing the first 75 centimeters of the small intestine by making a direct connection of the small pouch of the stomach to a loop of the small intestine, and thus reducing the area available for absorption.

Restrictive procedures allow normal digestion to occur, but they decrease the amount of solid foods patients can eat at one time by limiting the stomach size. After this surgery, the patient can usually only eat one cup of solid food at a time (at most) without nausea or stomach upset. However, the patient can still drink a lot of high-calorie liquids such as milkshakes if he or she chooses to do so with restrictive procedures. Thus, the potential for weight loss due to restrictive procedures is limited, and they may not be effective over the long term in many cases.

According to Brolin in his 2002 *Journal of the American Medical Association* article, the Roux-en-Y operation (which is a combination of a malabsorptive procedure, and a restrictive procedure) is the most effective form of bariatric surgery, giving patients high rates of weight loss compared to the other techniques. In addition, some studies have shown that after having the Roux-en-Y surgery, a majority of patients who had been diagnosed with diabetes or impaired glucose tolerance before their surgery experienced an improvement of their blood glucose level subsequent to the surgery.

In contrast, many patients who have had gastric restrictive surgical procedures have experienced relapses. There are reports of a failure rate as high as 80 percent with vertical banded gastroplasty, and it is falling out of favor. Adjustable gastric banding procedure (Lap-Band) as of this writing is approved by the FDA as a restrictive procedure.

### Advantages of Bariatric Surgery

The most obvious advantages of weight reduction surgery are the decreased weight and enhanced self-esteem and health experienced by many patients who had previous failures with many different types of diets and prescriptions and over-the-counter diet pills and other weight loss remedies. Patients with diabetes, prediabetes, and hypertension usually improve after bariatric surgery. In addition, patients with sleep apnea may enjoy a remission from this problem, which frequently disappears completely after surgery.

There are other advantages of bariatric surgery for obese patients, according to Brolin:

> In women, weight loss resulting from bariatric surgery has a salutary effect on sex hormone balance, menstrual regularity, fertility, and urinary stress incontinence. Women who had previously been infertile have become pregnant and delivered

healthy infants following bariatric operations; nutritional status can be maintained for both mother and developing fetus.

However, bariatric surgeons recommend that patients not become pregnant for at least one year after surgery.

### Disadvantages of Surgery

All forms of bariatric surgery carry risks for infection and vitamin deficiencies, such as deficiencies of iron, folate, calcium, and vitamin $B_{12}$, as well as other postoperative medical problems. If the banded gastroplasty is used, the band may break or slip and the surgery has to be redone. There is a risk of death with bariatric surgery, as with all surgeries, although the mortality rate is less than 1 percent, depending on the type of surgery used.

Some patients who have had bariatric surgery may experience dumping syndrome after surgery, developing abdominal cramps, nausea, and diarrhea, as well as sweating, dizziness, and even hypotension, particularly after eating carbohydrates. The incidence of dumping syndrome appears to be low after the Roux-en-Y procedure.

A rapid weight loss predisposes patients to gallstone formation, and thus, patients who have had bariatric surgery also have an increased risk for development of gallstones after surgery. Many surgeons check for gallstones before performing bariatric surgery, and if gallstones are found, they may offer patients elective simultaneous cholecystectomy at the time of bariatric surgery. Some physicians give patients medications preventive against the formation of gallstones.

Some patients may require further surgery after their weight reduction surgery, for example, to correct a complication, such as an abdominal hernia.

### The Postoperative Period

After the surgery, if the patient eats more than the now-smaller stomach can hold, she or he usually feels nauseous and sick. Most patients benefit by joining a support group of others who have had the surgery, so that they can gain practical tips as well as moral support from people who can identify with and fully understand what they are going through.

Interestingly, some physicians have found that the blood levels of ghrelin are significantly lower after patients have had Roux-en-Y surgery. Ghrelin is a hormone that is released by the stomach and that apparently affects hunger and satiety, or the feeling of fullness that a person experiences during and after eating. The researchers David E. Cummings, M.D., and his colleagues reported on their findings in 2002 in the *New England Journal of Medicine*.

They compared obese subjects who lost weight through dieting as well as subjects who lost weight through gastric surgery. The subjects who had gastric surgery had significantly lower levels of ghrelin. In contrast, the rates of ghrelin rose in the patients who lost weight through dieting. As a result, the dieters were much hungrier than were the patients who had the gastric bypass.

Said the researchers:

In summary, 24-hour plasma ghrelin levels increase in response to diet-induced weight loss, suggesting that ghrelin may play a part in the adaptive response that limits the amount of weight that may be lost by dieting. We also found that ghrelin levels are abnormally low after gastric bypass, raising the possibility that this operation reduces weight in part by suppressing ghrelin production. These data suggest that ghrelin antagonists [blocking medications] may someday be considered in the treatment of obesity.

### Criticisms of Weight Reduction Surgery

Bariatric surgery is considered controversial by many experts, and most physicians prefer that patients lose weight through limiting their caloric intake and increasing their levels of exercise; however, such methods may not work well for the morbidly obese person. Another criticism of bariatric surgery is that it causes digestive problems that were not present before the surgery, such as GASTROESOPHAGEAL REFLUX DISEASE (GERD), GALLSTONES, GASTROPARESIS, DUMPING SYNDROME, nausea, and malabsorption of micronutrients such as iron. Death is a rare complication.

Some forms of the surgery may be less likely to cause GERD than others, although every type of bariatric surgery has some effects on the digestive

system, since most bariatric surgery involves severely limiting the capacity of the stomach and hence the amount of calories that can be consumed.

For further information, contact the following organizations:

American Society for Bariatric Surgery
7328 West University Avenue
Suite F
Gainesville, FL 32607
(352) 331-4900
http://www.asbs.org

American Society of Bariatric Physicians
5453 East Evans Place
Denver, CO 80222
(303) 770-2526
http://www.asbp.org

See also DIET PILLS; GHRELIN; OBESITY; ROUX STASIS SYNDROME.

Brolin, Robert E., M.D. "Bariatric Surgery and Long-Term Control of Morbid Obesity." *Journal of the American Medical Association* 288, no. 22 (December 11, 2002): 2,793–2,796.

Cassell, Dana K., and David H. Gleaves, Ph.D. *Obesity and Eating Disorders*. 2d ed. New York: Facts On File, 2000.

Cummings, David E., M.D., et al., "Plasma Ghrelin Levels after Diet-Induced Weight Loss or Gastric Bypass Surgery." *New England Journal of Medicine* 346, no. 21 (May 23, 2002): 1,623–1,630.

MacDonald, Kenneth G., Jr., M.D., et al. "Bariatric Surgery: A Review." *General Surgery News*. Available online at http://www.upmc.edu/obesity surgery/presentations/gensurgNews.pdf. Posted April 2001. Downloaded January 26, 2003.

Personal electronic mail communication with Georgann Mallory, American Society for Bariatric Surgery, March 31, 2003.

**barium studies**  Tests that involve the ingestion or the rectal instillation of barium, a contrast dye, to allow the patient's gastrointestinal tract to show up well under a fluoroscope so that the doctor can identify medical problems. Barium may be given orally in a drink, as with an upper gastrointestinal (GI) test and a small bowel series, or may be introduced rectally, as with a barium enema. Barium studies are done when a gastrointestinal illness is suspected. A barium study is one of the preferred tests to screen for colorectal cancer; however, a COLONOSCOPY is usually recommended by gastroenterologists for that specific purpose. Biopsy samples cannot be taken during the barium study. If an abnormality is seen during the test, it is frequently followed up with an endoscopy, at which time a biopsy specimen can be taken.

See also CANCER, COLORECTAL.

**Barrett's esophagus**   A precancerous condition that is generally caused by long-standing ACID REFLUX due to GASTROESOPHAGEAL REFLUX DISEASE (GERD). In this case, GERD causes the esophageal lining to become changed to an intestinal type; the abnormality is called an intestinal metaplasia.

### Risk Factors

Some individuals have a greater risk of development of Barrett's esophagus than others; for example, white males appear to have the greatest risk of development of this condition. Other people at risk are smokers and those who have had acid reflux symptoms for many years.

### Symptoms

Barrett's esophagus itself does not cause any symptoms and must be looked for by endoscopy. A physician may suspect the condition if the patient has long-term GERD.

### Diagnosis and Treatment

Barrett's esophagus is diagnosed with an endoscopic examination of the esophagus. The normally pale lining of the esophagus is altered to a salmon color. The physician takes biopsy samples to examine them under the microscope. If the doctor who is examining the biopsy specimen locates cells that are known as goblet cells, which are not normally found in the esophagus or the stomach but are found in the small intestine, this finding is definitive proof of the presence of Barrett's esophagus.

When Barrett's esophagus is identified, treatment usually takes the form of medications, such as PROTON PUMP INHIBITOR drugs that control the acidity of the refluxed food, theoretically to prevent further damage. Unfortunately, medication does not cure or reverse the disease. The goal of treatment is damage control, so that the situation does not further worsen to esophageal cancer.

Some physicians may recommend surgery as a treatment for GERD, such as laparoscopic fundoplication, which is performed on the stomach and esophagus to prevent the food from moving back up the esophagus from the stomach. However, as with medical treatment, surgery has not been shown to reverse Barrett's esophagus or to reduce the progression to cancer.

Patients with Barrett's esophagus need periodic surveillance by endoscopy. The interval between endoscopies depends on the presence or the absence of dysplasia. If high-grade dysplasia is found, most physicians recommend an esophagectomy (removal of the esophagus), since the presence of high-grade dysplasia suggests the high likelihood of progression to cancer in the near future; in fact, cancer cells may already be present in some cases. An aggressive surveillance program of endoscopy every three months is an alternate option for patients with high-grade dysplasia.

In cases of low-grade dysplasia, physicians may order an endoscopy every six months for a year, and if the condition is stable, once every year thereafter. In patients with Barrett's esophagus without any evidence of dysplasia, the endoscopy is done at one year and thereafter every three years.

See also CANCER, ESOPHAGEAL; ESOPHAGITIS; ESOPHAGUS; HOARSENESS.

Sampliner, Richard E., M.D. "Barrett's esophagus." In *GI/Liver Secrets*. 2d ed. (Philadelphia, Pa.: Hanley & Belfus, Inc., 2001).

Spechler, Stuart Jon, M.D. "Barrett's Esophagus." *New England Journal of Medicine* 346, no. 11 (March 14, 2002): 836–842.

**Behçet's syndrome**   A rare multisystemic inflammatory disorder that causes lesions and ulcers in the mouth and the genitals. The tissues of the eyes may also be affected. The joints, the digestive tract, the central nervous system, the heart, the kidneys, the skin, the brain, and the blood vessels of patients may be affected as well. The cause of Behçet's syndrome is unknown.

### Diagnosis and Treatment

Behçet's syndrome is treated on the basis of the organ that is involved. Medications used to treat Behçet's syndrome include immune suppressant drugs such as prednisone, azathioprine, methotrexate, cyclophosphamide, and cyclosporine; however, a side effect of such treatment is that patients are more prone to infections. Colchicine may be used by patients who have arthritis.

For further information, contact the following:

American Behçet's Disease Association
P.O. Box 19952
Amarillo, TX 79114
(800) 723-4238 (toll-free)
http://www.behcets.com

Sakane, Tsuyoshi, M.D., et al. "Behçet's Disease." *New England Journal of Medicine* 341, no. 17 (October 21, 1999): 1,284–1,291.

**belching**   The oral release of gas from the stomach, also known as burping. The gas has usually been inadvertently swallowed into the digestive tract. Burping may be further enhanced during times of anxiety and stress. In some cases, the swallowed air may not even reach the stomach before it is expelled by belching. Belching may be seen in patients with GASTROESOPHAGEAL REFLUX DISEASE.

An endoscopy or an upper gastrointestinal X ray is frequently done for patients with chronic belching in order to exclude any serious underlying illness, such as gastric outlet obstruction. In most cases, no cause can be identified. In such cases, the treatment of chronic belching is frequently unsatisfactory.

**beriberi**   A severe deficiency of thiamine (vitamin $B_1$), a condition that is usually only found among children in poor countries. Dry beriberi is a disorder of the peripheral nerves that leads to such symptoms as numbness, tingling, and a burning sensation in the hands and feet, as well as leg cramps. Wet beriberi predominantly involves the heart, leading to heart failure. Cerebral beriberi occurs as a result of an acute illness that is superimposed on a chronic deficiency of thiamine. Cerebral beriberi leads to mental changes and brain damage, and sometimes even to death.

See also MALNUTRITION; VITAMIN DEFICIENCIES/ EXCESSES.

**beta blockers**   Medications that are used to treat patients who have heart disease and hypertension. Beta blockers are also useful for the prevention of the bleeding caused by esophageal varices seen in liver CIRRHOSIS. Varices are enlarged dilated veins that usually occur in the esophagus and stomach. The most common cause of varices is liver cirrhosis, and they occur in about one-third to half of patients who have cirrhosis. Bleeding is more likely to occur if the varices are large.

Beta blocker medications may also contribute to the development of GASTROESOPHAGEAL REFLUX DISEASE in some patients. Beta blockers also slow the heart, and some people take a dose of a beta blocker to calm themselves before an anticipated stressful situation, such as before going up to a podium to give a speech to a large crowd.

See also ACID REFLUX.

**bile**   A substance that is produced by the liver and that comprises bile acids, electrolytes, bilirubin, cholesterol, and phospholipids plus water. Bile aids in the digestion of food by assisting in breaking down fats as well as by absorption of nutrients. About half of the bile is stored in the gallbladder between meals. The gallbladder is stimulated by individuals' eating food; eating results in the release of bile into the small intestine, where the bile acts on the food to aid digestion and absorption of nutrients.

See also JAUNDICE; LIVER; LIVER FAILURE.

**bilirubin**   A substance that is formed by the breakdown of heme, present in hemoglobin as well as that in some other proteins. Most bilirubin that is produced (250 to 400 mg per day in adults) is derived from hemoglobin; the remaining 20 percent is contributed by other hemoproteins. Increased levels of bilirubin production are found in disorders that are associated with an increased red cell turnover, such as hemolytic anemia.

Bilirubin is potentially toxic, and it is detoxified by the body and then excreted in both the stool and the urine. Increased levels of bilirubin cause JAUNDICE, which is a yellowing of the skin. The presence of jaundice may indicate HEPATITIS, liver CIRRHOSIS, PANCREATIC CANCER, or other diseases. Bilirubin level may also be elevated among patients who have excessive breakdown of their red blood cells beyond the capacity of their liver to control, as in hemolytic anemia.

## bleeding, gastrointestinal

Loss of blood, usually from the stomach or colon, although other parts of the gastrointestinal system may also bleed. Gastrointestinal bleeding may be due to a simple case of hemorrhoids or may indicate a severe disease, such as a peptic ulcer or diverticulosis. It may also indicate colorectal cancer or another cancer. Bleeding from esophageal or gastric varices due to liver cirrhosis is usually massive.

Varices are enlarged dilated veins that usually occur in the esophagus and stomach and are most commonly caused by liver cirrhosis. Other causes of varices include hepatic and splenic vein thrombosis. Varices may also occur elsewhere in the gastrointestinal tract, including the duodenum, colon, and rectum.

Bleeding due to varices is more likely to occur if the varices are large. In such cases, BETA BLOCKER medications may be given to prevent bleeding. Once bleeding has occurred, medications such as octreotide are given and an endoscopic band ligation or sclerotherapy of the varices is performed to control the bleeding. This ligation is followed by banding at regular intervals, along with continued administration of beta blocker medications.

Similarly, diverticulosis also causes massive and painless bleeding. Abnormal blood vessels (arteriovenous malformations) in the gastrointestinal tract may ooze slowly or may cause massive bleed-

ing. One of the screening tests that are done for colon cancer is checking of the stool for occult blood. Colon polyps usually do not bleed unless they are either large or cancerous.

See also CANCER, COLORECTAL; OCCULT GASTROINTESTINAL BLEEDING.

## blue rubber bleb nevus syndrome

A rare sporadic or inherited disorder of the skin and the digestive tract. It is characterized by abnormal blood vessels in the gastrointestinal tract and by compressible nodules on the skin, with fewer nodules on other parts of the body. These nodules can cause gastrointestinal bleeding, ANEMIA, and even fatal bleeding.

The condition was first noted in 1860; it was named *blue rubber bleb nevus syndrome* in 1958 by Dr. W. Bean. (Some individuals also refer to this medical problem as Bean's syndrome, although that is not its common or official name.) The name *blue rubber bleb nevus syndrome* was chosen by Dr. Bean because of the color and appearance of the blood vessels, and their rubbery feeling to the touch.

### Diagnosis and Treatment

The signs of blue rubber bleb nevus syndrome are seen when an individual is as young as age two and continue throughout the patient's life. The malformed blood vessels can be found in any part of the body. Once a diagnosis is made, a search for these lesions in other parts of the body, using various imaging and endoscopic modalities, should be undertaken.

If the lesions cause anemia through slow bleeding, then iron treatment can usually resolve the problem. Smaller lesions may be corrected with minor surgery, but large lesions may require very severe treatments, such as extensive, and at times disfiguring, surgery.

The condition is considered very difficult to treat. Gastrointestinal areas that are affected can be treated with laser or with photocoagulation. The illness cannot be cured at the present, and at best the symptoms are managed.

For more information, contact the following organizations:

National Arthritis and Muscoloskeletal and Skin
  Diseases Information Clearinghouse
One AMS Circle
Bethesda, MD 20892
(301) 495-4484

Nevus Outreach, Inc.
1601 Madison Blvd.
Bartlesville, OK 74006
(918) 331-0595
http://www.nevus.org

**body mass index (BMI)**  A measurement that
takes into account both height and weight, using
various equations to provide tables that help physicians, patients, and others to determine whether
particular individuals are underweight, normal
weight, overweight, or obese. If patients are 100
pounds or more overweight, they are said to be
severely obese, as indicated in BMI tables.

Using BMI criteria, 54.7 percent of adults in the
United States were overweight and 19.5 percent
were obese in 1997. Recent estimates suggest that
about two-thirds of obese adults have a BMI
greater than 25, and 30 percent have a BMI
greater than 30, whereas as many as 5 percent
have a BMI exceeding 40. The prevalence of obesity amongst American children has more than
doubled over the last 20 years. Because OBESITY is
associated with many serious digestive problems
and other medical problems, such as DIABETES
MELLITUS, GASTROESOPHAGEAL REFLUX DISEASE, and
NONALCOHOLIC FATTY LIVER DISEASE (NAFLD), BMI
is an important concept. (See Appendix IX for
BMI tables for adults.)

### Problems with BMI

One problem with the concept of BMI is that it
does not take into account that some people are
heavily muscled, such as athletes or weightlifters.
In addition, the BMI does not factor in ethnic or
racial differences; for example, some Asian populations generally have smaller body frames and
weigh less than non-Asian people in the United
States and other countries. As a result, if physicians
rely upon BMI charts alone, some Asians who are
categorized as "normal" on the BMI charts may

actually be overweight and may be at risk for diabetes and other serious medical problems. On the
other hand, some muscular athletes, such as
Shaquille O'Neal, may be considered obese on the
basis of BMI tables alone.

However, despite these drawbacks, the body
mass index concept is considered by most experts
to be a useful one in helping to determine whether
most individuals are at a healthy weight.

### Children and BMI

Because children are rapidly growing, the BMI
concept is more complicated and requires consid-
eration of the child's age and sex as well as height
and weight. BMI tables for children have also
been developed, and they are helpful to parents
and physicians. (See Appendix X for BMI tables
for children.) Children whose BMI for age is considered to indicate risk of overweight have a BMI
between the 85th and the 94th percentiles. If
their BMI is in the 95th percentile or higher for
their age and sex, then they are considered to be
overweight.

It is also important to keep in mind that a BMI
that is normal or overweight at one age would not
be normal or overweight for an older child. For
example, according to the Centers for Disease
Control and Prevention (CDC), a male child with
a BMI of 19.3 at age two years would be in the
95th percentile: that is, 95 percent of children
have a lower BMI. The child's BMI could actually
drop to 17.8 by the time he is four years old, but
he would still be in the 95th percentile. The percentiles continue to change; for example, a boy
nine years in age who has a BMI of 21 would be
in the 95th percentile. When the boy reached the
age of 13, if his BMI were 25.1, he would still be
in the 95th percentile.

See also ANOREXIA NERVOSA; BARIATRIC SURGERY;
BULIMIA; DIET PILLS; OBESITY.

Schoenborn, Charlotte A., Patricia F. Adams, and Patricia
  M. Barnes. "Body Weight Status of Adults: United
  States, 1997–1998." *Advance Data from Vital and Health
  Statistics* no. 330 (September 6, 2002).

**Botox**  See BOTULINUM TOXIN.

**botulinum toxin** A very dangerous toxin (poison) that is produced by *Clostridium botulinum* bacteria, rare food-borne bacteria in the CLOSTRIDIUM family, which can cause the sickness that is known as botulism. The death rate for botulism is about 5 percent.

The toxin is sometimes transmitted in home-canned foods, particularly in foods that are not acidic and that have a pH level of greater than 4.6, at which spores germinate. Botulinum toxin may occur in a variety of foods, vegetables, and fish. Raw honey is especially implicated.

The toxin itself has no taste or smell. Botulinum toxin can produce severe reactions in untreated patients, including, at its most extreme, paralysis and death. Botulinum poisoning cases are not common in the United States; experts estimate that only about 110 cases occur per year.

### Symptoms of Food-Borne Botulism

In general, symptoms occur 12 to 36 hours after the infected food is consumed; however, in some cases, symptoms may occur only six hours after eating the food or as long as 10 days later. Wound infection by botulinum toxin may occur in injection drug users.

The following are the most common symptoms:

- Slurring of speech
- Drooping eyelids and double vision
- Difficulty in swallowing and dry mouth
- Weakened muscles
- Absence of fever

### Diagnosis and Treatment

Physicians can usually identify the disease on the basis of symptoms and results of laboratory tests done on the patient's stool, vomit, or blood.

The outcome of treatment is best when the disease is identified and treated immediately. Physicians administer botulism antitoxins. In addition, if the doctor thinks that some of the contaminated food may still be in the digestive system, he or she may induce vomiting or administer laxatives or enemas to get rid of it.

Patients affected by botulinum toxin generally require hospitalization for several weeks to months. The recovery period from this disease is at least several weeks with treatment, although steady improvement can usually be noted over that period (assuming that the person is getting better).

### Therapeutic Uses of Botox

Ironically, some forms of the botulinum toxin actually do have therapeutic uses. Generally referred to as Botox, botulinum toxin type A, which is a protein produced by *Clostridium botulinum,* has been used since 1989 as a treatment for several eye muscle disorders and since 2000 for cervical dystonia, a disease causing severe neck and shoulder spasms.

Botox is used for treatment of ACHALASIA as well as GASTROPARESIS, especially diabetic gastroparesis, when spasms of the pylorus may prevent the outflow of stomach contents into the duodenum. The injection of Botox into the lower esophageal sphincter and pylorus relaxes it, providing relief for some cases of patients with achalasia and gastroparesis respectively. Some physicians have also used Botox injections to provide temporary relief for patients who have FIBROMYALGIA or other illnesses that may cause chronic muscle pain, although those are not U.S. Food and Drug Administration–approved treatments as of this writing.

See also CONTAMINATED FOOD; FOOD-BORNE ILLNESSES.

**botulism** See BOTULINUM TOXIN.

**bowel movement** Expulsion of stool from the rectum and out through the anus. Some people have difficulties with constipation, which is the passage of difficult, infrequent or hard stools. If constipation becomes severe, the individual may suffer from fecal impaction. Other individuals may have chronic loose stools. People who have irritable bowel syndrome (IBS) may have intermittent constipation and/or diarrhea.

Most people have a bowel movement daily or about every other day; however, it is not essential to good health to have a bowel movement every single day, as some people believe. The normal frequency of bowel movements varies over a wide range of three per day to three per week.

See also CONSTIPATION; DEFECATION; DIARRHEA; FECAL IMPACTION; IRRITABLE BOWEL SYNDROME; LAXATIVE ABUSE; LAXATIVES.

**brain-gut axis**   The bidirectional neuronal interaction between the central nervous system (the brain and the spinal cord) and the enteric nervous system of the digestive system. These interactions regulate the biorhythms of intestinal movements and the secretions that are integral to normal digestion, absorption, and assimilation of food and the expulsion of waste through feces.

**breath tests**   Generally tests that utilize the breath to test for the patient's digestive function and the presence of diseases.

A breath test may be given to determine whether a person is infected with *Helicobacter pylori*, bacteria that are generally harbored within the gastrointestinal system when present in the body. After ingesting a specific meal labeled with a small amount of radioactivity, the patient breathes into a device, which measures the level of radioactivity released with radiolabeled carbon dioxide that is present in the breath. If the test result is positive for *H. pylori*, treatment is initiated.

Breath tests may also test for lactose intolerance and small bowel bacterial overgrowth.

Breath tests are also administered by police officials to individuals who are suspected of driving while under the influence of alcohol. The breath test reveals whether the driver has a level of alcohol that is above the allowable level in his or her state.

See also *HELICOBACTER PYLORI*.

**Budd-Chiari syndrome**   A rare disease that causes the clotting of the veins of the liver (hepatic vein) and may consequently cause liver damage. Budd-Chiari syndrome is associated with abdominal trauma, lupus, pancreatic cancer, liver cancer, and kidney cancer. It is also associated with preg-nancy as well as the use of oral contraceptives. In many cases, the cause of this medical problem is unknown.

People who have Budd-Chiari syndrome may have an excessive buildup of fluid in the abdomen (ascites), abdominal pain, jaundice, tenderness in the upper right abdomen, and an abnormally enlarged liver and spleen. The diagnosis is based on the patient's medical history and physical examination results plus a doppler ultrasound of the hepatic veins. CT scan or an MRI scan venography can be used to confirm the diagnosis and to plan therapeutic interventions. A liver biopsy may occasionally be performed.

The treatment of Budd-Chiari syndrome depends upon the cause. For example, among patients experiencing clotting of the vein of recent onset, blood thinners such as heparin and clot busters such as tissue plasminogen activator (TPA) are used.

The prognosis is not good for Budd-Chiari syndrome patients. Most patients die in less than four years. More than 60 percent of patients survive longer than five years after liver transplantation.

See also ASCITES; JAUNDICE; LIVER FAILURE.

**bulimia nervosa**   An eating disorder in which the individual binges (eats excessively) and then purges (forces herself or himself to vomit) at least twice a week for three or more months. Patients report that they feel that they have no control when they are overeating. The cause of bulimia nervosa is unknown, but a combination of psychological, biological, family, genetic, environmental, and social factors appear to play roles.

Most people with bulimia nervosa are females obsessed about their weight (although ironically, almost none is obese), although males may also occasionally exhibit these symptoms. Bulimia nervosa affects about 1 to 1.5 percent of adult females and about one to two million women in the United States. About half of the patients who have anorexia nervosa at first subsequently have bulimia.

Bulimic individuals may also abuse laxatives in their efforts to stay slim and suffer from abdominal cramping or diarrhea as a consequence. They may also abuse diuretics (water pills). Patients with bulimia may also exercise compulsively and feel very distressed if their daily exercise routine cannot be fulfilled, for example, if they cannot run because of extremely bad weather.

Bulimia patients may have abnormal blood electrolyte levels, for example, low levels of potassium. Bulimic patients may have esophagitis caused by constant self-induced vomiting.

Bulimic patients need psychological treatment and may also need to be hospitalized if their weight drops to a very low level and/or if severe fluid and electrolyte abnormalities develop.

For further information, contact the following organizations:

Anorexia Nervosa and Related Eating Disorders, Inc.
P.O. Box 5102
Eugene, OR 97405
(503) 334-1144

National Association of Anorexia Nervosa and Associated Disorders
P.O. Box 7
Highland Park, IL 60035
(847) 831-3438
http://www.anad.org

See also ANOREXIA NERVOSA; EATING DISORDERS; LAXATIVE ABUSE.

**cachexia** An abnormal metabolic state causing a wasting away of the body's muscle mass as well as body weight. It is due to an inadequate intake of nutrition to meet the individual's metabolic needs or the severe stress of illness, which then results in increased metabolic demands that the body is unable to meet. Cachexia is found among severely ill patients with such diseases as acquired immuno-deficiency syndrome (AIDS), advanced stages of cancer, congestive heart failure, chronic kidney failure, and other extremely serious illnesses and medical conditions.

### Symptoms

The following are the primary symptoms of cachexia:

- A lack of appetite
- Extreme fatigue
- A weight loss of 10 percent or more of body weight
- Weakness

Some patients also experience an early satiety (feeling full after eating only a small amount of food), as well as an impaired sense of taste, nausea, and constipation.

### Diagnosis and Treatment

Patients in a state of cachexia are treated with small, frequent high-fat meals and with nutritional supplements and drugs to stimulate the appetite, such as megestrol acetate, dronabinol (synthetic marijuana), or cyproheptadine.

Patients with cachexia may also be given recombinant growth hormone. Some patients are given drugs in the cytokine modulator class, such as thalidomide. (Thalidomide was a drug that caused pregnant woman to have deformed children in the mid-20th century, but researchers are now finding some use for the drug in treating severely ill patients who are not pregnant.)

Eicosapentaenoic acid (EPA) also known as alpha-3 omega fatty acid may be helpful in some cases. Anabolic steroids are frequently used. Patients with a functioning gut who are unable to eat because of their poor appetite or nausea may receive nutrition through feeding tubes. In some cases, nutrition may be administered intravenously, as a last resort.

Exercise may also help to increase appetite and inhibit cachexia.

See also ACQUIRED IMMUNODEFICIENCY SYNDROME; CANCER; FEEDING TUBE.

Corcoran, Colleen, and Steven Grinspoon, M.D. "Treatments for Wasting in Patients with the Acquired Immunodeficiency Syndrome." *New England Journal of Medicine* 340, no. 22 (June 3, 1999): 1,740–1,750.

Kotler, Donald P., M.D. "Cachexia." *Annals of Internal Medicine* 133, no. 8 (2000): 622–634.

**Campylobacter** A common and infectious form of bacteria that is responsible for many FOOD-BORNE ILLNESSES. The disease caused by *Campylobacter* bacteria is called campylobacteriosis. Few people in the United States die of this infection.

There are several varieties of *Campylobacter* bacteria that can cause people to become sick, including *Campylobacter jejuni* and *C. coli*. *Campylobacter jejuni (C. jejuni)* is the most common form of these bacteria. The Centers for Disease Control and Prevention (CDC) reports that *C. jejuni* is the primary cause of bacterial diarrhea in the United

States, infecting an estimated 2.4 million people per year, most of whom are either younger than age five or are young adults, aged 15 to 29 years. *C. jejuni* is also responsible for 5 to 14 percent of all the diarrhea that occurs on the globe.

### Causes of Transmission

*Campylobacter* organisms may be transmitted from raw or undercooked poultry products, as well as from contaminated water. These bacteria may also be transmitted by handling of waste from infected humans, animals, or birds. Pets may be carriers of *Campylobacter* bacteria, and pet owners should take special care when removing their pets' fecal material. Pet owners should always wash their hands after changing cat litter, scooping up dog waste, or cleaning a bird's or other pet's cage.

### Symptoms

Some people have no symptoms of *Campylobacter* infection. The key symptoms of campylobacteriosis are as follows:

- Diarrhea (frequently bloody)
- Abdominal pain and cramping
- Nausea and vomiting
- Fever
- Tiredness and overall weakness

Less common symptoms may include

- The development of Reiter's syndrome, which causes arthritis and painful urination, as a result of the infection
- Rarely, development of Guillain-Barré syndrome (GBS), a paralytic condition that usually occurs two to four weeks after the time of infection and requires hospitalization

In general, infected people are ill for two to five days, although individuals in a weakened condition may be ill for longer periods.

### Diagnosis and Treatment

The physician observes the symptoms of the patient and may order a stool specimen to identify *Campylobacter* bacteria.

In general, no medications are required in most cases, and simple hydration is all that is necessary. The physician may in some cases prescribe ciprofloxacin (Cipro) or erythromycin, especially for those patients who have an impaired immune system.

### Preventing Campylobacteriosis

In general, experts recommend the following actions to prevent this food-borne illness:

- Washing hands before food preparation
- Washing hands after handling raw meat or poultry
- Cooking meat thoroughly
- Drinking pasteurized milk and clean water
- Washing hands after cleaning animal feces or visiting a petting zoo

See also CONTAMINATED FOODS; DIARRHEA; FOOD-BORNE ILLNESSES.

**cancer**    A malignant tumor. Cancer may be diagnosed in any and all parts of the digestive system, including the mouth (oral cancer), the esophagus (esophageal cancer), the gallbladder (gallbladder cancer), the stomach (stomach cancer), the liver (liver cancer), the pancreas (pancreatic cancer), the colon and rectum (colorectal cancer), and the anus (ANAL CANCER). In addition, a cancerous tumor may develop in virtually any other part of the body.

### Causes of Cancer

The causes of cancer vary and are usually multifactorial. Smoking is a risk factor for ORAL CANCER and lung cancer, and smoking may also be implicated in many other forms of cancer. Similarly, alcohol use and smoking each increase the risk for esophageal cancer, and when both are present, the risk is increased exponentially. There is also a genetic predisposition to some forms of cancer, such as colorectal cancer and stomach cancer. In many cases, however, the cause of a particular cancer is unknown.

A study reported in a 2003 issue of the *New England Journal of Medicine* found that overweight and OBESITY increased the risk of death of many forms of cancer, including colorectal cancer, esophageal cancer, gallbladder cancer, pancreatic cancer, and kidney cancer, as well as non-Hodgkin's lymphoma. The researchers stated, "We estimate that current patterns of overweight and obesity in the United States could account for 14 percent of all deaths from cancer in men and 20 percent of those in women." They also concluded that 90,000 deaths each year that are caused by various forms of cancer could be averted in the United States if men and women achieved normal weight.

A few patients may have cancer in more than one site simultaneously; for example, they may have colon cancer at two different sites in the colon.

### Treatments for Digestive Cancers

Researchers performing clinical studies are actively seeking medications and treatments to treat existing cancer more effectively and to prevent cancer whenever possible. Often the cancer is surgically removed. If surgery is not possible because the cancer is advanced or is not a feasible option for another reason, chemotherapy and/or radiation therapy may be used to treat the patient.

Patients with advanced cancer who are not candidates for curative treatments may undergo palliative surgery or other therapeutic procedures to relieve their pain and/or to improve their quality of life. Some patients join clinical trials so that they have an opportunity to try treatments and medications that would not otherwise be available to them. Some patients whose cancers are otherwise nonresectable may receive chemotherapy and/or radiation therapy in order to shrink the tumor enough to get it down to a stage where it would be surgically resectable, as with cancer of the rectum.

The prognosis of cancer varies with the stage of detection and the type of cancer. For example, less than 10 percent of patients with esophageal cancer are alive after five years. In contrast, the five-year survival rate for all oral cancer patients is 56 percent. About 65 to 80 percent of patients with anal cancer survive five years or more. Colon cancer detection in the early stages is usually curative; however, when it is detected in the advanced stages, colon cancer leads to death in a few months to years.

For more information on cancer and treatments, contact the following organizations:

American Cancer Society
1599 Clifton Road NE
Atlanta, GA 30329
(404) 320-3333 (800) 227-2345 (toll-free)
http://www.cancer.org

Cancer Research Foundation of America
1600 Duke Street
Suite 110
Alexandria, VA 22314
(703) 836-4412 (800) 227-2732
http://www.preventcancer.org

National Cancer Institute
Division of Cancer Epidemiology and Genetics
6120 Executive Boulevard, MSC-7234
Executive Plaza South, 7th Floor
Rockville, MD 20852
(301) 496-1691

See also CANCER, ANAL; CANCER, COLORECTAL; CANCER, ESOPHAGEAL; CANCER, GALLBLADDER; CANCER, LIVER; CANCER, ORAL; CANCER, PANCREATIC; CANCER, STOMACH; OBESITY.

Calle, Eugenia E., et al. "Overweight, Obesity, and Mortality from Cancer in a Prospectively Studied Cohort of U.S. Adults." *New England Journal of Medicine* 348, no. 17 (April 24, 2003): 1,625–1,638.

**cancer, anal**   A tumor that occurs in the anus, which is the outlet of the bowel. Anal cancer is not common: fewer than 4,000 new cases are diagnosed each year in the United States and about 500 deaths result per year from this disease. Of all large bowel cancers, anal cancer represents only 1 to 2 percent of the cases. About 65 to 80 percent of patients with anal cancer survive five years or more.

### Causes of Anal Cancer

Unlike most other forms of digestive cancer, which are adenomacarcinomas, most anal cancer (about 70 percent) is of the squamous cell carcinoma type. Anal cancer is often also identified as a sexually transmitted disease because it is associated with the human papillomavirus (HPV), which may be transmitted by anal sex. As a result, one cause of anal cancer is unprotected anal sex. However, not all patients with anal cancer have participated in anal sex.

### Risk Factors

Most patients with anal cancer (about 80 percent) are ages 50 to 60 years old. Smoking is associated with an increase in anal cancer rate. Kidney transplantation patients have approximately 100 times greater risk of development of anal cancer. There are no known racial or genetic risks associated with development of anal cancer.

There is a slight preponderance of females over males, except for anal cancer that is associated with human immunodeficiency virus (HIV) infection. While the risk of anal cancer is higher in the HIV population, it is unclear if HIV/AIDS is an independent risk factor for anal cancer.

Studies of females and heterosexual males have indicated that people who have had 10 or more sexual partners, as well as those who have had genital or anal warts, have the highest risk of development of anal cancer. In addition, women with sexual partners who have been diagnosed with sexually transmitted diseases also have an increased risk of anal cancer. Studies also indicate that women with anal cancer are more likely to be diagnosed with vaginal or cervical cancer as well.

The presence of hemorrhoids, fissures, and fistulae does not increase the risk of development of anal cancer.

### Symptoms of Anal Cancer

The primary symptoms of anal cancer are pain and bleeding, itching and discharge, and a lump around the anus; however, sometimes there are minimal or no symptoms.

### Diagnosis and Treatment

Many of the symptoms of anal cancer can be seen with other illnesses, and consequently, a person who has these symptoms should not assume that he or she has anal cancer. Only a physician can make that determination, usually with a visual inspection of the anal region, digital rectal examination (DRE), anoscopy, and a biopsy to remove tissue from the area to check for cancer cells. If anal cancer is diagnosed, the physician usually also orders a pelvic computed tomography (CT) scan and may also order an ultrasound of the anal area. The cancer is staged as to how advanced it is and whether it has spread beyond the anal area.

The treatment of anal cancer depends on the type of the tumor and its location, as well as whether it arises from the anal margin or the anal canal and whether it is an adenocarcinoma or squamous cell carcinoma. The treatment modalities for anal cancer include resection, radiation, or chemotherapy plus radiation therapy. Adenocarcinoma is treated by the methods used for cancer of the rectum.

Treatment usually includes surgery. In some cases, the tumor alone may be removed; in others, extensive surgery may be undertaken. Patients may also receive preoperative radiation therapy and chemotherapy. Adenocarcinomas of the anal canal behave similarly to rectal cancers, and they are treated as such.

After treatment has been completed, patients should be seen at regular intervals as determined by their doctors.

### Treatment If Anal Cancer Has Spread

Anal cancer usually does not spread to distant sites (less than 20 percent spread). When it does spread, the liver is the most frequent site of the distant spread. Such patients are treated with chemotherapy.

See also CANCER, COLORECTAL; CONDYLOMA ACUMINATUM.

Abraham, Jame, M.D., and Carmen Allegra, M.D. *Bethesda Handbook of Clinical Oncology.* New York: Lippincott Williams & Wilkins, 2001.

Ryan, David P., M.D., Carolyn C. Compton, M.D., and Robert J. Mayer, M.D. "Carcinoma of the Anal Canal." *New England Journal of Medicine* 342, no. 11 (March 16, 2000): 792–800.

**cancer, colorectal**   A malignant tumor of the colon and/or rectum. Colorectal cancer does not include ANAL CANCER, which is a separate disease. Colorectal cancer is also simply referred to as colon cancer. The colon is the large intestine, also known as the large bowel. The rectum is the passage that connects the colon to the anus.

Colorectal cancer is the second leading cause of all cancer deaths in the United States, representing 10 percent of all deaths of cancer. In 1999 57,222 Americans died of colorectal cancer: 28,313 men and 28,909 women. In Canada, an estimated 6,400 people died of colorectal cancer in 2001, and 17,200 new cases of colorectal cancer were diagnosed.

### Risk Factors

Seventy-five percent of those diagnosed with colorectal cancer have no known family history of the disease. However, a family history and personal history of colon cancer are considered risk factors. A strong family history would place the person in a high-risk category, for example, if a first-degree relative is diagnosed with colon cancer, especially when the relative is younger than age 60. A personal or family history of polyps (adenoma type) is another risk factor for colon cancer, since precancerous polyps such as adenomas can proceed to cancer. Other risk factors are overweight and obesity. A large study reported in a 2003 issue of the *New England Journal of Medicine* revealed that overweight and obese people had a significantly increased risk of development and death due to colorectal cancer compared to the risk of people of normal body weight.

State by state death statistics in the United States in 1999 that were reported to be caused by colorectal cancer indicated that Maine had the highest rate of deaths, or 25.1 per 100,000 people. The lowest rate of deaths from colorectal cancer was found in Hawaii, at 13.6 per 100,000 people. The average for all states was 21.1 per 100,000 people.

Although it is unknown why Hawaiians had a significantly lower death rate of colorectal cancer than people in other states, it is possible that the high concentration of Asians and nonwhites and nonblacks may account at least in part for this very low rate, since whites and blacks have the highest rates of colorectal cancer. It is also possible that the higher level of physical activity in Hawaiians may

**ADJUSTED RATES OF DEATH DUE TO COLORECTAL CANCER,\* BY STATE RANK, 1999**

| Rank | State | Rate† |
|------|-------|-------|
| 1 | Maine | 25.1 |
| 2 | West Virginia | 24.6 |
| 3 | District of Columbia | 24.5 |
| 4 | Pennsylvania | 24.2 |
| 5 | Ohio | 24.2 |
| 6 | Delaware | 24.0 |
| 7 | Louisiana | 24.0 |
| 8 | New Hampshire | 23.9 |
| 9 | Rhode Island | 23.8 |
| 10 | New Jersey | 23.6 |
| 11 | Indiana | 23.6 |
| 12 | South Dakota | 23.2 |
| 13 | Illinois | 23.1 |
| 14 | Nevada | 23.0 |
| 15 | Vermont | 23.0 |
| 16 | Massachusetts | 22.7 |
| 17 | Nebraska | 22.6 |
| 18 | Maryland | 22.6 |
| 19 | New York | 22.5 |
| 20 | Kentucky | 22.4 |
| 21 | Arkansas | 22.3 |
| 22 | Missouri | 22.2 |
| 23 | Mississippi | 22.0 |
| 24 | South Carolina | 21.9 |
| 25 | Iowa | 21.8 |
| 26 | Virginia | 21.4 |
| 27 | Wisconsin | 21.3 |
| 28 | Connecticut | 21.2 |
| 29 | Michigan | 21.2 |
| 30 | Wyoming | 21.1 |
| 31 | Oklahoma | 21.0 |
| 32 | Kansas | 20.8 |
| 33 | Alaska | 20.6 |
| 34 | North Carolina | 20.3 |
| 35 | North Dakota | 20.1 |
| 36 | Tennessee | 20.0 |
| 37 | Texas | 19.9 |
| 38 | Florida | 19.8 |
| 39 | Oregon | 19.7 |
| 40 | Idaho | 19.4 |
| 41 | Alabama | 19.2 |
| 42 | Montana | 19.2 |
| 43 | Minnesota | 19.0 |
| 44 | Georgia | 18.7 |
| 45 | Washington | 18.7 |
| 46 | Arizona | 18.3 |
| 47 | Colorado | 17.9 |
| 48 | California | 17.8 |
| 49 | New Mexico | 17.4 |
| 50 | Utah | 16.2 |
| 51 | Hawaii | 13.6 |
| | **United States** | **21.1** |

\*ICD-10 codes: C18–C20, C26.0.

†Deaths per 100,000, age adjusted to 2000 total U.S. population.

## PERCENTAGE OF ADULTS WHO REPORTED NO LEISURE-TIME PHYSICAL ACTIVITY,* BY STATE RANK, 2000

| Rank | State | Percentage |
|---|---|---|
| 1 | Kentucky | 41.1 |
| 2 | Louisiana | 36.2 |
| 3 | Oklahoma | 34.4 |
| 4 | Arizona | 34.2 |
| 5 | West Virginia | 33.6 |
| 6 | Mississippi | 33.3 |
| 7 | Tennessee | 32.7 |
| 8 | Alabama | 31.6 |
| 9 | Ohio | 31.3 |
| 10 | Illinois | 30.9 |
| 11 | North Carolina | 30.4 |
| 12 | Kansas | 30.4 |
| 13 | Nebraska | 29.6 |
| 14 | New York | 29.4 |
| 15 | Georgia | 29.0 |
| 16 | Missouri | 28.8 |
| 17 | Florida | 28.8 |
| 18 | New Jersey | 28.6 |
| 19 | Texas | 28.5 |
| 20 | South Carolina | 28.1 |
| 21 | Arkansas | 28.1 |
| 22 | Delaware | 28.0 |
| 23 | Rhode Island | 27.5 |
| 24 | Iowa | 27.3 |
| 25 | Maine | 27.2 |
| 26 | South Dakota | 26.7 |
| 27 | New Hampshire | 26.7 |
| 28 | California | 26.5 |
| 29 | Indiana | 25.4 |
| 30 | Connecticut | 25.2 |
| 31 | Virginia | 25.0 |
| 32 | Nevada | 24.9 |
| 33 | Minnesota | 24.8 |
| 34 | Massachusetts | 24.6 |
| 35 | New Mexico | 24.4 |
| 36 | North Dakota | 24.3 |
| 37 | Maryland | 24.2 |
| 38 | Montana | 23.3 |
| 39 | Vermont | 23.2 |
| 40 | Hawaii | 23.2 |
| 41 | Pennsylvania | 23.0 |
| 42 | Michigan | 22.9 |
| 43 | Wyoming | 22.6 |
| 44 | Wisconsin | 22.1 |
| 45 | District of Columbia | 20.8 |
| 46 | Oregon | 20.1 |
| 47 | Alaska | 20.0 |
| 48 | Idaho | 19.8 |
| 49 | Colorado | 19.8 |
| 50 | Washington | 16.9 |
| 51 | Utah | 15.5 |
| | **Median** | **26.7** |

*No exercise, recreation, or physical activity (other than regular job duties) during the previous month.

Source: CDC, Behavioral Risk Factor Surveillance System.

provide some protective factor against development of colorectal cancer; for example, in 2000, only 23.2 percent of adults in Hawaii reported having *no* leisure-time physical activity, compared to 27.2 percent of adults living in West Virginia. Other factors may be involved as well in causing a lower than normal death rate of colorectal cancer; for example, Hawaiians who are age 50 and older are more likely than individuals in many other states to have either colonoscopy or sigmoidoscopy. Although colorectal cancer has a high fatality rate, when considered in terms of the frequency of diagnosis alone, colorectal cancer follows prostate, and lung cancer for men in the United States. For women in the United States, colorectal cancer diagnosis follows breast, and lung cancer in frequency of diagnosis. Overall, colorectal cancer is the second leading cause of cancer-related death in the United States.

Men have a higher risk of colorectal cancer than women, and African Americans, both men and women, have a significantly higher risk for colorectal cancer than that faced by whites in the United States. According to the National Cancer Institute, white men have a rate of 20.1 cases of colorectal cancer per 100,000 and black men have a rate of 27.2 per 100,000. White women have a rate of colorectal cancer of 13.7 per 100,000, compared to African American women, who have a rate of 19.5 per 100,000.

The risk for development of colorectal cancer increases with age; about 90 percent of all patients with colorectal cancer are older than age 50 years. Therefore, screening of people who are age 50 and older is very important. Patients who have INFLAMMATORY BOWEL DISEASE (IBD) have a greater risk of development of colorectal cancer than those without IBD. The risk of colorectal cancer in IBD patients depends upon the extent and duration of the disease.

Tobacco users have more than double (2.5) the risk of development of colorectal cancer of nonusers.

Other risk factors for the development of colorectal cancer include the following:

- A family or personal history of colorectal cancer or polyps

- Obesity
- A past history of the adenoma type of polyps in the colon (detected in a prior colonoscopy)
- A high-fat and low-fiber diet
- Alcohol abuse or alcoholism
- Physical inactivity/sedentary lifestyle

### Causes of Colorectal Cancer

Colorectal cancer is apparently caused by mutations that occur in the cellular deoxyribonucleic acid (DNA) and that then result in excessive and unregulated cell growth. Researchers have identified some of these mutations, but it is unknown what triggers normal cells to mutate. However, there is clearly a genetic factor at work, and the risk of development of colorectal cancer is increased if one or more family members have had polyps or colorectal cancer. About 25 percent of patients report a family history of colorectal cancer. Researchers are also studying the impact of diet and nutrition, OBESITY, and other factors that may cause or contribute to the development of colorectal cancer.

One factor that is known about colorectal cancer is that polyps, which are small to large outgrowths of the colon, are significant in the development of colorectal cancer. In fact, 95 percent of colon cancer occurs in preexisting adenoma-type polyps. Clinical studies, particularly the National Polyp Study in the United States, have shown that the presence of adenoma polyps is actually an interim step to the subsequent development of most colorectal cancer. When these polyps are detected and then removed by physicians (usually during a COLONOSCOPY, which is an internal investigation of the entire colon), the incidence of colorectal cancer is actually reduced by about 70 to 90 percent of the cases. Clearly the colonoscopy is an important diagnostic and preventive tool. (The colonoscopy is described in more detail later in this entry.) New developments with the noninvasive virtual colonoscopy should increase the number of patients who are screened.

On the basis of clinical research to date, it appears that in most cases, precancerous polyps take about seven to 10 years to develop into cancerous tumors. For this reason, and because colorectal polyps and cancer are more prominently found among middle-aged and older people, it is recommended that people who are age 50 and older undergo colon cancer screening. The various options are sigmoidoscopy, barium studies, the fecal occult blood test and colonoscopy although gastroenterologists prefer a colonoscopy to detect the presence of any precancerous polyps. If any polyps are found during the colonoscopy, they can be removed, and thus, they cannot develop into colorectal cancer. Further surveillance by physicians is undertaken on the basis of the type of polyps identified and removed. It should also be noted that not all polyps are precancerous or cancerous.

According to the National Center for Chronic Disease Prevention and Health Promotion, a division of the CENTERS FOR DISEASE CONTROL AND PREVENTION (CDC), at least one-third of all deaths of colorectal cancer in the United States could be prevented if everyone 50 years and older had regular screening tests for the disease.

### Symptoms

There are often no symptoms in the early stages of colorectal cancer. The presence of symptoms is not a good sign, because in about half of cases, by the time that symptoms arise, the cancer has usually spread. When symptoms do occur, the most frequently occurring symptoms are the following:

- Blood in the stool
- A change in bowel habits
- Diarrhea or constipation
- Unexplained weight loss
- Stools that are more narrow than usual for a person
- Sustained and unexplained fatigue

Laboratory tests may show the presence of a microscopic amount of blood in the stool, and blood tests may show the presence of iron deficiency anemia.

Many other illnesses can also cause these nonspecific symptoms, and patients who experience them should see their doctor for an evaluation.

### Diagnosis of Colorectal Cancer

There are several ways that doctors screen for and diagnose colorectal cancer. The simplest technique is the digital rectal examination, in which the doctor inserts a lubricated finger into the rectum to feel for any abnormalities. If an abnormality is detected in this examination, the doctor orders further studies. The primary care physician can perform the rectal examination. However, the digital examination can only examine a very small part of the rectum that is within the reach of the finger, whereas the colon is about five feet long. Therefore, the rectal examination can help to detect only a small fraction of colorectal cancers.

The fecal occult blood test is another screening tool, as are the colonoscopy and the sigmoidoscopy.

**Fecal occult blood test** There are laboratory tests for colorectal cancer, of which the most commonly used test is the fecal occult blood test (FOBT); however, a lack of occult (hidden) blood does not definitively rule out colorectal cancer. Nor does the presence of blood prove that the person has colorectal cancer. Blood in the stool may be caused by hemorrhoids, infection, or another cause. However, when there is blood in the stool, colorectal polyps and/or cancer should be ruled out. As a result, if the FOBT result is positive for occult blood, the doctor usually orders a colonoscopy.

The FOBT test detects microscopic blood in the stool that may indicate colorectal cancer. Individuals are given special cards on which to collect their own small stool specimens. The physician then checks the specimens on the cards for invisible blood (not visible to the patient but visible upon testing with special reagent). It should be noted that not all polyps bleed; only large polyps and cancerous tumors are likely to bleed.

Because the risks for development of colorectal cancer increase with age, people older than age 50 should have the FOBT every year. Unfortunately, according to the CDC, only about 21 percent of whites and African Americans have annual FOBTs, and the percentages of those having annual FOBTs are even lower for Hispanics (11 percent) and Asians/Pacific Islanders (10 percent).

**Invasive screening procedures** There are also several invasive procedures that are undertaken to detect the presence of colorectal cancer, including the barium enema, the flexible sigmoidoscopy, and the colonoscopy. A gastroenterologist, a physician who is an expert in diagnosing and treating digestive diseases and disorders, usually performs the flexible sigmoidoscopy or preferably the colonoscopy, whereas a radiologist performs the barium enema. The sigmoidoscopy and even the colonoscopy may also be performed by physicians who are not gastroenterologists.

During the double-contrast barium enema, patients are fully conscious. They are administered through the rectum a barium dye that bathes and highlights the colon, making it appear opaque on X rays. Air is then introduced, to give a double contrast and to make the X ray view more clear. (In a single-contrast barium enema, only the barium is used and the air is not introduced, but the test result is less accurate.) If an abnormality is found by the barium enema, a colonoscopy is then performed. The barium enema does not visualize the lower colon and the rectum well, and an additional sigmoidoscopy is required to perform a more complete evaluation.

The most extensive procedure to check for colon cancer is the colonoscopy, in which the doctor visually inspects the entire colon. In the United States, patients are usually sedated, although sedation is often not used in other countries. The colonoscopy is the best procedure to detect colorectal cancer because it inspects the entire colon.

A sigmoidoscopy is similar to a colonoscopy; however, with a sigmoidoscopy, the doctor inspects only the lower third of the bowel. This procedure may be chosen because it is less expensive than the colonoscopy. However, most experts, such as Dr. Minocha, believe that having a sigmoidoscopy to detect colorectal cancer or precancerous polyps is comparable to having a mammogram for breast cancer on one breast. This is not surprising, since sigmoidoscopy is less effective than full colonoscopy.

Many famous people have undergone colonoscopy, which has detected either polyps or colorectal cancer, including President Ronald Reagan, President George W. Bush, and the baseball player Darryl Strawberry.

The virtual colonoscopy is another procedure that has been developed in recent years. This procedure involves radiological imaging of the colon without actually introducing a scope into the rectum. Recent data suggests that the efficacy of the virtual colonoscopy is similar to colonoscopy. However, any abnormality that is seen in the virtual colonoscopy requires a follow-up colonoscopy, which does use the scope and as such, as of this writing, is a virtual colonoscopy that has not been endorsed by gastroenterologists as a screening option.

The actions that the surgeon can take as a result of the findings during the procedure are also dependent on the type of procedure performed. For example, polyps (precancerous growths) can be detected during a sigmoidoscopy, but they cannot be removed by electrocautery unless the colon is completely cleaned out ahead of time, whereas normally it is not. Also, if any precancerous polyps are identified during a sigmoidoscopy, the doctor then orders a subsequent colonoscopy so that the entire colon can be checked for polyps, which can then be removed. As a result, the patient has to have two major procedures instead of one.

The physician's goal is another factor in determining which test is ordered. For example, if the doctor wants to remove any tissue to check for cancer (a biopsy), this procedure cannot be performed during a barium enema or virtual colonoscopy. The doctor may, however, perform a biopsy during either a colonoscopy or a sigmoidoscopy.

Unfortunately, many people who are 50 years and older do not have a sigmoidoscopy every five years or do not have colonoscopy once every 10 years, and in some of them, colorectal cancer that could have been prevented with such tests develops. More frequent examinations are required for patients who have a higher than average risk of development of colorectal cancer.

In a state-by-state analysis in the United States, the highest percentage of individuals older than 50 who had *not* had either a sigmoidoscopy or a colonoscopy in the past five years, as of 1999, was found in Nebraska: 77.4 percent had not had either test. The lowest percentage was found in Delaware, where 53.8 percent of adults age 50 and older had had neither screening procedure. Thus, Delawarans were the best screened for colorectal cancer. (See the state-by-state chart of people ages 50 and older who had had neither a sigmoidoscopy nor a colonoscopy in the preceding five years.)

Because colorectal cancer is a major killer, it is essential that physicians convey to their patients that early diagnosis and treatment are life savers, and especially that colonoscopy is not only an important preventive test to screen for colorectal cancer, but also a cost-effective test.

### Staging of Cancer

If colorectal cancer is identified, doctors determine how advanced the cancer is and how fast it is growing. This is called staging. They then further categorize the cancer, using the Tumor–Node–Metastasis or TNM system, developed by the American Joint Committee on Cancer, which is used to stage all forms of cancer. Staging is important because it helps physicians to determine the recommended course of treatment and assess the prognosis.

With colorectal cancer, the TNM system provides a method of classification that is based on determinations of how deeply the tumor has penetrated through (which is the *T*) the walls of the colon, as well as whether it has spread to nearby (the *N*) lymph nodes, and whether it has metastasized (the *M* for metastasis) to distant tissues.

For example, if the finding is that the tumor is categorized as T is N0 M0, this means that the cancer is in its earliest stage. (T is not a 0 or a 1, it simply stands alone in this stage.) This cancer is also known as carcinoma in situ or intramucosal carcinoma and has a 100 percent five-year survival rate. (Nobody dies within five years of colorectal cancer if it is identified in this stage.) A bit more serious stage of tumor but one that still has an excellent prognosis is T1 N0 M0. There are other components of T-staging colorectal cancer, such as T2, T3, and T4. When the cancer is considered to be at the T4 level, it has spread through the colon wall and extended into nearby organs or tissues.

The worst stage of colorectal cancer is M, irrespective of the T or N stage, which indicates the cancer has spread to distant sites, such as the liver or lungs. At that point, doctors cannot cure the cancer, and they can only take palliative measures to ease the pain of the patient until death occurs.

**PERCENTAGE OF ADULTS AGED 50 YEARS OR OLDER WHO REPORTED NOT HAVING HAD A SIGMOIDOSCOPY OR COLONOSCOPY IN THE LAST 5 YEARS, BY STATE RANK, 1999**

| Rank | State | Percentage |
|------|-------|------------|
| 1 | Nebraska | 77.4 |
| 2 | Kentucky | 74.3 |
| 3 | West Virginia | 73.8 |
| 4 | Missouri | 73.4 |
| 5 | Nevada | 72.0 |
| 6 | Oklahoma | 71.8 |
| 7 | Mississippi | 71.6 |
| 8 | Louisiana | 71.1 |
| 9 | Kansas | 71.0 |
| 10 | Arkansas | 70.5 |
| 11 | Idaho | 70.3 |
| 12 | Tennessee | 70.2 |
| 13 | Alabama | 70.1 |
| 14 | Montana | 69.6 |
| 15 | North Dakota | 69.6 |
| 16 | Arizona | 69.5 |
| 17 | Pennsylvania | 69.4 |
| 18 | North Carolina | 69.0 |
| 19 | Maine | 69.0 |
| 20 | Colorado | 69.0 |
| 21 | Iowa | 68.8 |
| 22 | Utah | 68.6 |
| 23 | Indiana | 68.4 |
| 24 | South Carolina | 67.9 |
| 25 | Vermont | 67.9 |
| 26 | South Dakota | 67.7 |
| 27 | New Mexico | 67.6 |
| 28 | Texas | 67.4 |
| 29 | Ohio | 67.4 |
| 30 | Oregon | 66.7 |
| 31 | Wyoming | 66.0 |
| 32 | Illinois | 65.9 |
| 33 | Virginia | 65.6 |
| 34 | Florida | 65.2 |
| 35 | New York | 65.1 |
| 36 | Massachusetts | 65.0 |
| 37 | New Jersey | 64.7 |
| 38 | Hawaii | 64.6 |
| 39 | Alaska | 64.5 |
| 40 | Georgia | 64.4 |
| 41 | Wisconsin | 63.8 |
| 42 | Minnesota | 63.5 |
| 43 | Washington | 63.0 |
| 44 | New Hampshire | 62.4 |
| 45 | California | 61.7 |
| 46 | Connecticut | 61.0 |
| 47 | Rhode Island | 60.6 |
| 48 | Michigan | 60.1 |
| 49 | Maryland | 59.3 |
| 50 | District of Columbia | 57.4 |
| 51 | Delaware | 53.8 |
| | **Median** | **67.7** |

Source: CDC, Behavioral Risk Factor Surveillance System.

There are three basic stages of N information on the nodes. N0 means there is no lymph involvement, N1 means there are cancer cells in one to three lymph nodes, and N2 means cancer is found in four or more lymph nodes.

As for M categories, either there is no spread to distant tissues or organs (M0) or there is spread (M1).

### Treatment of Colorectal Cancer

*Surgery*   Surgery is the only viable cure for colorectal cancer. Other options, such as chemotherapy and radiation therapy, are both considered secondary treatments. They are important adjuvant treatments for rectal cancer. Chemoradiation therapy may also be used to downstage (shrink) a rectal tumor in an effort to convert it from an inoperable one, or, in some cases of resectable tumors to reduce the extent of the surgery to be done. In general, chemotherapy and radiation therapy are used to extend the patient's life but not to cure colon cancer. Patients with late stage colorectal cancer may also wish to join a clinical study to participate in the most advanced research available, enabling them to use drugs or treatments that would not otherwise be available to them.

In surgery, doctors remove all or part of the cancerous colon/rectum and also any lymph nodes that are found in the area. Usually the colon's functioning can be maintained through reconnections that the surgeon creates; however, if this is not possible, the patient may need a temporary or a permanent colostomy, with which the waste material goes directly into a bag that is external to the body and is periodically emptied by the patient. In about 15 percent of cases, a permanent colostomy is required.

Advances in surgery have allowed surgeons to attempt curative resection, even for those patients for whom there is limited spread of cancer to the liver.

*Chemotherapy*   Some patients receive chemotherapy for colorectal cancer. It is generally only used in colon cancer if the cancer is advanced but is often used in rectal cancer. Chemotherapy may be used in rectal cancer to shrink an otherwise nonresectable tumor in order to downstage it to a surgically resectable one, in an effort to improve the prognosis.

Anticancer drugs are usually introduced through an intravenous lines or sometimes with a catheter that is placed into the portal vein connecting to the liver. Some forms of drugs are available in pill form. Chemotherapy may cause the patient to feel nauseous, tired, and dizzy, and anticancer drugs may also cause hair loss.

*Radiation therapy*    Another treatment option is to irradiate the cancerous tissue. Radiation may be given through a machine in a hospital or an outpatient center. In some cases, radiation pellets may be internally inserted into the rectum. Radiation therapy may cause loss of appetite, nausea, fatigue, and irritation at the site of the radiation, as well as diarrhea that may be bloody.

*Clinical trials*    Another treatment option is to join a clinical trial in which new medications or other therapies are being tested. Frequently, this choice is made when the cancer is in an advanced stage and all other treatment options are exhausted.

See also CANCER, ANAL; COLOSTOMY; FIBER; OBESITY; OCCULT BLEEDING; POLYPS; SIGMOIDOSCOPY.

Bond, John H., M.D. "Polyp Guideline: Diagnosis, Treatment, and Surveillance for Patients with Colorectal Polyps." *American Journal of Gastroenterology* 95, no. 11 (November 2000): 3,053–3,063.

Calle, Eugenia E., et al. "Overweight, Obesity, and Mortality from Cancer in a Prospectively Studied Cohort of U.S. Adults." *New England Journal of Medicine* 348, no. 17 (April 24, 2003): 1,625–1,638.

Calvert, Paula M., M.D., and Harold Frucht, M.D. "The Genetics of Colorectal Cancer." *Annals of Internal Medicine* 137, no. 7 (2002): 603–612.

Kim, George P., Chris H. Takimoto, and Carmen Allegra. "Colorectal Cancer." In *Bethesda Handbook of Clinical Oncology.* Philadelphia: Lippincott, Williams & Wilkins, 2001.

Lieberman, David A., M.D., et al. "Use of Colonoscopy to Screen Asymptomatic Adults for Colorectal Cancer." *New England Journal of Medicine* 343, no. 3 (July 20, 2000): 162–168.

Minocha, Anil, M.D. *The Gastroenterology Resident Pocket Survival Guide.* McLean, Va.: International Medical Publishing, 1999.

National Center for Chronic Disease Prevention and Health Promotion. "The Burden of Chronic Diseases and Their Risk Factors: National and State Perspectives." Centers for Disease Control and Prevention, 2002.

Toribara, Neil, M.D. "Colorectal Cancer." In *GI Liver Secrets.* 2d ed. Philadelphia: Hanley & Belfus, 2001.

Weinberg, David S., and Christine Laine. "Colorectal Cancer Screening." In *20 Common Problems in Gastroenterology.* New York: McGraw-Hill Medical Publishing Division, 2002.

**cancer, esophageal**    A malignant tumor of the esophagus, the food tube that lies between the throat and the stomach. The esophagus is sited behind the trachea (the windpipe) and travels downward; the average length of the adult esophagus is 10 inches. Esophageal cancer represents about 1.5 percent of all cancers and 7 percent of all gastrointestinal cancers.

According to Devesa, Blot, and Fraumeni, Jr., in their 1998 article in the medical journal *Cancer,* the incidence of esophageal cancer among white males has increased by greater than 350 percent since the 1970s, possibly because of the combined factors of smoking and obesity. The survival rate is still poor.

About 250,600 new cases of esophageal cancer were diagnosed in the United States in 2002, according to the American Cancer Society. In 2002, there were an estimated 12,600 deaths of esophageal cancer: 9,600 deaths of men and 3,000 deaths of women.

The five-year survival rate over the period 1992–97 for esophageal cancer among all races was less than 10 percent.

There are two basic types of esophageal cancer: squamous cell carcinoma and adenocarcinoma. Squamous cell carcinoma is more common among African Americans in the United States who have been diagnosed with esophageal cancer, and adenocarcinoma is more commonly found among whites diagnosed with this disease. Squamous cell esophageal cancer is associated with heavy and chronic alcohol consumption as well as with smoking. Squamous cell esophageal cancer also has a high incidence among people living in China and Southeast Asia.

Most cases of esophageal adenocarcinoma are preceded by BARRETT'S ESOPHAGUS, a precancerous condition that occurs after years of untreated GAS-TROESOPHAGEAL REFLUX DISEASE.

### Risk Factors

In the United States, men are about three times more likely to have esophageal cancer than women. Among racial groups, African Americans have the highest rate of esophageal cancer (15.0 per 100,000) and Filipinos (people who originally immigrated from the Philippines) have the lowest rate of all groups, at 2.0 per 100,000.

According to Morris Brown, Devesa, and Fraumeni, in their chapter on the epidemiology of esophageal cancer in *Atlas of Clinical Oncology: Cancer of the Upper Gastrointestinal Tract*, the lifetime risk of being diagnosed with esophageal cancer in the United States is 0.99 percent for African American males, 0.67 for white males, 0.43 percent for African American females, and 0.25 percent for white females.

Age is another factor in the development of esophageal cancer, and the risk is greatest for individuals between the ages of 50 and 70 years.

In developed countries, other risk factors for the development of esophageal cancer include ALCOHOLISM, cigarette SMOKING, and use of smokeless tobacco (tobacco that is chewed or stuffed into the cheek). The more a person smokes, the greater his or her risk for development of esophageal cancer. When individuals drink and smoke, the combined factors further increase the risk of the development of esophageal cancer.

The presence of Barrett's esophagus, a chronic alteration of the lining of the wall of the esophagus that is usually caused by gastroesophageal reflux disease, increases the risk of the development of esophageal cancer. Cancers that arise from Barrett's esophagus are adenocarcinomas rather than squamous cell carcinomas.

Patients who have had other forms of head and neck cancer have an increased risk for development of esophageal cancer.

In looking at esophageal cancer around the world, the highest rates worldwide are found in China, Iran, France, and South Africa.

Overweight and obesity are also linked with esophageal cancer, according to research published in a 2003 issue of the *New England Journal of Medicine*.

Other factors that are associated with esophageal cancer are a low intake of fresh fruits and vegetables, achalasia, the presence of the human papillomavirus, and lye-induced strictures of the esophagus. Environmental exposure to radiation or asbestos may also play a role in the development of esophageal cancer.

The differences in risk factors for squamous cell and adenocarcinoma include the following:

1. Alcohol is an increased risk for squamous cell cancer but not adenocarcinoma.
2. Adenocarcinoma is more common among whites; squamous cell cancer is found more often among blacks.
3. Barrett's esophagus is not a risk factor for squamous cell cancer.

### Signs and Symptoms

Many patients have no symptoms in the early stages of esophageal cancer. When symptoms occur, they may include some or all of the following indicators:

- Difficulty in swallowing (dysphagia)
- Weight loss
- Anemia
- Pain in the throat or between the shoulder blades of the back
- Chronic cough
- Chronic hoarseness
- Vomiting
- Vomiting of blood

### Diagnosis of Esophageal Cancer

Physicians diagnose esophageal cancer on the basis of the patient's symptoms, the findings of the physical examination, and the results of tests. The most frequently appearing symptom is DYSPHAGIA, which is difficulty with swallowing foods or even liquids that may be accompanied by pain when eating or drinking is attempted. Initially, the dysphagia occurs with solids only. Progressively, it gets worse and difficulty in swallowing liquids indicates a more severe dysphagia than is found when patients have difficulty with eating solid foods only. The patient may also be hoarse and constantly clear the throat. Another indicator is weight loss when a patient has not tried to lose weight. In this case, weight loss is usually caused by the patient's difficulties with eating as well as the effect of meeting the increased metabolic demands due to cancer.

The presence of esophageal cancer may be suggested by an abnormal result found with barium swallow of the esophagus, in which barium is swallowed by the patient and the physician observes its passage down the esophagus by using a fluoroscope. In the case of abnormal barium swallow results, and in many cases without a barium swallow, the doctor usually recommends an ENDOSCOPY, in which a slender tube with a camera lens is inserted down the patient's throat. The endoscopy enables the physician to view the interior of the esophagus on the monitor and he/she can also take biopsy specimens (small tissue samples) to check for cancer.

Other tests may include a computed tomography (CT) scan, endoscopic ultrasound, and a bone scan to determine whether cancer has spread beyond the esophagus.

If the test results and the subsequent biopsy findings reveal that the patient has esophageal cancer, the disease is staged: The physician determines how advanced the cancer is and how fast it is growing. They also seek to determine whether the cancer has spread (metastasized) to other organs; if it has, the disease is usually not curable, although patients may try treatments in attempts to delay any further spread of cancer, as well as to provide symptomatic relief.

Physicians also check for any spread to nodes in the surrounding area; if there is spreading, the prognosis is not good. Lymph nodes are tiny immune organs that work to remove toxins from the body. However, once cancer involves the lymph nodes, this indicates a poorer prognosis.

### How Esophageal Cancer Is Treated

Assuming that the cancer has not reached a stage in which treatment would be futile, as it often does, the most common form of treatment is surgical resection, which is removal of the part of the esophagus that is cancerous. The stomach may be pulled up and hooked to the remaining healthy esophagus, or the removed part may be replaced with a part of the patient's colon. Even if the disease is thought to be in its early stages, experts report that only about 15 percent of patients survive for three years or more after the surgery.

After surgery, the patient may need to receive nutrition intravenously, at least for a while, because swallowing is difficult or painful. Some patients are given a feeding tube, which is a tube that is inserted through the nose and goes directly into the stomach. Alternatively, the tube may be inserted into the small intestine, directly through the abdominal wall. Liquid nutrition is provided until patients can eat without it again.

Physicians may also use radiation therapy to attempt to shrink the tumor. They may combine radiation therapy with chemotherapy, which is the use of drugs given to destroy cancer cells. At times, chemoradiation may be done to shrink a nonsurgically resectable tumor to a resectable one. In general, chemotherapy for esophageal cancer is given through an intravenous line rather than in the form of a pill.

In patients in whom cancer has spread beyond the limits of a curative resection, a stent (tubing that is made of synthetic material) may be placed into the esophagus to keep it open so that the patient may swallow. Laser treatments may also be used.

The patient may also be encouraged to join a clinical trial, a formal study of drugs or treatments that are being tested for their effectiveness in combating esophageal cancer (or other cancers or diseases). When a patient with an advanced form of cancer joins a clinical trial, he or she may have access to an experimental medication or treatment that is not otherwise available.

See also ESOPHAGUS.

Calle, Eugenia E., et al. "Overweight, Obesity, and Mortality from Cancer in a Prospectively Studied Cohort of U.S. Adults." *New England Journal of Medicine* 348, no. 17 (April 24, 2003): 1,625–1,638.

Devesa, Susan S., William J. Blot, and Joseph F. Fraumeni, Jr., M.D. "Changing Patterns in the

Incidence of Esophageal and Gastric Carcinoma in the United States." *Cancer* 83 no. 10 (November 15, 1998): 2,049–2,053.

Lewey, Scott M., and Peter R. McNally. "Endoscopic Cancer Screening and Surveillance." In *GI/Liver Secrets.* 2d ed. Philadelphia: Hanley & Belfus, 2001.

Tierney, Lawrence M., Jr., M.D., Stephen J. McPhee, M.D., and Maxine A. Papadakis, M.D. "Malignant Esophageal Lesions (Cancer of the Esophagus)." In *Current Medical Diagnosis and Treatment 2002.* New York: Lange Medical Books, 2002.

McCarthy, Nicole, and Jean Grem. "Esophageal Cancer." In *Bethesda Handbook of Clinical Oncology.* New York: Lippincott Williams & Wilkins, 2001.

Morris Brown, Linda, and Susan S. Devesa. "Epidemiologic Trends in Esophageal and Gastric Cancer in the United States." *Surgical Oncology Clinics of North America* 11 (2002): 235–256.

Morris Brown, Linda, Susan S. Devesa, and Joseph F. Fraumeni, Jr., M.D. "Epidemiology of Esophageal Cancer." In *Atlas of Clinical Oncology: Cancer of the Upper Gastrointestinal Tract.* London: B. C. Decker, 2002.

**cancer, gallbladder**    Malignant tumor of the gallbladder or the bile duct. About 5,000 people are diagnosed with gallbladder cancer each year in the United States. Many cases of gallbladder cancer are detected by chance during surgery for other gallbladder problems, such as gallstones.

### Risk Factors

Gallbladder cancer is two to three times more commonly found among women than men. (There are no gender differences found among people with cancer of the bile duct.) There are also racial and ethnic differences in risks: Native Americans have the highest risk for gallbladder cancer, followed by natives of Israel, Mexico, Chile, and northern Japan.

A study of more than 42,000 Danish patients with gallstone disease over the period 1977 to 1989, which was reported in a 1999 issue of the *British Journal of Cancer,* found a linkage between gallstones and later development of digestive cancer. Patients with gallstone disease who did not have a CHOLECYSTECTOMY (the removal of the entire gallbladder) had an increased risk for gallbladder cancer, liver cancer, and cancers of the extrahepatic duct and the pancreas. Patients who did have cholecystectomy had an increased risk for cancers in the ampulla of Vater, which is also known as the hepatopancreatic ampulla. This is a dilation of the major duodenal papillae that receive the common bile duct and pancreatic duct.

Patients who have had pancreatic cancer may also be at an increased risk for development of gallbladder cancer.

In general, patients who have previously had the following diseases, disorders, or exposures have the greatest risk of development of gallbladder cancer:

- Those with existing gallstones
- Those who have a calcified wall of the gallbladder
- People who are carriers of typhoid bacteria
- People who have polyps in the gallbladder
- Obese individuals

### Symptoms

Patients with gallbladder cancer are usually asymptomatic or have nonspecific symptoms until the disease is advanced. The symptoms and signs, when present, include the following:

- Pain in the upper right abdomen
- Nausea and vomiting
- Lack of appetite
- Jaundice
- Pruritus (very itchy skin)
- Hepatomegaly (enlarged liver)
- Ascites (fluid buildup in the abdomen)
- Weight loss
- Dark urine (the color of cola)
- Intolerance of fatty foods

### Diagnosis and Treatment

The patient who has symptoms indicative of gallbladder disease is usually evaluated with an ultrasound, which can rule out gallstones. If gallbladder cancer is present, the ultrasound may show localized thickening and irregularity of the wall of the gallbladder. An ENDOSCOPIC ULTRASOUND (an ultrasound done through the endoscope rather than through the skin and the abdominal wall) is superior but is not widely available as of this writing. A computed tomography (CT) scan may also be done for diagnosis as well as identification of spread of the cancer to other adjacent organs.

If the cancer has not advanced beyond the gallbladder, surgery is usually considered to be the best treatment for most patients. For T1 tumors (the earliest stage of gallbladder tumors), the five-year survival rate is about 80 to 90 percent. Survival rates drop with advance in the level of the tumor.

See also CANCER; CANCER, LIVER; CANCER, PANCREATIC; ESOPHAGUS; HEPATOCELLULAR CARCINOMA.

Chow, W. H., et al. "Gallstones, Cholecystectomy and Risk of Cancers of the Liver, Biliary Tract and Pancreas." *British Journal of Cancer* 79, no. 3/4 (1999): 640–644.

De Groen, Piet C., M.D., et al. "Biliary Tract Cancers." *New England Journal of Medicine* 341, no. 18 (October 28, 1999): 1,368–1,378.

Hegde, Upendra, and Jean Grem. "Biliary Tract Cancer." In *Bethesda Handbook of Clinical Oncology.* New York: Lippincott Williams & Wilkins, 2001.

**cancer, liver**  A malignant tumor that originates in the liver or frequently is a fatal cancer that has spread from other parts of the body to the liver. Unless the patient is a candidate for surgical removal of the cancerous part of the liver, he or she cannot survive without liver transplantation. The term *cancer of the liver* broadly includes cancer of the bile duct (bile duct cancer) as well as of the liver itself, although when physicians specifically state that a patient has liver cancer, they are usually not referring to bile duct cancer or to the cancer that has spread to the liver from cancer of other organs, like colon cancer.

Patients with liver cancer have a poor survival rate. The median survival is six to 20 months. (This means that half of the individuals who are diagnosed with liver cancer live less than six to 20 months and half live longer.) The American Cancer Society reports that only about 6 percent of people who are diagnosed with liver cancer in the United States survive for five or more years, primarily because liver cancer is usually not diagnosed until a late stage, when the disease is no longer treatable. There are few or no symptoms in the early stages of liver cancer, when the disease might be treatable with surgical excision of the cancerous part of the liver.

According to the American Cancer Society, there were about 16,600 new cases of cancer of the liver and the intrahepatic bile duct in the United States in 2002. Of these cases, 11,000 patients were men, and 5,600 were women. There were also 14,100 deaths of liver cancer and intrahepatic bile duct cancer in 2002, 8,900 men and 5,200 women who died of these diseases.

Liver cancer is not common in the United States: it accounts for only about 1.5 percent of all cancer diagnoses. However, liver cancer is much more common among people in many poor countries. Globally, liver cancer is the fifth most common cancer in the world and the fourth most common cancer killer worldwide.

### Risk Factors

An estimated 80 percent of the cases of liver cancer occur in developing countries, especially in sub-Saharan Africa and Southeast Asia. Hepatitis B and C and high alcohol consumption are common in these areas. In addition, food contamination with aflatoxin, which may be a factor, is common.

Liver cancer occurs about 10 times more frequently in poor countries in Africa and Asia than in the United States. The key reason for this prominence of liver cancer is the heavy incidence of viral hepatitis in these countries. Obesity and overweight are also risk factors for development and death from liver cancer, according to a 2003 study in the *New England Journal of Medicine.*

There are several different types of liver cancer. HEPATOCELLULAR CARCINOMA (HCC) is the most common form, representing about 70 percent of all liver cancers. It is also known as malignant hepatoma or simply hepatoma. HCC is usually associated with cirrhosis of the liver, stemming from chronic HEPATITIS B and C infection or from chronic alcoholism. (Chronic hepatitis B carriers may have hepatoma without development of cirrhosis.) Hepatitis B and C are viruses that can be spread through blood products, sexual contact, or sharing of needles used to inject drugs.

It is also possible for cancers that arise in other parts of the body to spread to the liver, particularly cancers originating in the breast, colon, lung, pancreas, and stomach. This is known as metastatic cancer.

Of those liver cancer cases that are not hepatocellular carcinomas, the largest single cause, representing less than 10 percent of all liver cancers originating in the liver, are cholangiocarcinomas. These are cancers that develop in branches of the bile ducts from the liver. This form of cancer may be caused by liver parasites, especially in people who have liver cancer in Southeast Asia.

Another form of liver cancer is angiosarcoma, which is a very rare cancer that occurs within the blood vessels of the liver. Angiosarcoma is associated with exposure to chemical carcinogens such as vinyl chloride and arsenic. Many patients have secondary or metastatic liver cancer, cancer that originates elsewhere and spreads to the liver.

People who have cirrhosis of the liver, particularly those who are also alcoholics or who have viral hepatitis, are at the greatest risk for development of liver cancer. Individuals who have HEMOCHROMATOSIS, a disease of iron overload, have an increased risk for development of liver cancer.

Liver cancer is more common among people older than 55 to 60 years old. In the United States, African Americans and Hispanics have twice the risk of development of liver cancer of whites. Some Asian groups have a high rate of incidence; men who have emigrated from Vietnam have a very high rate of occurrence, primarily because of the associated high rate of viral hepatitis in Vietnam.

In looking at the incidence of liver cancer by ethnicity in Los Angeles, California, over the period 1988 to 1992, researchers considered trends and patterns among liver cancer patients and reported their findings in the 2001 issue of the *International Journal of Cancer*. The researchers found that white males in Los Angeles had a liver cancer rate of 2.9 per 100,000 people, followed by a rate of 5.1 for black men. The rate increased to 5.8 for Japanese men and further increased to 6.5 per 100,000 for Hispanic men. Chinese men had a much higher

rate, of 16.1 per 100,000, and Korean men had the highest rate of all: 23.9 cases per 100,000 men.

Women also had an increased risk for liver cancer based on their ethnicity, but it was a much lower rate than found among men. For example, white women in Los Angeles had a rate of 1.1 cases of liver cancer per 100,000 women. The rate increased to 2.2 per 100,000 for black women. The highest rates of liver cancer were found among Chinese women (4.4 per 100,000) and Korean women (5.5 per 100,000).

In very rare cases, liver cancer can be caused by aflatoxin, which is a substance that can occur in some forms of mold. In this case, aflatoxin leads to mutations of the p53 tumor suppressor gene. The type of fungus that generates aflatoxin can sometimes be found on peanuts, corns, and nuts, and aflatoxin contamination is a serious problem in countries in Asia and Africa; however, in the United States, the Food and Drug Administration (FDA) prohibits the sale of foods that have high levels of aflatoxin.

A family history of liver cancer also constitutes an increased risk for the development of liver cancer.

### Symptoms and Signs

Most people in the early stages of liver cancer have no symptoms; that is one key reason for the high rate of fatalities. When symptoms occur, they may include the following:

- Weight loss
- Abdominal swelling
- Appetite loss
- Pain in the upper right abdomen
- Yellow jaundice of the skin or eyes
- Darkened urine (caused by jaundice)
- Nausea and vomiting
- Fever
- Ascites (fluid buildup in the abdomen)

### Diagnosis and Treatment

Liver cancer diagnosis is based on the patient's symptoms as well as on results of diagnostic tests, such as blood tests of a patient's liver enzymes and function as well as a test for alpha fetoprotein (AFP). High AFP blood level may indicate liver cancer. Doctors may also order a liver scan, a bone scan (in the event that the cancer may have spread to the bones), X rays, a liver ultrasound, and a computed tomography (CT) scan. Magnetic resonance imaging (MRI) is also sometimes used. If cancer is present, these diagnostic imaging tools (MRI, CT, ultrasound) also help the doctor to stage the cancer, to determine its severity.

A biopsy, which is the removal of a small amount of tissue to check for cancer, is usually used to confirm definitively the presence of liver cancer, although in some cases, very high alpha-fetoprotein level laboratory test findings and characteristic CT findings may be considered adequate tools for diagnosis. Physicians may decide that the risks to the patient of performing a liver biopsy outweigh the benefits, because of the potential for fatal bleeding, and because of the low risk of inadvertently spreading any existing cancer cells. Sometimes a diagnostic biopsy is obtained by the physician by using a laparoscope, a device that can be inserted through a small incision in the abdomen, to inspect the liver and surrounding organs visually.

If only part of the liver is involved, as mentioned earlier, that part can be surgically removed. Liver cancer can also be treated with radiation and chemotherapy to extend the patient's life, although not to cure the liver cancer. Many patients with liver cancer are advised to join a clinical trial, which is an ongoing study of diseases. Joining a clinical trial may enable patients to try drugs or treatments that are being tested and that are not available to the general public.

If the cancer has not spread beyond the liver, and it is not widespread within the liver itself, patients may be candidates for a liver transplantation, assuming that a donor liver can be located in time.

In the case of advanced cancer, patients are treated with radiation therapy or chemotherapy, and some patients may receive both forms of treatment.

### Prevention of Liver Cancer

Hepatoma may be prevented by avoidance of the underlying conditions with which it is associated, such as viral hepatitis B and C, and treatment of chronic viral hepatitis if it has been contracted.

Hepatitis B vaccination is now universally recommended in children.

### Screening for Liver Cancer

Screening for hepatocellular carcinoma is recommended for patients with liver cirrhosis due to any cause as well as those with chronic hepatitis B carrier state without cirrhosis. It is usually accomplished by a regular check of the patient's alpha-fetoprotein level and ultrasound screenings of the liver.

See also HEMOCHROMATOSOSIS; HEPATITIS; LIVER; LIVER ENZYMES/FUNCTION TESTS; LIVER FAILURE; LIVER TRANSPLANTATION; OBESITY.

Calle, Eugenia E., et al. "Overweight, Obesity, and Mortality from Cancer in a Prospectively Studied Cohort of U.S. Adults." *New England Journal of Medicine* 348, no. 17 (April 24, 2003): 1,625–1,638.

Lawrence, Steven P., M.D. "Evaluation of Focal Liver Masses." In *GI/Liver Secrets*. 2d ed. Philadelphia: Hanley & Belfus, 2001.

McGlynn, Katherine A., et al., "International Trends and Patterns of Primary Liver Cancer." *International Journal of Cancer* 94 (2001): 290–296.

**cancer, oral**  Malignant tumor of the mouth, the oropharynx (part of the throat that is in the back of the mouth), the lips, the lining inside the lips and cheeks, the floor of the mouth that lies under the tongue, the tongue itself, and the tonsils. Oral cancer is the sixth most common cancer worldwide. Most oral cancers are squamous cell carcinomas rather than adenocarcinomas. According to the American Cancer Society, there were about 29,000 new cases of oral cancer diagnosed in the United States in 2002. There were also an estimated 1,600 deaths caused by oral cancers in 2002, 1,200 men and 400 women. The five-year survival rate for oral cancer patients is 56 percent, according to the American Cancer Society; however, the five-year survival rate for blacks is much lower, only 34 percent.

### Risk Factors

Oral cancer is more commonly found among people ages 45 and older, but younger individuals may also be diagnosed with oral cancer. Smoking greatly increases the risk of development of oral cancers, as does the use of smokeless (chewing) tobacco or pipe tobacco, and an estimated 80 percent of all oral cancers are attributed to smoking. Chronic or heavy alcohol use, poor oral hygiene, and immune suppression in organ transplantation patients can also lead to oral cancers. When individuals both smoke and consume alcohol regularly, their risk for development of oral cancer is greatly increased.

Chronic and heavy sun exposure may cause cancer of the lip, as may pipe smoking.

### Symptoms and Signs of Oral Cancers

An oral cancer may occur without symptoms in the early stages. Symptoms that may occur (at any stage) include the following:

- A sore throat that does not heal
- Dysphagia (pain or difficulty with swallowing)
- Trouble with moving the tongue or the jaw
- Changes in the sound of the voice
- Ear pain
- A sore in the mouth or on the lip or another area of the oral cavity that does not heal
- A lump on the mouth
- White or red patchy areas on the gums, tongue, or lining of the mouth

Note: These symptoms may also occur with other diseases, and only a physician can diagnose an oral cancer.

### Diagnosis of Oral Cancers

If physicians suspect the presence of an oral cancer, on the basis of a patient's symptoms and/or the appearance of the oral cavity or mouth, they refer the patient to either an oral surgeon or an ear, nose, and throat specialist. The expert performs a biopsy, which is the removal of a small amount of tissue, to check for cancer.

If cancer is found, then the cancer is staged: the pathologist who analyzed the biopsy result and the doctor (who may order other tests) determine how advanced the cancer is and how aggressively it is growing. Dental X rays and X rays of the head, neck, and chest can help in staging the cancer. The physician may also order a computed tomography (CT) scan, ultrasound, or magnetic resonance imaging (MRI) scan to obtain more information about the tumor. The positron emission tomography (PET) scan may also be used to detect early stages of oral cancer. These tests may help doctors to determine the location and size of the tumor and to detect whether cancer has spread (metastasized) to other parts of the body.

### Treatment of Oral Cancers

The treatment depends on how advanced the cancer is and whether it has spread beyond the oral cavity. Regardless of the treatment chosen, doctors may advise patients to have any needed dental work performed first, because having it done later may be too difficult. In addition, a feeding gastrostomy tube may be placed endoscopically (in a percutaneous endoscopic gastrostomy [PEG]) or radiologically before surgery.

The treatment may include surgery, radiation therapy, or both. In addition to the surgeon and the oncologist (cancer doctor), physicians also often recommend that patients receive treatment by other specialists, such as a dentist, a plastic surgeon (because surgery may cause facial deformities), and a dietitian (because surgery and the cancer itself may make eating difficult).

Patients with advanced oral cancer may be treated with chemotherapy, which is administration of cancer-killing drugs. Patients who have advanced oral cancer are also often encouraged to join a clinical trial. Clinical trials are studies in which physicians test experimental medications and other therapies on people who have specific diseases and medical problems. These drugs and treatments are generally not available to patients unless they are enrolled in clinical trials.

See also SMOKING.

**cancer, pancreatic**    Malignancy of the pancreas, a pear-shaped organ that is about six inches long and is surrounded by the stomach and intestines in close proximity to the spleen, the liver, and the gallbladder. The pancreas produces insulin, which controls blood sugar level. The pancreas also generates pancreatic juices, which help to digest food. When cancer is diagnosed in the pancreas, it usually appears in the head of the pancreas (75 percent of the time); it appears in the body or tail of the pancreas in the remaining cases. Most forms of pancreatic cancer start in the ducts carrying the pancreatic juices.

According to the American Cancer Society, there were an estimated 30,300 new cases of pancreatic cancer diagnosed in the United States in 2002, 14,700 men and 15,600 women. There were also an estimated 29,700 deaths, 14,500 men and 15,200 women. About 40,000 people in Europe die of pancreatic cancer each year, and the disease occurs about equally among men and women.

Pancreatic cancer is the fourth leading cause of cancer among men and the fifth leading cause of cancer among women in the United States, and it is also responsible for about 5 percent of all cancer deaths. Pancreatic cancer is the most lethal form of all the cancers, and the majority of people who are diagnosed with this disease die within twelve months. The five-year survival rate is less than 5 percent among patients who are diagnosed with pancreatic cancer.

### Risk Factors

Age is a key risk factor for pancreatic cancer, and most people in whom this disease develops are above age 60. The presentation of painless jaundice with weight loss in an elderly individual is an ominous sign.

Gender is another factor. The incidence of pancreatic cancer in women is increasing, whereas it has stabilized among men. In a national and state-by-state analysis of deaths from pancreatic cancer in the United States, the national death rate for men over the 1994–98 period was 8.7 per 100,000 men and 7.2 per 100,000 women.

According to the American Cancer Society, in the United States, the District of Columbia had the highest rates of pancreatic cancer: 11.7 per 100,000 men and 8.6 per 100,000 women. Utah had the lowest rate of pancreatic cancer among the states: 7.4 per 100,000 men and 5.0 per 100,000 women. The reasons for this geographic difference are unknown.

Health habits can lead to pancreatic cancer, and smoking is a known risk factor for the development of pancreatic cancer. Smokers who stop SMOKING decrease their risk for pancreatic cancer within several years.

Other risk factors for developing pancreatic cancer are as follows:

- A family history of pancreatic cancer (the disease is more likely if a parent or sibling has had pancreatic cancer)
- A diagnosis of diabetes, especially long-standing type 2 diabetes
- The presence of chronic pancreatitis, an inflammation of the pancreas
- Chronic occupational exposure, such as with exposure to petrochemicals
- A diet that is very high in fat and meat consumption

### Symptoms and Signs

Most patients have no symptoms until the disease is very advanced. The most common symptom is abdominal pain, which may radiate into the patient's back.

Other symptoms of pancreatic cancer are as follows:

- Diarrhea
- A yellowish tinge to the skin and the whites of the eyes (JAUNDICE)
- Abdominal and upper back pain or discomfort
- Appetite loss
- Unintended weight loss
- Nausea and vomiting
- Weakness
- Very dark (cola-colored) urine
- Pale, chalky stool
- Itchy skin

### Diagnosis

The doctor who suspects pancreatic cancer orders blood tests involving the liver, as well as imaging studies. Laboratory tests reveal increased level of bilirubin, a substance that is produced by the liver. Normally, bilirubin travels from the liver to the gallbladder to the intestine. When a bile duct is blocked by a tumor in the pancreas, bile cannot be normally excreted through the bile ducts; thus the bilirubin may accumulate instead in the blood and bilirubin levels are elevated in the blood and urine. This accumulation of bilirubin causes the yellow skin color that is characteristic of JAUNDICE. Stools, on the other hand, appear pale and chalky because of the absence of bile. The use of genetic markers in diagnosis (such as mutations of the K-*ras* gene and p53 tumor suppressor gene) is investigational as of this writing.

Other diagnostic tests that are commonly ordered by most physicians when they are suspicious of the presence of pancreatic cancer are computed tomography (CT) testing and/or MAGNETIC RESONANCE IMAGING (MRI), as well as ultrasound imaging or other tests to help with diagnosis. An endoscopic retrograde cholangiopancreatography (ERCP) (an endoscope test of the bile ducts and the pancreas) and an endoscopic ultrasound study may also be undertaken.

Ultimately, a biopsy determines whether cancer is present. The biopsy is performed by inserting a needle through the abdomen or inserting an endoscope in the throat for performing an ERCP. Doctors seek to determine whether the cancer has spread to neighboring organs, such as the gallbladder or even farther afield, such as to the kidney or bones. CT scans, an endoscopic ultrasound (EUS), and MRI scans can help doctors to determine the size of the primary tumor and to pinpoint its exact location. If endoscopic ultrasound is available, it may further help doctors to diagnose and stage pancreatic cancer. In the case of a typical finding on imaging studies when a lesion is deemed to be surgically resectable, the surgeon may proceed directly to surgery without undertaking a biopsy.

### Treatment of Pancreatic Cancer

Most patients with pancreatic cancer are treated by a GASTROENTEROLOGIST, as well as an oncologist, or cancer specialist, and by surgeons as well as by their regular physicians. The most common and effective treatment for pancreatic cancer is surgery to remove part of the pancreas and the surrounding tissue, including parts of the stomach and the small intestine, a procedure that is known as the Whipple resection; however, this surgery is very difficult to perform, and to date, the prognosis for patients remains poor, despite surgical advances.

Doctors may also use radiation therapy to irradiate the cancerous area or chemotheraphy to destroy the cancer cells.

As of this writing, because the probability of successful treatment is so low among patients with pancreatic cancer, many doctors recommend that patients whose cancer is surgically nonresectable participate in a clinical trial, in which they receive medication or treatment that is otherwise not available to them because it has not yet been approved for general public use.

See also LIVER ENZYMES/FUNCTION TESTS; PANCREAS; SMOKING; WHIPPLE PROCEDURE.

American Cancer Society. "Cancer Facts and Figures, 2002." 2002.
Gulley, James, and Chris H. Takimoto. "Pancreatic Cancer." In *Bethesda Handbook of Clinical Oncology*. New York: Lippincott Williams & Wilkins, 2001.

**cancer, stomach**   A malignancy that is found in the stomach, a major organ of the digestive system, and is also known as gastric cancer. Most stomach cancers are adenocarcinomas. According to the American Cancer Society, about 21,600 new cases of stomach cancer were diagnosed in 2002 in the United States. There were an estimated 12,400 deaths from stomach cancer in the United States in 2002: 7,200 men and 5,200 women. The five-year survival rate for stomach cancer in the United States is about 10 percent, and there is little difference between races in terms of survival rate.

In looking at the global population, an estimated 600,000 people worldwide die of stomach cancer each year. The highest incidences of stomach cancer are found in Asia, South America, and Scandinavian countries. The highest incidence of stomach cancer worldwide is found in Japan, followed by Costa Rica, China, Brazil, the former Yugoslavia, and Finland. Interestingly, Japanese people who leave Japan continue to have a high rate of gastric cancer; however, their children and grandchildren have a rate of stomach cancer that is more consistent with that of the people in the country to which they have relocated. It is unknown why this is true; it may be related to diet.

Early gastric cancer is diagnosed when the cancer remains within the superficial layers of the stomach wall. Advanced gastric cancer is cancer that has spread deep beyond the stomach's submucosal layer. Most people in North America (80 to 95 percent) who are diagnosed with stomach cancer have advanced gastric cancer. However, in contrast, about 30 percent of Japanese people who are diagnosed with gastric cancer have early gastric cancer. The difference occurs because Japanese undergo screening for gastric cancer on a regular basis, whereas it is not done in the United States because of the low incidence.

### Causes of Stomach Cancer

Some studies indicate that the common stomach bacterium *Helicobacter pylori* may be implicated in some cases of gastric cancer, because some clinical studies have demonstrated that people who are infected with *H. pylori* have two to six times the risk of development of stomach cancer than do others. *H. pylori* is the same bacterium that causes most peptic ULCER.

A study of 1,246 Japanese patients with *H. pylori* and 280 patients who were not infected was reported in a 2001 issue of the *New England Journal of Medicine*. All of the subjects had duodenal ulcers, gastric ulcers, or other stomach problems. In about 3 percent of the *H. pylori* group stomach cancer developed but in none of the uninfected persons in the control group. As a result, researchers concluded that *H. pylori* was implicated in gastric cancer.

### Risk Factors

Age is a key risk factor, and most stomach cancer patients are older than age 50. Gender is another risk factor: most stomach cancer victims are male in a ratio of about 1.7 males to 1.0 female. Race is another risk factor for stomach cancer: African Americans have about a 1.5 higher risk of development of stomach cancer than whites. There may also be a genetic risk involved in stomach cancer, although research continues on that subject to identify the chromosomal location of the gene that triggers stomach cancer; however, it is known that those with a family history of stomach cancer have

a two to three times greater risk of development of stomach cancer. The emperor Napoleon, his father, and his grandfather all died of gastric cancer.

The risk for stomach cancer is increased two- to threefold among patients who have PERNICIOUS ANEMIA; in a small fraction of these patients stomach cancer will develop.

The use of tobacco increases the risk of development of gastric cancer, and tobacco users have a 1.5 to three times greater risk of development of stomach cancer than nonusers.

Other risk factors include the following:

- Presence of Menetrier's disease
- Type A blood
- Deficiencies of vitamins A, C, E, beta-carotene; selenium; or fiber
- Diets rich in complex carbohydrates (such as fava beans), as well as heavy consumption of salted, pickled, or smoked foods; dried fish; and cooking oil (Note: a diet rich in fiber, fresh fruits, and vegetables leads to a *decreased* risk for stomach cancer)

### Symptoms

Patients who have stomach cancer may have a few nonspecific or no symptoms in the early stages. If symptoms do occur, they may be vague or easily ignored by the patient, and sometimes by the physician. Some symptoms that may occur with stomach cancer are the following:

- Abdominal pain or discomfort
- Weight loss
- Chronic indigestion or heartburn
- Nausea and vomiting
- Ulcerlike pain
- Constipation or diarrhea
- Extremely bloated feeling after eating
- Appetite loss
- Gastrointestinal bleeding
- Dysphagia (difficulty in swallowing)
- Early satiety (sensation of being very full soon after starting to eat)

- Excessive belching
- Weakness and fatigue
- Vomiting of blood or presence of blood in the stool

Important note: not everyone who has these symptoms has stomach cancer; such symptoms may indicate a temporary gastric problem or another health problem altogether. However, people with such symptoms should consult their physician for a complete physical examination and should also have any diagnostic tests that the doctor recommends.

### Diagnosing Stomach Cancer

An UPPER GASTROINTESTINAL X RAY of both the esophagus (the food tube leading to the stomach) and the stomach can help by highlighting the stomach to detect possible tumors. The patient swallows liquid barium (which tastes like chalk), so that the stomach and esophagus can be seen on a fluoroscope and any serious abnormalities can often be detected.

An endoscopy is another procedure in which a special tube is passed through the mouth and into the esophagus and then the stomach. Using this device, the doctor can see inside the stomach and can remove tissue for biopsy. The endoscopy is preferred to the upper gastrointestinal (GI) X ray test because the doctor can obtain a biopsy specimen with the endoscopy. If cancer is present, a biopsy (removal of tissue for examination by a pathologist) also helps the doctor to determine how aggressive the cancer is at the time of the biopsy. Staging of the tumor is important because it helps the doctor determine the treatment to recommend.

Most countries, including the United States, rely on the Tumor-Node-Metastasis (TNM) system of staging all forms of cancer. This system uses various tests and parameters to evaluate the depth of the tumor invasion into the stomach wall (T), whether it has advanced into the lymph nodes (the *N* part of the TNM system), and whether it has spread beyond the stomach, or metastasized (M0 or M1).

Routine screening for stomach cancer is not recommended in the United States.

### Treatment for Stomach Cancer

Patients with stomach cancer may be treated with surgery, chemotherapy, and radiation treatment.

*Surgery*    The most common form of treatment for stomach cancer is surgery, in which the surgeon removes all or part of the stomach (a GASTRECTOMY or partial gastrectomy). At least 80 percent of patients have an advanced case of stomach cancer at the time of diagnosis, and curative surgery is not indicated in those cases; however, palliative surgery (surgery that is performed not to cure the patient, but to alleviate the symptoms) may be done to relieve obstructions.

A gastrectomy is a major operation. Patients may need to change their diet considerably and permanently after the surgery. Patients who have had total gastrectomy often also need injections of vitamin $B_{12}$, because they can no longer absorb the vitamin naturally through the food that they eat.

Some patients who have had gastric surgery may experience DUMPING SYNDROME, a condition that occurs when the food enters the small intestine too quickly. The primary symptoms of dumping syndrome are weakness, dizziness, palpitations, sweating, cramps, nausea, as well as vomiting that occurs shortly after eating. Chronic diarrhea is another complication experienced by patients who have had a gastrectomy. Eating smaller and more frequent meals may help resolve this problem, as well as avoiding foods high in sugar content.

*Chemotherapy*    Another treatment option for stomach cancer is chemotherapy. Cancer-killing drugs for stomach cancer patients may be administered in oral form or by injection, depending on the particular patient and the treatment regimen. Chemotherapy may cause nausea, vomiting, and hair loss, which usually end when the chemotherapy is completed.

*Radiation therapy*    Radiation therapy is another treatment for stomach cancer. High-energy rays are directed at the cancerous part of the body. The appropriate time frame for radiation therapy is best determined by the radiation oncologist (cancer radiotherapy doctor). Radiation therapy patients may experience nausea and vomiting, and the irradiated area may become reddened and sore.

Patients receiving radiation therapy may also be very fatigued and have diarrhea.

See also HELICOBACTER PYLORI; RADIATION THERAPY.

Avunduk, Canan. *Manual of Gastroenterology.* 3d ed. Philadelphia: Lippincott Williams & Wilkins, 2002.

Deutsch, John C., M.D. "Gastric Cancer." In *GI/Liver Secrets.* 2d ed. Philadelphia: Hanley & Belfus, 2001.

Fuchs, Charles S., M.D., and Robert Mayer J., M.D. "Gastric Cancer." *New England Journal of Medicine* 331 (July 6, 1995): 32–41.

Kim, George P., and Chris H. Takimoto. "Gastric Cancer." In *Bethesda Handbook of Clinical Oncology.* New York: Lippincott Williams & Wilkins, 2001.

Mayne, Susan T., et al. "Nutrient Intake and Risk of Subtypes of Esophageal and Gastric Cancer," *Cancer Epidemiology, Biomarkers & Prevention* 10 (October 2001): 1,055–1,062.

Uemura, Naomi, M.D., et al. "*Helicobacter Pylori* Infection and the Development of Gastric Cancer." *New England Journal of Medicine* 345, no. 11 (September 13, 2001): 784–789.

**Candida**   A common yeast that is found in the body. It is a commensal yeast (living with another organism from which they derive a benefit) that is normally seen in the oral cavity, gastrointestinal tract, and vagina. *Candida* are not harmful unless an infection occurs. *Candida* organism can cause infections in the skin, mouth, throat, or internal organs when the normal balance of bacteria is disrupted or the person's immune system is suppressed (such as patients who have received organ transplantation, patients with cancer, and patients with ACQUIRED IMMUNODEFICIENCY SYNDROME [AIDS]). A mouth infection of candida is also called THRUSH. The infection may also spread into the bloodstream, especially in immunosuppressed patients. *Candida* infections of other organs, such as the esophagus and kidneys, may also develop.

### Risk Factors

People who have some diseases, such as DIABETES MELLITUS, are more prone to development of *Candida* infections than others. Sometimes taking antibiotics can cause *Candida* infections, particularly vaginitis in women. An extended dosage of antibiotics is more likely to cause such an infection than is one short course of drugs that is taken for just three to five days.

In rare cases, a *Candida* infection can become systemic, causing the individual to feel very sick and lethargic, and this condition can be fatal.

### Symptoms

Oral thrush may cause no symptoms or may cause a cottony feeling in the mouth, the loss of taste, and painful eating and swallowing. If *Candida* organisms are found on the skin or in the genital area, they usually cause intense itching and may also cause pain. Vaginal candidiasis causes itching and discharge and, in some cases, pain during urination and during sexual intercourse. A cottage cheese–like substance in the vagina is characteristic of *Candida* infection, and the infection also produces a distinctive odor.

### Diagnosis

Oral thrush may be suspected during physical examination and later confirmed by examining oral scrapings with a potassium hydroxide (KOH) preparation. A vaginal examination reveals redness and swelling in the area when *Candida* infection is present, with a curdlike discharge. The presence of vaginal *Candida* organisms can be confirmed as with oral thrush.

### Treatment

Antiyeast creams or drugs are usually effective in combating a yeast infection, and oral antiyeast medications are also efficacious. Some doctors use both oral and topical (used on the skin) medications or intravaginal preparations. Some people, especially patients who are immunocompromised, experience chronic fungal infections and may need to take a "low-maintenance" dose of antiyeast medication. There are also oral drugs that combat fungal infections. Patients in whom *Candida* infection has spread may require intravenous antifungal medications. Patients usually need treatment for about two weeks or more.

See also LACTOBACILLUS; THRUSH; YEAST.

**canker sores** Painful small mouth sores that usually spontaneously resolve in a few days. Various factors have been implicated in causing canker sores, including stress, hormonal factors, food allergies, an altered immune system, heredity, vitamin deficiencies (of $B_1$, $B_2$, $B_6$, and $B_{12}$), and deficiencies of iron, folic acid, and zinc.

Larger canker sores may require six weeks to heal. Most patients get these ulcers two to four times per year. Occasionally, some patients have canker sores almost all the time. Canker sores are more common during childhood and adolescence and are seen less frequently in adulthood.

Canker sores may also result from infections (herpes), chemotherapy, and systemic illnesses such as CROHN'S DISEASE.

**Caroli's disease** A rare congenital disease in which the ducts that transport bile from the liver to the intestine are abnormally widened (also called cystic) in one or more places. Caroli's disease may run in families. This condition may result in inflammation, infection, or GALLSTONES. Typical symptoms of Caroli's disease include abdominal pain, jaundice, and fever. Patients with Caroli's disease may experience periodic flare-ups of CHOLANGITIS, which is the inflammation of the bile duct. They may also experience liver abscesses.

Those who have Caroli's disease have a greater risk than others of development of cancer of the bile ducts (cholangiocarcinoma): an estimated 2 to 15 percent of Caroli's disease patients have this form of cancer.

The treatment of choice for Caroli's disease is surgery, which can reduce, but not eliminate, the risk of cancer. The complication of CHOLANGITIS is treated with antibiotics. In refractory cases, liver transplantation offers the only hope for patients who have no evidence of cancer.

For further information, contact

American Liver Foundation
75 Maiden Lane
New York, NY 10038
(800) 465-4837 (toll-free)
http://www.liverfoundation.org

**celiac disease/celiac sprue** A severe food allergy that is caused by an allergic reaction to gluten, a substance that is found in wheat, rye, or barley and leads to damage to the small intestine. The role of oats is controversial, and as of this writing, it appears that pure oats are not a problem; however, pure oats are difficult to obtain, and hence oats should be avoided in patients with celiac sprue. Affected individuals are treated with a strict gluten-free diet.

As indicated by antibody testing, celiac sprue affects an estimated one in every 200 to 300 people in North America and Europe. About one in 4,700 people in the United States has actually been diagnosed with celiac disease; however, according to the National Institutes of Health, there is clear evidence that the disease is underdiagnosed in the United States, as indicated by blood samples drawn from Americans by the Red Cross and then tested for celiac disease. As a result, as many as one in 200 to one in 500 Americans may actually have the disease.

### Causes of Celiac Sprue

This disease is caused by an inappropriate immune cell response to the presence of gluten in some foods. In affected people, the immune system perceives gluten in the same way as a foreign invasion. This excites an inflammatory response that causes damage to the intestinal lining of the small intestine, leading to impaired absorption.

### Risk Factors

Celiac sprue is usually diagnosed in children or young adults, although about 20 percent of the cases are diagnosed among people older than age 60. Celiac sprue may also be diagnosed during or after pregnancy, especially among women who are severely anemic after the delivery of the baby. This medical problem is found among all races and ethnicities, although it is rare among Asians and blacks.

People who have celiac sprue are more likely to have other associated autoimmune illnesses, such as type 1 (insulin-dependent) diabetes or autoimmune thyroiditis. An estimated 3 to 8 percent of type 1 diabetes patients also have celiac sprue.

### Symptoms

Children with celiac sprue may have an enlarged abdomen, chronic diarrhea, and delayed growth. Infants may be very pale. Some children have constipation rather than diarrhea. If the condition is not diagnosed and treated, children may have delayed puberty, short stature, and ANEMIA. Older children with celiac sprue may have chronic abdominal pain, defects in the enamel of the teeth, and even emotional disorders, such as depression or irritability.

Celiac sprue usually develops in early childhood, but many cases are identified during adulthood. As mentioned, it may appear for the first time in pregnancy. Adults with celiac sprue have symptoms of diarrhea, weight loss, and excessive gas (flatulence). They may also experience LACTOSE INTOLERANCE. About half of all adult patients have iron deficiency anemia. They may also have other vitamin deficiencies, including deficiencies in vitamins $B_{12}$, D, and K. Many patients have no symptoms at all and may instead have asymptomatic and unexplained iron deficiency anemia.

Other symptoms that may occur in patients with celiac sprue are as follows:

- Pale skin
- Muscle pain and cramps
- Joint pain
- Anemia
- Edema (excessive retention of water weight)
- Extensive bruising (due to insufficiency of vitamin K)

A skin condition known as dermatitis herpetiformis may also be seen. An itchy and burning rash develops and can become blisters that rupture. A rash may be seen on the elbows, knees, buttocks, back, face, neck, and abdomen. Some patients have a deficiency of immunoglobulin A (IgA) antibodies.

### Diagnosis

Special blood tests of the immune system can be used to detect celiac sprue when physicians suspect that the condition is present. Specifically, the patient's blood is tested for antibodies to gliadin plus antibodies to endomysium and/or tissue transglutaminase. The antitissue transglutaminase testing is less expensive than the antiendomysial antibody test, but the tests are equally accurate. An antireticulin test is also available, but it is usually not needed and not performed. Physicians also perform a small bowel biopsy, which is considered the definitive test to look for damage to the intestinal lining caused by celiac sprue.

Patients are also tested for iron deficiency anemia, since it is a very common medical problem among people with celiac sprue. They may also be tested for deficiencies of calcium and vitamin D, which are also frequently seen among patients who have celiac sprue. As mentioned earlier, a vitamin $B_{12}$ deficiency may also be present, although it is less commonly found than are the other types of deficiencies. Some patients with celiac sprue are also deficient in vitamin K.

### Treatment

Doctors put children or adults with celiac sprue on a very strict gluten-free diet. Patients are instructed to avoid all foods that contain any wheat, barley, rye, or oats. Some dessert items and ice creams, and even some vitamin pills, contain wheat fillers, and these items must be completely avoided.

An estimated 70 percent of patients with celiac sprue significantly improve on a gluten-free diet, which is the only treatment for celiac sprue. Patients who do not respond to a gluten-free diet may require corticosteroids and other immunosuppressive medications in order to suppress the inflammatory damage that is caused by sprue. Patients with celiac sprue have an increased risk for gastrointestinal cancers.

Patients or the parents of children with celiac sprue must be especially vigilant in reading food labels and asking questions about food preparation when not eating at home. The majority of patients respond well to a gluten-free diet.

For support group information, contact the following organization:

Celiac Sprue Association
P.O. Box 31700
Omaha, NE 68131

(402) 558-0600
http://www.csaceliacs.org

See also ALLERGIES; FOOD.

Farrell, Richard J., M.D., and Kelly P. Ciaran, M.D. "Celiac Sprue." *New England Journal of Medicine* 346, no. 3 (January 17, 2002): 180–188.

**Chagas' disease** An infectious tropical disease caused by the protozoan parasite *Trypanosoma cruzi* that is transmitted through an insect bite or a blood transfusion. It is also known as American trypanosomiasis. About 18 million people worldwide are affected with *T. cruzi,* with an annual mortality rate of about 50,000 patients.

In Latin America, the disease has also been transmitted through donated blood after organ transplantation. In the chronic form of the disease, the affected person's life expectancy may be decreased by about nine years.

Chagas' disease was discovered by Carlos Chagas, a physician in Brazil in the 19th century. Chagas' disease is primarily found in Central America and South America, where it is a common problem, and as many as a million people are infected each year. If not diagnosed and treated, Chagas' disease causes a condition known as MEGA-COLON, an abnormal enlargement of the colon, and can produce an enlargement of the esophagus (megaesophagus). It may also affect the heart and cause congestive heart failure.

### Risk Factors

People who live in rural areas in poorly constructed houses or huts have greater risk, particularly those who live in houses made of mud or adobe. The insects living in such houses, reduviid insects or "kissing bugs," spread Chagas' disease after biting an animal or human who is infected with the disease. Individuals living in the following countries are most at risk for development of Chagas' disease: Argentina, Belize, Bolivia, Brazil, Chile, Colombia, Costa Rica, Ecuador, El Salvador, French Guiana, Guatemala, Guyana, Honduras, Mexico, Nicaragua, Panama, Paraguay, Peru, Suriname, Uruguay, and Venezuela. Immigrants from these countries to the United States or other developed nations are also at risk as carriers of this disease.

### Symptoms

Chagas' disease may occur in an acute or chronic form. Most (70 to 90 percent) infected individuals never have any symptoms and are asymptomatic carriers of the parasite. However, when chronic disease occurs, the problems usually do not arise until patients are 40 to 50 years of age.

In the acute form of Chagas' disease, which is usually found more among children than adults, the patient has an enlarged spleen, enlarged lymph nodes, fever, rapid heartbeat, and swelling of the legs and face.

In the chronic phase of the disease, which can occur 10 to 30 years after the infection, patients experience a variety of problems. Some patients (about 27 percent) have incurable heart disease. Others (about 6 percent) have enlargements in the digestive tract, which cause severe constipation or swallowing problems (dysphagia). Other patients (about 3 percent) experience neurological symptoms.

### Diagnosis and Treatment

The diagnosis of Chagas' disease is based on the signs and symptoms, results of laboratory tests and imaging studies, as well as the geographical location of the patient. The parasite can only be detected in the acute stage.

In most cases, nifurtimox or benznidazole is used to treat a recently acquired infection. In addition, treatment should be given to all immune-suppressed patients. Drugs can eradicate the parasite in about 50 percent of the cases of acute Chagas' disease, but they cannot reverse the complications that are seen in the chronic form of the disease. As such, the role of treatment in the chronic stage when complications have occurred is controversial. (Contact the Centers for Disease Control and Prevention in Atlanta to obtain information about these drugs.) If the infection is chronic, treatment is symptomatic, depending upon the problems that are seen.

### Prevention of Chagas' Disease

The best prevention is avoidance of sleeping in poorly made houses in developing countries in

Latin America. In addition, insects should be promptly destroyed by people living or visiting such areas. Mosquito nets should be used when the person is asleep. Finally, it is important to remember that there are numerous problems associated with screening the blood supplies for Chagas' disease, and thus, if a blood transfusion is required, the patient may contract Chagas' disease from infected blood. One approach that is used to prevent this problem is to ask prospective blood donors questions that may identify potentially affected individuals and then to exclude those with high risk for infection from donating their blood to a blood bank facility.

See also PARASITIC INFECTION.

**chest pain, noncardiac**    Mild to severe discomfort that occurs anywhere in the rib area and is due to causes other than coronary artery disease. Chest pain may be caused by a heart attack; however, there are at least 200,000 cases of noncardiac chest pain in the United States each year. As many as 30 percent of those patients who undergo cardiac catheterization for acute chest pain are found to have normal angiogram results. According to Lee and Goldman in their 2002 article on acute chest pain in the *New England Journal of Medicine,* of all patients who enter emergency departments reporting acute chest pain, about 15 percent are found to be experiencing myocardial infarction (heart attack) and 30 to 35 percent have unstable angina (heart disease).

When they are not coronary in nature, chest pains may be caused by an ULCER or by the ACID REFLUX that is generated by GASTROESOPHAGEAL REFLUX DISEASE (GERD). Noncardiac chest pains may also be caused by a musculoskeletal problem, such as FIBROMYALGIA, osteoarthritis, rheumatoid arthritis, vertebral disk disease, or other musculoskeletal problems. Musculoskeletal causes may represent up to 20 percent of all noncardiac chest pain causes.

Some patients with chest pains are suffering from ESOPHAGITIS, an inflammation of the esophagus. They may also have other esophageal problems.

Patients may also have emotional disorders, such as panic disorder or anxiety disorder, which can cause a racing heart as well as chest pains. As many as one-third of all patients who experience noncardiac chest pains may actually be experiencing panic disorders. In addition, the psychological stress of fearing that the chest pains are caused by a heart attack can further accelerate the patient's emotional dismay and distress, worsening the chest pains.

The term *noncardiac chest pain* is actually a misnomer, since it does not exclude all cardiac causes, but only those that are related to coronary artery disease. Thus, noncardiac chest pains also include pains due to microvascular angina of the heart or syndrome X. The role of mitral valve prolapse is controversial, but it appears not to contribute to chest pain in most cases.

### Patient Confusion over Noncardiac Chest Pains

Chest pains cause nearly all patients to suffer extreme anxiety, because they believe they are having a heart attack. Patients go to the emergency room of the nearest hospital and are shocked to have a normal electrocardiogram with or without additional test results and to be told that their heart is fine. Often the pattern repeats itself, and the patient with severe chest pains returns to the emergency room weeks or months later, again convinced that he or she is having a heart attack.

If patients with chest pain are also told that the cause of their problem is unknown, they may become very confused. They may also be offended, thinking that the doctor is accusing them of hypochondria. They are also often uncertain about what to do if the problem occurs again, as it often does. It is best if doctors can help patients to determine a possible cause for the problem. If the doctor thinks that the problem may be digestive in nature, the patient should be referred to a gastroenterologist. In all cases, a cardiac cause must be first excluded before the physician looks for other causes, because a heart attack can kill.

### Diagnosis

Anyone having chest pain should see a doctor to determine the cause of the pain and should not assume that the problem is solely digestive in nature. Even experienced physicians have had difficulty determining whether their own chest pain indicated a heart condition or a digestive problem. Guessing wrong could mean the difference between life and death.

In most cases, physicians order an electrocardiogram of the heart as well as blood tests for cardiac enzymes. Further testing depends upon the results of these tests as well as the patient's risk factors for coronary artery disease. In addition, a coronary angiogram or a myocardial perfusion imaging study with thallium-201 may be ordered. The physician may also order a stress test.

If the results of all of these cardiac tests are negative, further diagnostic evaluation is then needed, including a gastrointestinal evaluation. The physician may need to order 24-hour pH monitoring and/or endoscopy to determine whether the noncardiac chest pains are caused by a digestive disorder. A therapeutic trial of a double-dose proton pump inhibitor such as omeprazole (Prilosec) taken twice a day for eight to 12 weeks may be undertaken. A subsequent reduction in the severity and frequency of symptoms would suggest that the chest pains were related to GERD. In some cases, a referral to a rheumatologist and/or a psychiatrist may be needed.

### Treatment of Noncardiac Chest Pains

If the physician is convinced that the problem is musculoskeletal in nature, he may order antiinflammatory medications or painkillers and may also recommend physical therapy.

When patients appear to have emotional disorders that are causing their noncardiac chest pains, doctors may order benzodiazepine (antianxiety) medications or antidepressants. Sometimes beta blocker drugs can help with panic attacks that cause a racing of the heart. A psychologist can also provide assistance by providing cognitive–behavioral therapy, which is a form of therapy that helps patients identify irrational thought patterns and replace them with logical thoughts.

If the patient has GERD, medications such as proton pump inhibitors and histamine-2 receptor blockers can help alleviate the problem. Patients will be advised to give up smoking and to lose weight if they are obese. They are also advised to avoid large fatty meals, as well as stay away from alcohol, mint, chocolate, onions, and orange juice. In addition, patients are advised to raise the head of their bed, since lying down can exacerbate the symptoms of GERD. They are also told to eat their evening meal at least three hours before retiring to bed.

Relaxation exercises can considerably help in easing the chest pains and acid reflux among patients with GERD.

See also PROTON PUMP INHIBITORS.

Lee, Thomas H., M.D., and Lee Goldman, M.D. "Evaluation of the Patient with Acute Chest Pain." *New England Journal of Medicine* 342, no. 16 (April 20, 2000): 1,187–1,195.

Minocha, Anil, M.D. "Noncardiac Chest Pain: Where Does It Start?" *Postgraduate Medicine* 100, no. 6 (December 1996): 107–114.

Minocha, Anil, M.D., and Abraham S. Joseph, M.D. "Pathophysiology and Management of Noncardiac Pain." *KMA Journal* 93 (May 1995): 196–201.

**children and digestive diseases**  Children may have many of the same digestive diseases as adults; however, infants are at particular risk for some diseases, such as necrotizing enterocolitis, and older children are more at risk for other diseases. Children in the United States also have an increasing problem with OBESITY. The body mass index (BMI) (a measure that considers height and weight) is further adjusted by age and gender for children. (See Appendix X for tables on the BMIs of boys and girls at different ages.)

Sometimes the same disease may result from a different cause in a child and in an adult. For example, "spitting up" or even GASTROESOPHAGEAL REFLUX DISEASE (GERD) is fairly common among babies less than one year old. In general, these problems resolve as the child grows. In some cases, however, treatment and even surgery are needed, for example, if the child is not gaining weight and is severely ill. On the other hand, the adult-onset form of GERD frequently does not resolve on its own.

Although not common, infants are at risk for some genetically transmitted diseases, such as

HIRSCHSPRUNG'S DISEASE. Children may also contract infectious diseases including PARASITIC INFECTIONS, particularly since they are less careful about cleanliness and personal hygiene than are most adults.

### Emotional Problems and Digestive Symptoms

Sometimes children report frequent digestive problems such as stomachaches, which may merit further investigation. If the stomachaches always or nearly always seem to center around the time of an activity that is undesirable to the child, such as going to school or doing housework or schoolwork, then the child may be consciously or unconsciously trying to avoid activities by reporting medical problems. The child is not necessarily lying about the stomachaches, and in fact, he or she may actually experience stomach pain when thinking about or preparing to perform an activity that is deemed unpleasant. Only a physician can make an appropriate diagnosis of a digestive disease or disorder.

It is also true that the child may have a physical basis for complaint; for example, it is possible for children to suffer from the symptoms of GERD, particularly if they are taking medication for asthma.

### Children at Risk for Digestive Disorders

Children with diabetes are at higher risk for development of digestive diseases and disorders than are nondiabetics. Children who have some other disorders, such as asthma, have a greater risk for development of digestive diseases, such as gastroesophageal reflux disease (GERD).

See also ADOLESCENTS; INFANTS.

Minocha, Anil, M.D., and Christine Adamec. *How to Stop Heartburn: Simple Ways to Heal Heartburn and Acid Reflux.* New York: John Wiley & Sons, 2001.

**cholangitis**  Inflammation and infection of the bile duct as a result of a blockage due to gallstones or stricture (narrowing) causing an obstruction to the normal flow of bile into the small intestine or to other causes. Patients experience fever, jaundice, and abdominal pain. Patients with cholangitis need to be hospitalized and given antibiotics and may need to undergo procedures such as endoscopic retrograde cholangiopancreatography (ERCP) to remove an existing blockage. Some patients need surgery.

A parasitic infection with roundworm (ascariasis), liver fluke (Clonorchis sinensis), or tapeworm (*Echinococcus granulosus*) in the bile duct may lead to cholangitis.

See also BILE; CHOLECYSTECTOMY; GALLSTONES; PARASITIC INFECTION.

**cholecystectomy**  The surgical removal of the entire gallbladder, usually because of the disease that is caused by GALLSTONES. Rather than relying upon one large incision in an "open" surgery, the laparoscopic cholecystectomy is currently the primary procedure of choice to remove the gallbladder. However, sometimes the open method of cholecystectomy is required; in it a long abdominal incision must be made rather than the multiple tiny incisions that are used in the laparoscopy. This type of open surgery is indicated if there are complications or the patient is obese or has a history of multiple abdominal surgeries.

### Risk Factors

Some people are especially at risk for development of gallstones and consequently need cholecystectomy, such as Native Americans and individuals who are obese. Patients who have had BARIATRIC SURGERY (weight reduction surgery) may also have an increased risk for development of gallstones, which is due to the rapid weight loss that they have experienced subsequent to the surgery.

### Decreasing the Risk of Development of Gallstones

Some studies have shown that regular exercise can decrease the risk of gallbladder disease that requires cholecystectomy in women; for example, in a study reported in 1999 in the *New England Journal of Medicine*, which was part of the Nurses' Health Study, researchers found that physical activity (or inactivity) is an independent risk factor for decreasing (or increasing) the risk of needing a cholecystectomy among women. This was true whether the women exercised vigorously or not. Any physical activity beyond merely sitting around for hours significantly decreased the risk of later gallbladder disease and the need for surgery.

Said the researchers:

In this prospective study of 60,290 women, increased physical activity was associated with a significant reduction in the risk of cholecystectomy. An average of 2 to 3 hours of recreational exercise per week appeared to reduce the risk by approximately 20 percent. The inverse association was not limited to a particular kind of activity but instead was found for a variety of activities and for a combination of several activities. In contrast, sedentary behavior as assessed by time sitting was positively associated with the risk of cholecystectomy. These associations were independent of other known risk factors, including relative body weight and recent weight change, a finding that suggests that physical activity may have an important role beyond its effect on weight control in the prevention of gallstone disease requiring cholecystectomy.

Women who spent 41 to 60 hours a week sitting down doing work or driving had a significantly greater risk of needing cholecystectomy than women who spent less than six hours a week sitting down.

### Increasing the Risk

Researchers have also found that rapid weight loss increases the risk of women for cholecystectomy. This is also a fact that is well known to most physicians who perform bariatric surgery on obese individuals and who frequently prescribe medications to prevent against the formation of gallstones.

In a study reported in a 1999 issue of the *Annals of Internal Medicine,* researchers looked at nurses in the Nurses' Health Study who had periods of weight loss and weight regain and their likelihood of needing cholecystectomy. They found that 55 percent of those who had undergone cholecystectomy had experienced one or more episodes of weight loss followed by weight regain. They also found that intentional weight loss increased the risk for development of gallstones and requirement for cholecystectomy more than unintentional weight loss:

Our results corroborate those of other studies of our cohort and other populations on the significance of obesity as a risk factor for gallstones. However, our findings reinforce the idea that in addition to avoidance of obesity, it is important to maintain stable weight in adulthood. These findings pose a problem for the obese patient. Because body mass index is the strongest observed risk factor for cholelithiasis and obesity is associated with many other adverse health outcomes, attainment of a lower body weight should not be discouraged in obese patients. However, our data suggest that obese persons should be advised about the risks of weight fluctuation and counseled to adopt lifestyle changes that have the greatest likelihood of achieving stable weight.

Clearly, a slow and steady weight loss is the safest, ideally, about one to two pounds per week, although it may not be the most personally appealing to the obese individual who wishes to lose weight as fast as possible.

Most patients with gallstones do not require surgery, unless there is a problem such as biliary colic, cholecystitis, or gallstone pancreatitis. Prophylactic cholecystectomy may be undertaken in cases when the risk of complication of gallbladder disease is high (as with a calcified gallbladder or a large gallbladder polyp or among young Native American females). Other categories of individuals who may need prophylactic cholecystectomy include those who have sickle cell anemia, those awaiting organ transplantation, and some individuals who plan prolonged travel to a remote area.

See also CHOLECYSTITIS; EXERCISE; GALLBLADDER; GALLSTONES.

Leitzmann, Michael F., M.D., et al. "Recreational Physical Activity and the Risk of Cholecystectomy in Women." *New England Journal of Medicine* 341, no. 11 (September 9, 1999): 777–784.

Syngal, Sapna, et al. "Long-Term Weight Patterns and Risk for Cholecystectomy in Women." *Annals of Internal Medicine* 130, no. 6 (March 16, 1999): 471–477.

**cholecystitis**    Inflammation and infection of the gallbladder, which are usually caused by an impaction of the gallbladder opening (the cystic duct) by GALLSTONES. Cholecystitis may also occur in the absence of any gallstones in patients who are otherwise very sick. This is known as acalculous cholecystitis. Acute cholecystitis usually requires CHOLECYSTECTOMY, which is the surgical removal of the entire gallbladder.

**cholecystokinin (CCK)**    A hormone that is involved in digestion. Cholecystokinin is produced by the wall of the small intestine. It is responsible for the secretion of the enzymes that are found in pancreatic juice and it also causes the gallbladder to empty. CCK is also seen in the nervous system and perhaps acts as a neurotransmitter. CCK is also used as part of diagnostic testing to evaluate gallbladder emptying. The other major digestive hormones are SECRETIN and GASTRIN.

**choledochal cyst**    An abnormal cystic dilation of the bile duct. Choledochal cysts are benign but may become cancerous. The choledochal cyst is a rare condition, which, when found, usually occurs during early childhood; however, it can also be seen in adulthood. The choledochal cyst may be a congenital birth defect or be acquired during life.

A choledochal cyst may prevent or slow the bile from going to the intestine, and it may also cause the bile to back up. Patients with choledochal cysts may suffer from episodes of abdominal pain, jaundice, and pancreatitis, although some patients experience no signs or symptoms.

Physicians may suspect choledochal cysts when the patient complains of pain and some laboratory tests, particularly liver enzyme tests, reveal abnormalities. An abnormal mass may rarely be felt by the physician during an abdominal examination. An ultrasound or computed tomography scan can reveal the presence of an abnormal duct. ENDOSCOPIC RETROGRADE CHOLANGIOPANCREATOGRAPHY (ERCP) helps confirm the diagnosis. Magnetic resonance cholangiopancreatography is a noninvasive option that may be used as an alternative to ERCP. Treatment of choledochal cysts is surgical, with excision of the cyst.

See also CAROLI DISEASE; LIVER ENZYMES/FUNCTION TESTS.

**choledocholithiasis**    A condition in which stones are lodged in the bile ducts. About 15 to 20 percent of patients who have GALLSTONES have choledocholithias, which can lead to CHOLANGITIS (inflammation and infection in the bile ducts), as well as development of PANCREATITIS.

**cholelithiasis**    Gallstone disease.
See also GALLSTONES.

**cholera**    An infectious and dangerous diarrheal disease of the small intestine. It is caused by the bacterium *Vibrio cholerae*, which is found in contaminated water. Cholera can cause severe digestive illness. The bacteria release a toxin that triggers the increased secretion of water and electrolytes in the intestine. Some cases of cholera are spread by contaminated shellfish, particularly bad oysters. If cholera is not treated, it can lead to dehydration and even death.

Cholera is not common in the United States and Canada, and it is primarily found in less developed countries that are located in Asia, Africa, the Mediterranean, both South and Central America, and Mexico. Most cases that have been identified in the United States can be traced to travelers who have recently returned from Asia or Africa.

### Some Historical Background

The underlying cause of cholera was first uncovered by Dr. John Snow, a British anesthesiologist in the mid-19th century, whose discovery, based on meticulous observations, was described in *Epidemiology* by Leon Gordis. Dr. Snow observed that in one week of 1854, 600 people who were living in several blocks around one particular pump had all died of cholera. Snow deduced that contaminated water was the cause of cholera, despite the prevailing theory of the time, which was that cholera was caused by a low-lying cloud.

Dr. Snow went from house to house, gathering data on deaths per household and information on where the family obtained their water. Snow found that in houses that were served by several water companies that obtained their water supply from a polluted part of the Thames River, the death rate was 315 deaths per 10,000 houses. But in homes that were supplied water from another company that obtained its water farther upstream, the death rate was only 38 deaths per 10,000 homes.

### Risk Factors

The key risk factors are an association with contaminated water or recent travel to a country where cholera often occurs.

### Symptoms of Cholera

Symptoms of cholera occur within several hours to about five days from the time of infection. The key symptoms of cholera are as follows:

- Watery diarrhea
- Stool that has flecks that look like rice (rice water stools)
- Manifestations of dehydration, (dry skin and dizziness) which may be rapid
- Extreme thirst and weakness
- Abdominal cramps
- Severe muscle cramps
- Nausea and vomiting

### Diagnosis and Treatment

Physicians may suspect cholera on the basis of the patient's symptoms and any recent exposure to known epidemics of cholera. If bacteria are collected in a stool sample or culture, they can be analyzed. The bacteria are often seen by specialized examination under the microscope in the procedure known as dark field or phase contrast microscopy of stool. Cholera organisms look like shooting stars.

A stool culture can confirm the presence of cholera. The patient's blood may also be checked for the presence of antibodies to cholera; however, the antibodies develop one to two weeks after infection and thus can only confirm the diagnosis retrospectively.

The primary treatment for cholera is to prevent dehydration or to reverse dehydration that is already present with rehydration, and that rehydration may be lifesaving. Most patients can be treated with oral hydration solutions. If the patient's condition is severe, hospitalization is needed and intravenous fluids are administered.

Physicians may also prescribe antibiotics, which are given to reduce the duration of the sickness and to help limit the spread. Antibiotics such as tetracycline or doxycline are frequently used. Tetracycline is usually not prescribed for children who do not yet have their permanent teeth, because it can permanently discolor teeth that are in the process of formation. Similarly, tetracycline is not used for pregnant women. With children and pregnant women, erythromycin is prescribed instead.

Doctors are particularly concerned about the rehydration of children who have cholera. Intravenous fluids are not necessary in the majority of cases. Most children with the disease can be treated with a formula that replaces the salt and water lost from dehydration, and such therapy can prevent the deaths of from one million to two million children worldwide per year. The World Health Organization has developed an inexpensive oral rehydration solution of sugar and electrolytes. Some studies have found that a rice-based oral rehydration solution is very effective.

### Prevention: Cholera Vaccines

In parts of the world where cholera is known to be a problem, residents may receive cholera vaccines. People traveling to areas where cholera is a problem may also receive a vaccine before they travel to that area.

In the United States and Canada, the vaccine is given by injection. However, the vaccine is only effective in about 50 percent of cases, and it is not required for travel to other countries. In addition, the vaccine may cause fever and headache, as well as pain at the injection site. If a patient has trouble with breathing or hives after an injection, he or she should seek immediate emergency medical attention.

### Travelers Who Wish to Avoid Cholera

Experts report that there are some basic actions that travelers to countries known to harbor cholera can take to limit their risk of contracting the disease.

- Avoiding unboiled water
- Avoiding ice
- Buying no food items from street vendors

- Eating no raw vegetables or salads while in the country
- Avoiding raw seafood
- Drinking only bottled water or treating water with either chlorine or iodine tablets
- Drinking carbonated soft drinks
- Drinking only hot tea or coffee that is made from boiled water
- Consuming only hot cooked foods

See also CONTAMINATED FOOD OR WATER; FOOD-BORNE ILLNESSES; TRAVEL.

Gordis, Leon, M.D. *Epidemiology*. 2d ed. Philadelphia: W. B. Saunders Company, 2000.
Rabbani, G. H., M.D. "The Search for a Better Oral Rehydration Solution for Cholera." *New England Journal of Medicine* 342, no. 5 (February 3, 2000): 345–347.

**cholestasis** A stagnation or an obstruction of the flow of bile from the liver to the intestines, which may result from a variety of conditions, including use of medications and bile duct blockage by GALL-STONES or CANCER. Patients with cholestasis may experience JAUNDICE, abdominal pain, and itching.

**cholesterol** A type of body fat (lipid) that is made in the body and is also found naturally in some types of animal foods, such as fish, meat, poultry, eggs, and dairy products. Cholesterol circulates in the body as lipoproteins, including low-density lipoproteins (LDL) and high-density lipoproteins (HDL). LDL, which leads to clogging of the blood vessels, is considered to be a "bad" cholesterol; HDL is a "good" form of cholesterol because it is associated with a lower risk of atherosclerosis and its complications, such as heart disease and stroke. Consequently, higher levels of HDL are desirable. If the blood vessels become excessively clogged, then the individual is at an increased risk for stroke or heart attack.

Cholesterol level can be measured in the blood, and if the levels of LDL or total cholesterol are considered too high by a physician, then the patient can be given a diet to follow. In many cases, patients are also given prescribed medications to help lower their LDL level. In general, the type of medication usually considered to treat patients with high LDL level is a drug such as atorvastatin (Lipitor), pravastatin (Pravachol), simvastatin (Zocor) or resuvastatin (Crestor). These medications can effectively lower LDL cholesterol levels by as much as 15 to 60 percent. Some patients with high cholesterol levels may be treated with niacin, but it is poorly tolerated because of its side effects.

**CLASSIFICATION OF LDL, TOTAL CHOLESTEROL, AND HDL CHOLESTEROL (MILLIGRAMS PER DECILITER)**

**LDL Cholesterol**

| | |
|---|---|
| Less than 100 | Optimal |
| 100–129 | Near optimal/above optimal |
| 130–159 | Borderline high |
| 160–189 | High |
| 190 and higher | Very high |

If patients have diabetes, then the recommended LDL is less than 100.

**Total Cholesterol**

| | |
|---|---|
| Less than 200 | Desirable |
| 200–239 | Borderline high |
| 240 or higher | High |

**HDL Cholesterol**

| | |
|---|---|
| Less than 40 | Low |
| 60 or higher | High |

Source: National Cholesterol Education Program. "Third Report of the National Cholesterol Education Program (NCEP) Expert Panel on Detection, Evaluation, and Treatment of High Blood Cholesterol in Adults (Adult Treatment Panel III)." NIH Publication no. 02-5215, September 2002.

### Risk Factors

Some individuals have a greater risk for development of health problems associated with their cholesterol level, including individuals with family members who have high cholesterol level or who have one or more of the following health problems or fit one or more of the following categories:

- Have diabetes
- Have hypertension

- Are obese
- Are sedentary
- Are black or Native American
- Consume a very-high-fat diet

### Recommended Levels of Cholesterol

In 2002 the National Heart, Lung, and Blood Institute released their new guidelines for cholesterol control, which are listed the table.

### Diagnosis and Treatment

As mentioned, cholesterol problems are diagnosed on the basis of blood levels of HDL and LDL, and patients who are diagnosed with cholesterol disorders are usually prescribed dietary modifications and exercise plans. In addition, in some cases, patients are also prescribed medications to help them to lower their LDL level.

Medications alone, however, should not be used to resolve the cholesterol problem, and patients must also make changes to their diet, such as decreasing their level of dietary fat and increasing their fiber consumption. Patients with diabetes as well as cholesterol disorders are urged to make their glucose level as close to normal as possible and patients with hypertension are advised to lower their blood pressure level to as close to normal as possible.

Regular exercise is also usually recommended for patients. It need not be strenuous or difficult, and a mere daily walk can often help to improve health, although strenuous exercise results in better outcomes than mild exercise. Obese patients should reduce their weight to the optimal range. As of this writing, preliminary data suggest that the Atkins Diet, in addition to lowering weight, reduces total cholesterol level and increases the levels of HDL (good cholesterol).

For further information on cholesterol levels, contact the following organization:

The National Heart, Lung, and Blood Institute
Building 31, Room 5A52
31 Center Drive MSC 2486
Bethesda, MD 20892
(301) 592-8573
http://www.nhlbi.nih.gov

See also FIBER; GALLSTONES.

National Cholesterol Education Program. "Third Report of the National Cholesterol Education Program (NCEP) Expert Panel on Detection, Evaluation, and Treatment of High Blood Cholesterol in Adults (Adult Treatment Panel III)." NIH Publication No. 02-5215, September 2002.

Pearlman, Brian L., M.D. "The New Cholesterol Guidelines: Applying Them in Clinical Practice." *Postgraduate Medicine* 11, no. 2 (August 2002): 13–26.

**chromoendoscopy**   A procedure in which an endoscopy is performed, and a special dye is sprayed on the gastrointestinal wall to the area of interest, using a spray catheter. The dye allows the highlighting of abnormalities on the gastrointestinal wall that may have been ambiguous or otherwise have escaped detection. This procedure is not commonly performed as of this writing because of the lack of good studies showing whether using these special dyes produces better clinical outcomes than using traditional endoscopy without the dyes.

See also ENDOSCOPY.

**Churg-Strauss syndrome**   A rare disease that involves inflammation of the blood vessels (vasculitis) affecting many organs of the body, primarily the lungs, and causing difficulty with breathing, coughing and wheezing, as well as asthma. However, it also affects the digestive system in that many Churg-Strauss syndrome patients also suffer from abdominal pain, appetite loss, diarrhea, gastrointestinal bleeding, colitis, and unintended weight loss. Other organs that may be affected by Churg-Strauss syndrome include the heart, the peripheral nerves, the kidneys, and the liver.

The cause of this medical problem is unknown, although it is suspected that there may be autoimmune factors at work.

For further information, contact the following organizations:

American Lung Association
1740 Broadway
New York, NY 10019
(212) 315-8700
http://www.lungusa.org

National Heart, Lung and Blood Institute
    Information Center
P.O. Box 30105
Bethesda, MD 20824
(301) 592-8573
http://www.nhlbi.nih.gov/health/public/heart/
    index.htm

National Institute of Allergy and Infectious
    Diseases
9000 Rockville Pike
Bethesda, MD 20892
(301) 496-5717
http://www.niad.nih.gov

See also VASCULITIS.

**cirrhosis**    Severe and potentially fatal scarring of
the liver. Many cases of cirrhosis are caused by
years of chronic ALCOHOLISM, although cirrhosis
can also occur in individuals who are not alcoholics
but instead have viral or autoimmune HEPATITIS or
other diseases. Whereas viral hepatitis C is a common cause of cirrhosis in the United States and
other countries in the West, hepatitis B is a major
cause of cirrhosis in some Asian and African countries. Hereditary disorders such as HEMOCHROMATO-
SIS (iron overload) and WILSON'S DISEASE (copper
overload) also lead to cirrhosis.

In addition, it should also be noted that most
alcoholics do not develop cirrhosis. Heavy alcohol
intake on a prolonged basis causes inflammation
(alcoholic hepatitis) and can lead to scarring of the
tissue in the liver, which is called cirrhosis. When
scar tissue becomes too pervasive, and the liver is
unable to function any more the individual
requires liver transplantation to stay alive.
Cirrhosis develops in those who have both hepatitis C and alcoholism earlier than in those who have
one of the conditions.

Malnutrition or viral hepatitis can also lead to
cirrhosis. Sometimes a severe reaction to prescription drugs, for example, a reaction to methotrexate, may cause cirrhosis.

### Risk Factors for Cirrhosis

Other than chronic heavy alcohol consumption,
there are other individual risk factors for the devel-

opment of cirrhosis; for example, cirrhosis death is
about 1.5 times more common among nonwhites
than among whites in the United States. Men are
more likely to have cirrhosis than women.

### Symptoms, Signs, and Complications of Cirrhosis

Although patients may have no symptoms or signs
when they are in the early stages of cirrhosis, indications do develop as the condition of the liver further deteriorates. The following are some of the
key indicators of cirrhosis:

- JAUNDICE (yellowing of the skin, caused by
  bilirubin)
- ASCITES (fluid buildup in the abdomen)
- Massive painless bleeding caused by increased
  pressure in the veins in the esophagus or stomach (varices) that then burst, which is further
  exacerbated because the patient may also have
  decreased clotting factors that do not permit
  bleeding to stop
- Nausea and fatigue (which may be mistaken as
  "normal" reactions of the body to excessive
  drinking)
- An increased sensitivity to drugs that are
  metabolized by the liver, which can no longer
  manage this metabolizing function well, such as
  a sensitivity to acetaminophen (Tylenol), which
  can cause severe liver failure in alcoholics at
  doses much lower than those that can be
  tolerated by nonalcoholics
- Liver cancer, caused by long-standing liver
  cirrhosis
- Altered mental status (hepatic encephalopathy)
- Infection in the ascitic fluid (spontaneous bacterial peritonitis)

### Diagnosis and Treatment

In a patient with chronic compensated liver disease
(in which the liver is diseased but still functioning
well enough to not cause problems to the body),
the exact diagnosis of cirrhosis can only be made by
examining a liver biopsy sample under a microscope. The body only needs a small part of the liver
to function. Complications do not occur until most
of the liver is gone. In advanced cases, physicians

can make a preliminary diagnosis based on a patient's symptoms and signs, such as the presence of jaundice or ascites. However, in early cases of cirrhosis, the patient may be asymptomatic and may also have no laboratory test abnormalities.

In the later stages of the illness, laboratory tests of liver function suggest diagnosis if cirrhosis is present. Imaging tests may also show an enlargement or scarring of the liver, as well as the presence of any complications such as ascites. At the same time, patients who have acute hepatitis due to alcohol or viruses may have deranged but reversible liver function, and these conditions may mimic cirrhosis.

Patients with cirrhosis who drink are advised that they must immediately stop drinking alcohol. If they are alcoholics, they may need hospitalization to undergo detoxification from alcohol. It is difficult for a long-term alcoholic simply to give up drinking; he or she is addicted to alcohol. In addition, the body often responds to the sudden ending of alcohol consumption with severe reactions, such as seizures and extreme vomiting and diarrhea.

If individuals who are alcoholics completely avoid alcohol, their liver cells may recover completely when the liver is only inflamed (hepatitis) rather than scarred. On the other hand, cirrhosis may be irreversible, although patients may live for years with cirrhosis that is not advanced. As such, the outcome depends on how severely damaged the liver is at the point when the patient becomes abstinent from alcohol. Patients with cirrhosis should also be vaccinated against hepatitis A and B if they have not been exposed to these infections in the past, in order to prevent contraction of viral hepatitis, which would cause further liver damage.

There is no known medical treatment for cirrhosis, and generally, treatment involves identifying and treating the cause of the illness as well as any complications that may arise. Liver transplantation is the only known definitive cure for cirrhosis. Some physicians recommend medications such as colchicine to help the cirrhotic liver, although this is an investigational therapy. There are also some reports that milk thistle, an herbal remedy, helps some patients with certain forms of liver disease.

The Mayo Clinic Model for End Stage Liver Disease (MELD) score is used to identify those patients who are at the highest risk for death over short term and thus also have the greatest need for liver transplantation. The higher the score, the higher the patient's priority.

See also ALCOHOL ABUSE AND DEPENDENCE/ALCOHOLISM; ASCITES; LIVER ENZYMES/FUNCTION TESTS; LIVER FAILURE; LIVER TRANSPLANTATION; PANCREATITIS.

**Clostridium**  A bacterium that causes food-borne illnesses. An illness caused by *Clostridium perfringens,* one of the *Clostridium* bacteria, is also known as the cafeteria germ because many disease outbreaks have resulted from foods left for long periods on steam tables or elsewhere at room temperature. *Clostridium* organisms are ubiquitous in the environment and are commonly found in dust, dirt, and sewage and in the intestinal tract of infected humans and animals.

An infection with *Clostridium perfringens* causes diarrhea and abdominal gas pains within eight to 24 hours of consuming the infected food. Generally, symptoms subside within a day or so, although some minor symptoms may continue for a week or longer. Most patients recover without treatment.

The *Clostridium botulinum* bacteria are extremely dangerous, primarily because they produce a powerful toxin that causes botulism, a severe form of food contamination that also causes food poisoning. However, fortunately, this form of the bacteria is not common.

Another species of the *Clostridium* bacterium, *Clostridium difficile,* is responsible for many cases of antibiotic-induced diarrhea. It is very common, especially among hospitalized patients. Symptomatic patients can be treated effectively with metronidazole or oral vancomycin. In a few cases, the infection cannot be eradicated and patients may suffer from relapse shortly after treatment is stopped.

See also BOTULINUM TOXIN; CONTAMINATED FOOD; DIARRHEA; FOOD-BORNE ILLNESSES.

**colic**  A term that is usually used to describe intermittent attacks of abdominal pain, probably characterized by spasms of a hollow organ such as the gut. There is no standard definition of the term *colic.* Frequently, the term is used by parents and physicians when infants cry for no apparent reason during the first three months of life, and the parents become concerned and seek medical help for this problem. It is a benign and usually self-limited condition.

Colic is a common condition of many infants. A colicky type of pain may also be due to biliary colic in GALLSTONE disease patients and in renal colic in patients who have kidney stones. However, the term *biliary colic* is a misnomer because the pain is steady and not colicky.

See also COLITIS; INFANTS.

**colitis**   Inflammation of the colon. Colitis may be due to a variety of causes. It may present as simple redness and swelling of the colon wall all the way to the presence of ulcers; for example, ulcerative colitis is a chronic disabling condition and one type of inflammatory bowel disease. Colitis may also be due to Crohn's disease, radiation therapy, medications such as aspirin, and infections such as AMEBIASIS. The treatment of colitis depends on the cause.

See also AMYLOIDOSIS; CHURG-STRAUSS SYNDROME; CROHN'S DISEASE; INFLAMMATORY BOWEL DISEASE; NECROTIZING ENTEROCOLITIS; ULCERATIVE COLITIS.

**colon**   The large bowel, which is a key part of the digestive system. The colon is the final processing component of digestion. It receives about two liters of unabsorbed food remnants, intestinal secretions, and debris in fluid form. Unabsorbed carbohydrates undergo bacterial fermentation in the colon. The colon also absorbs most of the water and then expels the waste in solid form through the rectum and anus.

See also CANCER, COLORECTAL; COLONOSCOPY.

**colonoscopy**   An endoscopic procedure that tests for colorectal cancer, POLYPS, and other malfunctions of the lower digestive system, such as DIVERTICULOSIS, INFLAMMATORY BOWEL DISEASE, or colitis that is caused by infections, radiation, or medications. The physician (frequently a gastroenterologist) uses a colonoscope to visualize the entire

colon. This procedure is in contrast with sigmoidoscopy, in which only the lower third of the colon is viewed by the doctor.

Some doctors are using virtual colonoscopies rather than actual colonoscopies for screening purposes. In virtual colonoscopy, a computed tomography (CT) scan is used instead of a colonoscope. The virtual colonoscopy is a noninvasive procedure that is performed by radiologists. If the virtual colonoscopy indicates a problem, colonoscopy is ordered. However, the virtual colonoscopy has not yet been endorsed as a screening option by the gastroenterology organizations as of this writing.

### Who Should Have Screening Colonoscopies and How Often

Most experts recommend that everyone age 50 and older have a baseline colonoscopy and subsequent colonoscopies at intervals that are determined by the doctor. For example, if a few minor precancerous polyps are detected in the colonoscopy, the doctor may recommend a surveillance colonoscopy in three to five years.

If the colonoscopy result is normal in a person with average risks for colorectal cancer, a surveillance colonoscopy 10 years later is recommended. However, if the findings are more serious, such as detection of COLORECTAL CANCER, a surgeon is usually consulted for the surgical removal of the cancerous area, and thereafter more frequent colonoscopies are scheduled.

In those patients who are at high risk for colon cancer, screening may begin at a much earlier age than 50 years old. Colonoscopy in high-risk individuals may be necessary at one- to three-year intervals between colonoscopies.

Most individuals have neither routine colonoscopies nor sigmoidoscopies, and consequently, many cases of colorectal cancer or precancerous polyps that could have been detected with screening procedures and treated are not identified, and thus patients may have a greater risk of colon cancer-related death.

### Preparation for the Colonoscopy

Before the procedure, patients are directed to take medications that completely cleanse the bowel, so that the physician has a clear and unoccluded view when performing the colonoscopy. If the doctor finds any evidence of polyps during the course of the colonoscopy, he or she can remove them. The doctor can also perform a biopsy of any abnormal area of the colon observed during the procedure. Stents may be placed in the cases of a narrowed colon caused by cancer or other illnesses.

### Patterns of Colonoscopies Ordered by Gastroenterologists

In a survey of 276 gastroenterologists nationwide in the United States on why they performed colonoscopies (and endoscopies) reported in a 2000 issue of *Gastroenterology* by David A. Lieberman and his colleagues, the researchers found that the most common reason for performing the colonoscopy was to evaluate a patient who had previously been diagnosed with colorectal cancer or with polyps (24 percent). The next most common reason for the procedure was to evaluate the cause of hematochezia (lower gastrointestinal bleeding), at 19 percent. In addition, 15 percent of the patients were given a colonoscopy because their FECAL OCCULT BLOOD TEST (FOBT) result was positive and 12 percent of the doctors performed colonoscopy on patients who had abdominal pain.

Only a small percentage of colonoscopies were done to screen for colorectal cancer, including 6 percent performed because of a history of colorectal cancer in the family and 3 percent done with no known family history of colorectal cancer.

### Virtual Colonoscopy

Imaging technology that was newly available to some physicians and patients in 2003 allows physicians to perform a virtual colonoscopy, using special computed tomography (CT) scan tools to look at the inside of the wall of the colon. If problems are identified in the virtual endoscopy, then an actual invasive endoscopy is performed. The pros and cons of the virtual endoscopy are described in a 2002 issue of *American Family Physician*.

**Advantages of the virtual colonoscopy** A key advantage of virtual colonoscopy is that it is noninvasive and no sedation is used. As of this writing, patients must still take medicine to clean out the bowel before having the procedure; however, improvement in the technology in the future may permit the test to be done without colon cleansing.

In one study of 100 patients who had virtual colonoscopies, none of the patients asked the examiners to stop the procedure. Another advantage is that if patients perceive the virtual colonoscopy as less frightening than the colonoscopy, more people will be willing to have them and more disease will be detected. At most, about 20 percent of Americans have ever had a colonoscopy, and yet it is the best way to detect colorectal cancer in the early treatable stages.

Experts also report that the virtual colonoscopy may be easier for the patient than the actual colonoscopy. In addition, the virtual colonoscopy surpasses the double-contrast barium enema in detecting colorectal polyps.

**Disadvantages of the virtual colonoscopy** The chief disadvantage of the virtual colonoscopy is its cost (known to be higher than the cost of an actual colonoscopy). Another disadvantage is that the virtual colonoscopy is less sensitive at detecting polyps that are smaller than one centimeter in diameter. In addition, sometimes fecal material that is retained in the colon can be misinterpreted as polyps in the virtual colonoscopy. There is also some radiation exposure in virtual colonoscopy, equivalent to that of several plain X-ray films. As of this writing, the expertise for interpreting the images obtained in the virtual colonoscopy is not widely available.

Another disadvantage of the virtual colonoscopy is that if any polyps are identified by the virtual colonoscopy, the patient subsequently has to have an actual colonoscopy so that the physician can remove them. Also, physicians can only biopsy tissue with an actual colonoscopy.

See also CANCER, COLORECTAL; CHROMOENDOSCOPY; ENDOSCOPY; POLYPS; SIGMOIDOSCOPY.

Lieberman, David A., et al. "Patterns of Endoscopy Use in the United States," *Gastroenterology* 118, no. 3 (2000): 619–624.

Wood, Bradford J., and Pouneh Razavi. "Virtual Endoscopy: A Promising New Technology." *American Family Physician* 66, no. 1 (July 1, 2002): 107–112.

**colorectal cancer**   See CANCER, COLORECTAL.

**colostomy**   Surgery that is performed after damage to the colon and/or to the rectum from cancer or other causes, such as diverticulitis. The colostomy creates an opening in the abdominal wall to the colon, through which stools enter either a temporary or a permanent collection bag.

The temporary colostomy allows healing to occur after surgery; later the colostomy is closed and the two disconnected parts of the colon are hooked back together again. In the meantime, patients are trained to empty the bag periodically.

In many cases, the colostomy may be permanent. See also CANCER, COLORECTAL.

**condyloma acuminatum (anal warts)**   The most commonly known venereal disease that is diagnosed in the United States. Most patients who have this disease (about 67 percent) are female. The disease is caused by infection with the human papillomavirus (HPV); more than 70 different types of HPV are currently known.

In women, condyloma acuminatum is primarily spread through vaginal intercourse, and the greater the number of sexual partners that a woman has, the higher her risk for contracting HPV and subsequent anal warts; for example, women who have five or more sexual partners over the course of five years have about 12 times the risk of infection of women who have had one sexual partner.

Among men, the disease may be spread through either heterosexual or homosexual contact. As with women, the risk of infection increases with the number of sexual partners. In addition, men who are positive for the human immunodeficiency virus (HIV) also have a greater risk for contracting HPV and subsequently having anal warts.

Some studies have shown that a history of anal warts increases the probability of development of anal cancer, such as a study reported in the *New England Journal of Medicine* in 1997, which was based on telephone interviews with hundreds of men and women who had been diagnosed with anal cancer.

In another interesting study, reported in a 1999 issue of the *Archives of Internal Medicine,* the researchers found that, contrary to popular perception, many lesbians have apparently had unprotected sexual encounters with males. In the sample of nearly 7,000 females who identified themselves as lesbians, 17.2 percent reported having had a sexually transmitted disease (STD). Among the most frequently occurring STDs, experienced by 4.8 percent, were anal or genital warts. Lesbians who said they had had six or more male sexual partners in their life were most likely to have had a sexually transmitted disease (STD). Said the researchers, "Lesbians who had engaged in anal intercourse reported higher rates of STDs and abnormal Pap smears than those who had not engaged in these activities."

### Symptoms and Signs
Patients may be asymptomatic or may have pain, bleeding, burning, and pruritus in the anal area.

### Diagnosis and Treatment
The diagnosis of anal warts can usually be made by a visual inspection by a doctor, although a biopsy may be needed in some cases. Physicians need to exclude condyloma acuminatum from other forms of the disease, such as hemorrhoids, cancer, and condlyoma latum, a disease that is linked to infection with syphilis, another venereal disease. Lesions that are present and that look suspicious to the physician can be biopsied to obtain further information and validate (or refute) the presence of condyloma acuminatum.

When condyloma acuminatum has been confirmed, there are various treatment methods. Doctors may choose chemical means to destroy the anal warts, using drugs such as podophyllin, trichloroacetic acid, or 5-fluorouracil/epinephrine gel. Podophyllin should not be used by women who are pregnant or may be pregnant.

Immune-modulating agents such as interferon alfa or iminquimod may be used to treat condyloma acuminatum. Imiquimod is a topical cream; interferon is injected. Patients may also be treated with ablative therapies, such as surgery, cryotherapy (freezing of the anal warts), or laser therapy.

Some physicians also use topical doses of antibacterial drugs such as cidofovir gel or Bacillus Calmette-Guérin (BCG).

Diamant, Allison L., M.D., et al. "Lesbians' Sexual History with Men: Implications for Taking a Sexual History." *Archives of Internal Medicine* 159 (December 13/27, 1999): 2,730–2,736.

Frisch, Morten, M.D., et. al. "Sexually Transmitted Infection as a Cause of Anal Cancer." *New England Journal of Medicine* 337, no. 19 (November 6, 1997): 1,350–1,358.

**conscious sedation** A medicated state that relaxes the individual and may cause him or her to fall asleep, but is less strong than "general" anesthesia. Even though they may be sleepy, patients who have had conscious sedation still breathe on their own and respond to verbal commands. Conscious sedation is used in some procedures that are relatively brief and/or nonsurgical, such as COLONOSCOPY or upper ENDOSCOPY. It is more commonly used in the United States for endoscopies than in other countries, where no sedation may be used for such procedures.

See also SURGERY.

**constipation** Difficult or infrequent bowel movements. Production of less than three bowel movements per week is often referred to as constipation, but constipation can also include passing very hard stools or frequently having the sensation of incomplete defecation. For example, patients may feel as if they are not "empty" after they do have a bowel movement, and they may feel they need to have another bowel movement. Constipation may cause back pain and abdominal pain, as well as a generalized feeling of discomfort. Some people struggle with chronic pain associated with constipation that may or may not alternate with diarrhea, a condition that is known as IRRITABLE BOWEL SYNDROME (IBS). Patients can also have IBS without constipation: IBS—diarrhea predominant.

### Risk Factors

Older people have a much greater risk of chronic constipation than younger people, in large part because they generally lead a far more sedentary life. Older people are also more likely to be taking medications that can cause constipation, as well as to have diseases that are linked to problems with constipation, such as DIABETES MELLITUS, Parkinson's disease, or thyroid disease, particularly hypothyroidism (below normal levels of thyroid hormone). Abnormal electrolyte levels, such as low blood levels of potassium, may also cause constipation.

A diet that is poor in FIBER or insufficient in fluids may cause constipation. A sluggish colon can also cause constipation. This particular condition is often seen among patients with diabetes.

### Treatment

A blockage should be excluded in patients who have constipation. Many cases of general constipation can be resolved by increasing the amount of fiber in the diet and increasing fluid consumption or adding a very mild LAXATIVE. Stool softeners may also help some patients to resolve their constipation. Often, EXERCISE, even as simple as regular walking, can help to resolve problems with constipation.

Doctors may recommend bowel retraining, in which patients are urged to set aside specific times to use the toilet, particularly after meals, when they are more likely to be able to have a bowel movement.

In the most extreme case, which may occur after several days without passing a stool, the feces may become impacted and need to be manually disimpacted by either the individual, a caregiver, or a medical person.

Chronic constipation and straining at bowel movements may lead to the development of hemorrhoids. Patients with constipation that is related to IBS may be treated with a medication called tegaserod (Zelnorm). Biofeedback is also helpful in many cases of constipation, especially those that are characterized by difficult or painful defecation.

See also BOWEL MOVEMENT; DEFECATION; FECAL IMPACTION; HEMORRHOIDS; LAXATIVE ABUSE; NARCOTIC BOWEL SYNDROME.

**contaminated food or water** Food that is overgrown with bacteria, viruses, or other substances that can cause illness or even death if consumed. Contaminated water is also the cause of the transmission of many diseases. Careful food preparation

## COLD STORAGE CHART

Following short but safe time limits helps consumers to prevent refrigerated food from either spoiling or becoming dangerous to eat. In general, according to the United States Department of Agriculture, freezing keeps most food safe indefinitely. As a result, the recommended storage times are provided for quality purposes only.

| Product | Refrigerator (40°F) | Freezer (0°F) |
| --- | --- | --- |
| **Eggs** | | |
| Fresh, in shell | 3 to 5 weeks | Do not freeze |
| Raw yolks & whites | 2 to 4 days | 1 year |
| Hard cooked | 1 week | Does not freeze well |
| Liquid pasteurized eggs, egg substitutes | | |
| opened | 3 days | Does not freeze well |
| unopened | 10 days | 1 year |
| **Mayonnaise** | | |
| Commercial, refrigerate after opening | 2 months | Do not freeze |
| **Frozen Dinners & Entrees** | | |
| Keep frozen until ready to heat | — | 3 to 4 months |
| **Deli & Vacuum-Packed Products** | | |
| Store-prepared (or homemade) egg, chicken, ham, tuna, & macaroni salads | 3 to 5 days | Does not freeze well |
| **Hot Dogs & Luncheon Meats** | | |
| Hot dogs | | |
| opened package | 1 week | 1 to 2 months |
| unopened package | 2 weeks | 1 to 2 months |
| Luncheon meats | | |
| opened package | 3 to 5 days | 1 to 2 months |
| unopened package | 2 weeks | 1 to 2 months |
| **Bacon & Sausage** | | |
| Bacon | 7 days | 1 month |
| Sausage, raw—from chicken, turkey, pork, beef | 1 to 2 days | 1 to 2 months |
| Smoked breakfast links, patties | 7 days | 1 to 2 months |
| Hard sausage—pepperoni, jerky sticks | 2 to 3 weeks | 1 to 2 months |
| Summer sausage—labeled "Keep Refrigerated" | | |
| opened | 3 weeks | 1 to 2 months |
| unopened | 3 months | 1 to 2 months |
| **Ham, Corned Beef** | | |
| Corned beef, in pouch with pickling juices | 5 to 7 days | Drained, 1 month |
| Ham, canned—labeled "Keep Refrigerated" | | |
| opened | 3 to 5 days | 1 to 2 months |
| unopened | 6 to 9 months | Do not freeze |
| Ham, fully cooked vacuum sealed at plant, undated, unopened | 2 weeks | 1 to 2 months |
| Ham, fully cooked vacuum sealed at plant, dated, unopened | "Use-By" date on package | 1 to 2 months |

*(continues)*

## COLD STORAGE CHART (continued)

| Product | Refrigerator (40°F) | Freezer (0°F) |
|---|---|---|
| **Ham, fully cooked** | | |
| whole | 7 days | 1 to 2 months |
| half | 3 to 5 days | 1 to 2 months |
| slices | 3 to 4 days | 1 to 2 months |
| **Hamburger, Ground & Stew Meat** | | |
| Hamburger & stew meat | 1 to 2 days | 3 to 4 months |
| Ground turkey, veal, pork, lamb, & mixtures of them | 1 to 2 days | 3 to 4 months |
| **Fresh Beef, Veal, Lamb, Pork** | | |
| Steaks | 3 to 5 days | 6 to 12 months |
| Chops | 3 to 5 days | 4 to 6 months |
| Roasts | 3 to 5 days | 4 to 12 months |
| Variety meats—tongue, liver, heart, kidneys, chitterlings | 1 to 2 days | 3 to 4 months |
| Prestuffed, uncooked pork chops, lamb chops, or chicken breasts stuffed with dressing | 1 day | Does not freeze well |
| **Soups & Stews** | | |
| Vegetable or meat added | 3 to 4 days | 2 to 3 months |
| **Cooked Meat Leftovers** | | |
| Cooked meat & meat casseroles | 3 to 4 days | 2 to 3 months |
| Gravy & meat broth | 1 to 2 days | 2 to 3 months |
| **Fresh Poultry** | | |
| Chicken or turkey, whole | 1 to 2 days | 1 year |
| Chicken or turkey, pieces | 1 to 2 days | 9 months |
| Giblets | 1 to 2 days | 3 to 4 months |
| **Cooked Poultry Leftovers** | | |
| Fried chicken | 3 to 4 days | 4 months |
| Cooked poultry casseroles | 3 to 4 days | 4 to 6 months |
| Pieces, plain | 3 to 4 days | 4 months |
| Pieces covered with broth, gravy | 1 to 2 days | 6 months |
| Chicken nuggets, patties | 1 to 2 days | 1 to 3 months |
| **Pizza, cooked** | 3 to 4 days | 1 to 2 months |
| **Stuffing, cooked** | 3 to 4 days | 1 month |

Credit: Food Safety and Inspection Service, "Food Safety Facts: Basics for Handling Food Safely," United States Department of Agriculture, July 2002.
Source: USDA Meat and Poultry Hotline

**MOLDY FOOD: WHEN TO USE, WHEN TO DISCARD**

*Note: Anyone who knows he or she is allergic to molds should discard the entire food item containing mold.*

| Food | Handling | Reason |
|---|---|---|
| **Luncheon meats, bacon, or hot dogs** | Discard | Foods with high moisture content can be contaminated below the surface. Moldy foods may also have bacteria growing along with the mold. |
| **Hard salami and dry-cured country hams** | Use. Scrub mold off surface | It is normal for these shelf-stable products to have surface mold. |
| **Cooked leftover meat and poultry** | Discard | Foods with high moisture content can be contaminated below the surface. Moldy foods may also have bacteria growing along with the mold. |
| **Cooked casseroles** | Discard | Foods with high moisture content can be contaminated below the surface. Moldy foods may also have bacteria growing along with the mold. |
| **Cooked grain and pasta** | Discard | Foods with high moisture content can be contaminated below the surface. Moldy foods may also have bacteria growing along with the mold. |
| **Hard cheese** (not cheese for which mold is part of the processing) | Use. Cut off at least 1 inch around and below the mold spot (keep the knife out of the mold itself so it will not cross-contaminate other parts of the cheese). After trimming off the mold, re-cover the cheese in fresh wrap. | Mold generally cannot penetrate deep into the product. |
| **Cheese made with mold** (such as Roquefort, blue, Gorgonzola, Stilton, Brie, Camembert) | Discard soft cheeses such as Brie and Camembert if they contain molds that are not a part of the manufacturing process.<br><br>If surface mold is on hard cheeses such as Gorgonzola and Stilton, cut off mold at least 1 inch around and below the mold spot and handle as with hard cheese (above). | Molds that are not a part of the manufacturing process can be dangerous. |
| **Soft cheese** (such as cottage, cream cheese, Neufchatel, *chevre,* Bel Paese)<br><br>**Crumbled, shredded, and sliced cheeses** (all types) | Discard | Foods with high moisture content can be contaminated below the surface. Shredded, sliced, or crumbled cheese can be contaminated by the cutting instrument. Moldy soft cheese can also have bacteria growing along with the mold. |
| **Yogurt and sour cream** | Discard | Foods with high moisture content can be contaminated below the surface. Moldy foods may also have bacteria growing along with the mold. |
| **Jams and jellies** | Discard | The mold could be producing a mycotoxin. Microbiologists recommend against scooping out the mold and using the remaining condiment. |

*(continues)*

**MOLDY FOOD: WHEN TO USE, WHEN TO DISCARD** *(continued)*

| Food | Handling | Reason |
|---|---|---|
| **Fruits and vegetables, firm** | Use. Cut off at least 1 inch around and below the mold spot (keep the knife out of the mold itself so it will not cross-contaminate other parts of the produce). | Small mold spots can be cut off fruits and vegetables with low moisture content (cabbage, bell peppers, carrots, etc.) It is difficult for mold to penetrate dense foods. |
| **Fruits and vegetables, soft** | Discard | Fruits and vegetables with high moisture content (cucumbers, peaches, tomatoes, etc.) can be contaminated below the surface. |
| **Bread and baked goods** | Discard | Porous foods can be contaminated below the surface. |
| **Peanut butter, legumes, and nuts** | Discard | Foods processed without preservatives are at high risk for mold. |

Credit: United States Department of Agriculture's Meat and Poultry Hotline. "Molds on Food: Are They Dangerous?" April 2002

can prevent many types of food contamination; for example, simply washing the hands after using the toilet gets rid of many contaminants that could otherwise contaminate food.

In addition, cross-contamination should be avoided. Cross-contamination occurs when a contaminated food is placed beside clean food, and the bacteria are able to contaminate it as well. To prevent cross-contamination of foods, items such as chicken, fish, and beef should not be placed near other food. In addition, after cutting up of meat, the cutting board should be thoroughly washed or another cutting board should be used before other items, such as fruits or vegetables, are cut.

It is also very important to discard food by its pass-by date, as well as to throw away food that has been in the refrigerator or freezer for an extended period. The Cold Storage Chart on pages 75–76, which is offered by the Food Safety and Inspection Service of the United States Department of Agriculture, provides helpful guidelines on when various types of foods should be discarded.

In most cases, moldy food should be discarded, because it may be dangerous and because many people are allergic to mold. However, in some cases, such as with some types of meats or cheeses, mold *can* be safely scraped off. The table on pages 77–78 from the Department of Agriculture provides guidelines on the types of food that should be

discarded when they have mold and those on which mold can be scraped off. People who are allergic to mold should avoid all moldy foods.

### International Consequences

Sometimes a case of food contamination can affect people in other countries because of the shipping of foods across countries. Reports of contaminated foods affecting Americans and Canadians have been traced back to *Salmonella* infection that was caused by Scandinavian alfalfa sprouts that were grown from imported seeds. In addition, *Shigella* infections in Europeans have been caused by prawns imported from Asia. Serious diseases can sometimes be spread in contaminated food; for example, people in the United States have contracted cholera by drinking fresh coconut milk that was imported from Asia.

Fortunately, the United States, Canada, and many other countries have strict rules regarding the inspection of imported foods, but occasionally problems still occur anyway.

See also BOTULINUM TOXIN; CHOLERA; FOOD-BORNE ILLNESSES; *ESCHERICHIA COLI; LISTERIA; SALMONELLA*.

Tauxe, Robert V., and James M. Hughes. "International Investigation of Outbreaks of a Disease." *British Medical Journal* 313, (November 2, 1996): 1,093–1,094.

**CREST syndrome** The acronym *CREST* represents a combination of five medical problems: calcinosis (the calcification of tissues), Raynaud's phenomenon (extreme skin color changes that occur in response to temperature changes), esophageal dysfunction, sclerodactyly (the thickening of the skin on the hands and feet), and telangiectasia (the presence of abnormally dilated blood vessels, usually in the face, upper body, or hands). CREST syndrome is also a subset of SCLERODERMA. Some CREST syndrome patients may also have musculoskeletal, cardiac, renal, neurologic, or pulmonary symptoms and signs of disease.

The cause of CREST syndrome is unknown. The diagnosis is based on the presence of the five medical problems that CREST syndrome comprises. Treatments are based on the patient's symptoms; for example, if patients have gastroesophageal reflux disease (GERD) as a component of esophageal dysfunction, they receive recommendations given to other GERD patients, such as raising the heads of their bed and avoiding large fatty meals and other foods that worsen reflux. In addition to using medications, such as acid blockers, patients with Raynaud's phenomenon may be advised to wear gloves and hats, both outdoors and indoors. Vasodilator and immunosuppressive drugs may be beneficial.

See also GASTROESOPHAGEAL REFLUX DISEASE.

Wemple, Mary A., M.D. "CREST Syndrome." eMedicine. Available online. URL: http://www.emedicine.com/derm/topic88.htm. Downloaded January 15, 2003.

**Crohn's disease** One of two severe chronic inflammatory bowel disorders. (The other form of INFLAMMATORY BOWEL DISEASE is ulcerative colitis.) Crohn's disease was named after Dr. Burrill B. Crohn, an American physician who first described the disease in 1932. Crohn's disease is uncommon, occurring in about 30 to 100 of every 100,000 people. It is not curable, but it is treatable. Crohn's disease is also known as regional enteritis.

Since clinical features vary widely, some experts believe that Crohn's disease may be more than one disease that has thus far been lumped into one.

Currently, Crohn's disease is subdivided by subtypes as

1. inflammatory
2. fistulous
3. obstructive

The clinical features of the subtypes tend to overlap in many cases.

The onset of Crohn's disease usually occurs in either adolescence or early adulthood. The cause of Crohn's disease is largely unknown, although some studies have found a genetic link on chromosome 16 among families with multiple members who have Crohn's disease, according to research reported in 2002 in the *New England Journal of Medicine*. In particular, mutations of the IBD1 gene, also called NOD2/CARD 15 gene have been identified as increasing the risk for certain types of Crohn's disease.

The disease may affect any section of the gastrointestinal system, from the mouth to the anus. It is a chronic disease of periodic flare-ups and remissions.

Some experts believe that Crohn's disease is an autoimmune disorder, but it is unknown whether this is true. Others believe that in a genetically predisposed individual, the disease may be triggered by infections or a toxin in the fecal stream; however, specific triggers have not been identified to date.

### Risk Factors

Crohn's disease is most frequently found among people who are between the ages of 12 and 40 years, although people of other ages may also be diagnosed with the disease. There is a genetic risk for the disease, and an estimated 12 to 18 percent of individuals diagnosed with Crohn's disease have other family members who have also been diagnosed with the disease.

People who smoke have higher risk of development of Crohn's disease. This is in contrast to ulcerative colitis, in which smoking is protective against the disease.

Stress does not cause Crohn's disease, but it can worsen the symptoms (as it frequently worsens the symptoms of many chronic diseases).

### Signs and Symptoms of Crohn's Disease

Individuals with Crohn's disease may have some or all of the following symptoms:

- Watery and persistent diarrhea
- Abdominal pain
- Weight loss
- Deep sores in the anal region
- Fever
- Irritations of the skin and/or eye
- Delayed growth and delayed puberty in children
- Malnutrition
- Rectal bleeding
- Arthritis

### Diagnosis of Crohn's Disease

The patient's medical history and symptoms are considered in diagnosing Crohn's disease. Physicians may also order a stool sample to rule out other diseases (such as parasitic or bacterial infections). Laboratory tests are usually ordered; many Crohn's disease patients have anemia caused by iron deficiencies or from deficiencies of vitamin $B_{12}$.

Physicians usually order a colonoscopy, both to rule out other diseases, such as IRRITABLE BOWEL SYNDROME (IBS), and to check for colonic inflammation and ulcers and other indications of chronic Crohn's disease; however, not all Crohn's disease occurs in the colon. Instead, the disease may be present in the small intestines, and thus a small bowel endoscopy, barium enema, and/or small bowel series may provide indications of the disease. A computed tomography (CT) scan of the abdomen is also a useful investigative tool, especially for the diagnosis of complications. Abdominal ultrasound and radionuclide scans are helpful in select cases.

### Treating Crohn's Disease

Patients who have Crohn's disease may be treated with dietary recommendations of foods to avoid (such as fiber and spicy foods), although dietary changes have not been shown to provide much improvement to most patients. The main nutrition-al problems are that patients may not eat enough, because the disease may induce anorexia (loss of appetite), or patients may be afraid to eat for fear of inducing diarrhea or pain. They also may not drink sufficient fluids, and dehydration may result. In addition, their ability to absorb nutrients is impaired.

Medications may be given to treat Crohn's disease, including anti-inflammatory drugs such as aminosalicylates like sulfasalazine (Azulfidine) and mesalamine (Asacol and Pentasa). Steroid drugs are frequently used for patients who have acute flare-ups. Steroids may have some distressing long-term side effects, which may end when the patient stops taking the drug, such as weight gain, acne, or difficulty in sleeping. Steroids also cause long-term side effects, especially bone loss. Both aminosalicylates and steroids may be given by mouth as well as in rectal suspensions by enema.

Antibiotics may also be used to treat the disease, especially metronidazole and ciprofloxacin (Cipro). Immune modulaters such as 6-mercaptopurine (6-MP) and azathioprine (Imuran) and methotrexate are also used for long-term treatment. Infliximab (Remicade) is a novel drug that is very effective in treating various types of Crohn's disease, even when conventional therapy has not been effective. It is effective in inducing and maintaining remission.

Some patients with Crohn's disease have shown improvement with the administration of growth hormone; a clinical study of 37 adults with Crohn's disease was described in 2000 in the *New England Journal of Medicine*. All of the subjects in the study had a moderate to severe case of Crohn's disease. The patients continued their regular medications during the study. They were all directed to increase their daily protein intake, because some studies have indicated that high-protein diets can improve symptoms.

The subjects who were given growth hormone had significant improvement in their symptoms when compared to the control group. The researchers concluded, "Our preliminary study demonstrates that growth hormone may be beneficial in the treatment of patients with chronically active Crohn's disease." As of this writing, the use of this drug for Crohn's disease is still investigational.

A 2003 study reported in the *New England Journal of Medicine* of 248 patients with Crohn's disease using the drug Antegren (natalizumab) found that the drug significantly increased the rate of remission and improved the patients' quality of life.

Most Crohn's disease patients may need surgery at some point in their lifetime to cope with the disease. There are many different types of surgeries that physicians may consider to relieve pain, obstructions, and symptoms of the disease.

For further information, contact the following organizations:

Crohn's and Colitis Foundation of America
386 Park Avenue South
New York, NY 10016
(800) 932-2423 (toll-free) or (212) 685-3440
http://www.ccfa.org

National Digestive Diseases Information
    Clearinghouse
National Institutes of Health
9000 Rockville Pike
Bethesda, MD 20892
(800) 891-5389 (toll-free) or (301) 654-3810
http://www.niddk.nih.gov

See also FISH OIL; ULCERATIVE COLITIS.

Ghosh, Subrata, M.D., et al. "Natalizumab for Active Crohn's Disease." *New England Journal of Medicine* 348, no. 1 (January 2, 2003): 24–32.

Minocha, Anil, M. J. Davis, and R. A. Wright. "Small Bowel Endometriosis Masquerading as Regional Enteritis." *Digestive Diseases Sciences* 39, no. 5 (1994): 1,126–1,133.

Minocha, Anil, et al. "Crohn's Disease Complicating Male Genitourinary Tract Without Overlying Cutaneous Involvement." *American Journal of Gastroenterology* 91 (1996): 1,463–1,464.

Slonim, Alfred E., M.D., et al. "A Preliminary Study of Growth Hormone Therapy for Crohn's Disease." *New England Journal of Medicine* 342, no. 22 (June 1, 2000): 1,633–1,637.

**cryoglobulinemia**  Usually refers to the presence in the blood of cryoglobulins, which are immuno-globulins or antibodies that precipitate in the cold and that dissolve after rewarming. Cryoglobulins are associated with numerous diseases, such as chronic HEPATITIS C, multiple myeloma, and lupus. Patients may experience skin rashes and kidney dysfunction due to cryoglobulinemia.

**Cryptosporidium**  A protozoon that is found and spread through CONTAMINATED FOOD OR WATER and that causes an illness called cryptosporidiosis. Once inside the body, this microbe infects the lining of the intestinal tract. A severe case was identified in Milwaukee, Wisconsin, in 1993, when over 400,000 people became infected with *Cryptosporidium* organisms that were transmitted in a contaminated public water supply.

*Cryptosporidium* infection is a very prevalent problem (although the Wisconsin case was unusually severe), and some experts believe that up to 2 percent of the population in the United States and Canada are infected with this microbe and another 80 percent have been infected at some time in the past. In healthy individuals, the disease is self-limited.

### Risk Factors

People who have a weakened immune system are more prone to become ill, including those with acquired immunodeficiency syndrome (AIDS), cancer, or other diseases that suppress the immune system. Individuals who deal frequently with farm animals are at risk, unless they wash their hands frequently. Even children visiting a petting zoo may contract cryptosporidiosis.

### Symptoms

After between five and 28 days from the time of infection, symptoms begin. (Some infected people do not have any symptoms.) They may include the following:

• Water diarrhea

• Abdominal cramps

• Nausea and vomiting

• Fever

- Headache
- Loss of appetite

### Diagnosis and Treatment

The disease is difficult to diagnose through symptoms only, since many diseases produce symptoms of diarrhea, abdominal cramps, and so forth. A stool sample can detect the disease, but only if the laboratory is specifically alerted to look for *Cryptosporidium* organisms. A routine stool test for ova and parasites may not screen for this protozoan.

Physicians may prescribe antibiotics and antidiarrheal medications. In severe cases, hospitalization is required and intravenous fluids are needed. Even if hospitalization is not required, it is important for patients to drink plenty of fluids to prevent dehydration.

The best treatment for immunodeficient patients (such as those with AIDS) is an improvement of their immune status, such as giving AIDS patients effective antiretroviral therapy that results in an improved immune system.

### Preventing Infection

Some simple actions can limit the risks of contracting *Cryptosporidium* infection, including the following:

- Filtering drinking water (chlorine does not kill this protozoan)
- Washing hands before and after preparing food
- Washing hands after changing diapers or working with small children
- Washing fruits and vegetables before eating them
- Avoiding unpasteurized milk

See also DEHYDRATION; PARASITIC INFECTIONS.

MacKenzie, William R., et al. "A Massive Outbreak in Milwaukee of *Cryptosporidium* Infection Transmitted through the Public Water Supply." *New England Journal of Medicine* 331, no. 3 (July 21, 1994): 161–167.

Chen, Xian-Ming, M.D., et al. "Cryptosporidiosis." *New England Journal of Medicine* 346, no. 2 (May 30, 2002): 1,723–1,731.

**cultures** Scientifically controlled growths of bacteria. Samples are taken from the patients' blood, sputum, feces, or urine, and then they are placed in a culture medium environment that is favorable to growth. The purpose of the culture is threefold: first, to determine whether bacteria are present; next, to identify the particular type of bacteria; finally, to ascertain the specific antibiotics most likely to destroy the bacteria that have been identified. Special culture media are required for certain pathogens.

A culture generally requires at least 24 to 48 hours before the laboratory results may be available to the physician. Some pathogens may take several days to weeks before definite results can be announced. Preliminary results are usually provided to physicians at 24 hours and an update given a day or two later.

If bacterial growth has occurred in the culture, the susceptibility to antibiotics is examined and that information guides the physician to use specifically targeted medications. Growth of some types of bacteria, such as tuberculosis, may take much longer than 48 hours to several days to weeks occur in a culture. In addition, results of antibiotic sensitivities may also take longer than 48 hours.

See also ANTIBIOTICS.

**cyclooxygenase-2 inhibitors** A class of medications that are prescribed to treat pain and arthritis inflammation, particularly that caused by chronic illnesses, such as rheumatoid arthritis. These drugs are generally less likely to cause stomach ulcers than are NONSTEROIDAL ANTI-INFLAMMATORY DRUGS, another class of medications used to treat similar illnesses. However, cyclooxygenase-2 (COX-2) inhibitor medications are not risk-free, and some patients experience ulcers and even gastrointestinal bleeding and other side effects as a result of taking these medications.

COX-2 inhibitor medications can also prevent the recurrence of colon polyps in some cases. The role of COX-2 inhibitors in preventing cancer of the colon, stomach and esophagus is being investigated. Some examples of COX-2 inhibitors are as follows: rofecoxib (Vioxx), valdecoxib (Bextra) and celecoxib (Celebrex).

See also GASTRITIS; OBESITY; PAIN; ULCERS, PEPTIC.

**cystic fibrosis  (CF)**    A very severe genetic disorder that results in a multisystem disease involving the sweat glands and the digestive, respiratory, and reproductive systems. Specifically, there are errors in the cystic fibrosis transmembrane conductance regulator (CFTR) gene. Cystic fibrosis (CF) causes the body to generate copious quantities of thick secretions that clog both the lungs and the pancreas and that also cause a high salt content of the perspiration. It is a disease that interferes with both breathing and digestion. Cystic fibrosis may also cause malabsorption in the intestines, generating an inability of the body to absorb needed nutrients.

Patients with cystic fibrosis have an increased risk of development of gastrointestinal cancers. They may also experience liver disease and even liver cancer. The gene for CF has been identified by researchers as appearing on chromosome 7.

### Risk Factors

Cystic fibrosis occurs predominantly among whites, although some Hispanics also have this disease. An estimated one in 3,300 Caucasians is diagnosed with cystic fibrosis, compared to one in 9,500 Hispanics. The incidence of cystic fibrosis is much lower in other racial and ethnic groups, although blacks in the United States are more likely to have cystic fibrosis than are blacks in other countries. Females with cystic fibrosis usually experience a delayed puberty as well as later problems with fertility. Nearly all (about 95 percent) men with cystic fibrosis are sterile.

### Symptoms and Signs of CF

The disease usually appears in infancy, and children with CF have frequent wheezing and coughing and are prone to development of frequent lung infections. However, some patients have few or no symptoms until they reach their teens or early adulthood. If symptoms and signs occur, the key symptoms are problems with respiration and delayed growth.

Other symptoms and signs include the following:

- Chronic coughing
- Poor weight gain

- Large foul-smelling stools
- Skin that tastes salty as a result of high level of salt in perspiration
- Frequent infections with pneumonia or bronchitis
- Failure to thrive in a child
- Pancreatitis
- Gallstones
- Infertility
- Sinusitis

### Diagnosis and Treatment

The classic symptoms of CF are usually evident to physicians. However, if the symptoms are mild, the patient may sometimes be misdiagnosed with asthma if further testing does not occur.

The sweat chloride test is generally used to diagnose cystic fibrosis. This test determines the presence of elevated chloride levels, an indicator of cystic fibrosis. In addition, results of sinus X rays and computed tomography (CT) scans are usually abnormal in cystic fibrosis patients. Genetic testing to identify the gene mutations can definitely identify the presence of cystic fibrosis.

Cystic fibrosis is not curable, although researchers are seeking a cure through gene therapy. At the present, physicians seek to treat the symptoms and the complications of the disease, whether they are infections, failure to thrive, or other medical problems. Patients may also be advised to eat high-calorie and high-fat diets, because of an underweight condition and their difficulty in attaining normal weight. Infections of the lung are treated with antibiotics. Patients should receive an influenza vaccine (flu shot) annually to limit their risk of development of flu. Pancreatic enzyme supplements are given in cases of PANCREATIC INSUFFICIENCY. Patients with cystic fibrosis are also advised to take vitamin and mineral supplements on a regular basis, as well as supplementation during periods of increased sweating, as needed.

For further information, contact the following organizations:

The Cystic Fibrosis Foundation
6921 Arlington Road

Bethesda, MD 20814
(301) 951-4422 or (800) FIGHT CF
http://www.cff.org

Canadian Cystic Fibrosis Foundation
2221 Yonge Street
Suite 601
Toronto, Ontario
M4S 2B4
(416) 485-9149
http://www.cysticfibrosis.ca

See also CANCER, LIVER; HEPATOCELLULAR CARCINOMA.

Ammer, Christine. *The New A to Z of Women's Health.* 4th ed. New York: Facts On File, 2000.

Knowles, Michael R., M.D., and Peter R. Durie, M.D. "What Is Cystic Fibrosis?" *New England Journal of Medicine* 347, no. 6 (August 8, 2002): 439–442.

Stern, Robert C., M.D. "The Diagnosis of Cystic Fibrosis." *New England Journal of Medicine* 3336, no. 7 (February 13, 1997): 487–491.

Wilschanski, Michael, et al. "Clinical and Genetic Risk Factors for Cystic Fibrosis–Related Liver Disease." *Pediatrics* 103, no. 1 (January 1999): 52–57.

Wynbrandt, James, and Mark D. Ludman. "Gilbert Disease." *The Encyclopedia of Genetic Disorders and Birth Defects.* 2d ed. New York: Facts On File, 2000.

**cytokines**  Hormonelike proteins that are produced by the activated immune cells to enhance the immune function by regulating it appropriately (up or down) in order to fight off disease. Cytokines allow immune cells to communicate with one another so that they can initiate, perpetuate and control the immune response. They are a necessary component of the immune system.

Numerous types of cytokines are produced; examples are interleukins, interferons, and tumor necrosis factor. However, at times, cytokines may function against the body itself and even worsen the disease process. Infliximab (Remicade), an antibody against tumor necrosis factor, is used as a treatment in rheumatoid arthritis and CROHN'S DISEASE.

**cytomegalovirus (CMV)**  An extremely common virus that rarely produces problems except among people who are immunocompromised, such as patients infected with the human immunodeficiency virus (HIV), those who have had organ transplantation, patients with advanced cancer, or others who are severely ill. Common symptoms are fever, fatigue, and swollen lymph glands. CMV may also cause ulcers in the esophagus, leading to painful swallowing. Involvement in the intestines can lead to perforation.

Foscarnet and ganciclovir are two key drugs that have been approved by the Food and Drug Administration (FDA) in the United States to treat patients with CMV. Some individuals who have acquired immunodeficiency syndrome (AIDS) require long-term maintenance therapy on medications for CMV.

Whitley, Richard J., M.D., et al. "Guidelines for the Treatment of Cytomegalovirus Diseases in Patients with AIDS in the Era of Potent Antiretroviral Therapy: Recommendations of an International Panel." *Archives of Internal Medicine* 158 (May 11, 1998): 957–969.

**defecation**   The act of having a bowel movement.

**dehydration**   A condition of an abnormally low level and imbalance of body fluids, usually also associated with electrolyte abnormalities, with the primary symptoms of thirst, dry skin and mucous membranes, and lightheadedness and nausea. The condition can at times be dangerous and even fatal. People with DIABETES MELLITUS are at a higher than average risk for experiencing dehydration; however, any person who consumes insufficient fluid or consumes too little fluid to meet increased fluid needs, as occurs with DIARRHEA, can become dehydrated.

Dehydration is a risk for those who are very physically active, and usually the summertime is when risk is greatest for active individuals (as well as inactive people) because of higher levels of perspiration due to the heat.

The primary causes of dehydration are as follows:

- Inadequate fluid intake
- Vomiting
- Diarrhea
- High fever
- Diuretic medications or other drugs
- Uncontrolled diabetes, causing high glucose levels (hyperglycemia) leading to increased urination
- Bleeding

### Signs and Symptoms

Weakness, dizziness, and skin pallor may indicate dehydration. Poor skin turgor is another indicator. (When the skin on the arm is pulled gently, it does not rapidly return to normal and remains pinched longer than usual.) Thirst may be a symptom of dehydration, although severely dehydrated people may occasionally be too ill to feel thirsty, and thus lack of thirst does not necessarily mean that a person is sufficiently hydrated.

### Diagnosis and Treatment

The diagnosis of dehydration is based on the medical history, symptoms and physician's observations of the signs of dehydration in the patient and can be verified by blood tests, including a test of electrolytes (sodium, potassium, chloride, and so forth) and blood urea nitrogen (BUN) levels. High BUN levels suggest that dehydration is present. Levels of electrolytes may be low or high. The elevated levels may occur because of a disproportionate loss of water content from the body.

Doctors treat patients with dehydration by seeking the cause of the problem, along with replacing their lost fluids and electrolytes to an adequate level. This is frequently done orally, and if needed, it is performed intravenously. The patient is also urged to consume liquids orally, whenever possible. Severely dehydrated individuals may require hospitalization for a day or longer. After discharge from the hospital, patients should continue to drink sufficient quantities of fluid for at least several days in order to prevent a recurrence of the dehydration. If the physician believes that individuals need antibiotics to fight off infection, they are prescribed. Similarly, treatment of the causes of dehydration, such as diabetes and diarrhea or bleeding also needs to be addressed.

See also ELECTROLYTES; NAUSEA AND VOMITING.

**diabetes mellitus**   A severe medical problem that is primarily characterized by the failure of the pancreas to create sufficient (or any) insulin or by the inability of the body to respond to the insulin that is produced (a condition that is also called insulin resistance). These problems with insulin regulation lead to high glucose level (hyperglycemia) and to multiple digestive problems as well as other medical problems. Sometimes people with diabetes also have hypoglycemia (low level of blood sugar) due to a decreased intake of nutrition while taking antidiabetic medication and urgently require the administration of glucose. Diabetes mellitus should not be confused with diabetes insipidus.

According to a report released by the National Center for Health Statistics in 2002, about 5 percent of the adult population in the United States reported having been diagnosed with diabetes. About 10 million people nationwide have diabetes. About 800,000 new cases of diabetes are diagnosed each year.

Many people who have diabetes have serious gastrointestinal problems, and some experts believe that as many as 75 percent of all patients with diabetes have such problems. According to two diabetes specialists, Wolosin and Edelman, in their 2000 article in *Clinical Diabetes:*

> The entire [gastrointestinal] GI tract can be affected by diabetes from the oral cavity and esophagus to the large bowel and anorectal region. Thus, the symptom complex that may be experienced can vary widely. Common complaints may include dysphagia, early satiety [fullness after eating], reflux [acid reflux], constipation, abdominal pain, nausea, vomiting, and diarrhea. Many patients go undiagnosed and undertreated because the GI tract has not been traditionally associated with diabetes and its complications.

People with diabetes may sometimes experience acutely severe digestive problems that may be life-threatening. Doctors Mesiya and Minocha explain further in their 1998–99 *Southern Medical Journal* monograph: "Acute problems include stress gastritis during ketoacidosis, acute pancreatitis and acute cholecystitis. Most problems are, however, chronic, and may manifest with remissions and relapses."

People who have diabetes are not only more likely to suffer from gastrointestinal problems than nondiabetics, but they are also directly affected by the degree of blood sugar control that they maintain. Good control reduces the risk for digestive diseases and disorders.

One article illustrates both points very clearly. In a study of thousands of subjects, including 423 diabetics (nearly all having type 2 diabetes), reported in a 2001 issue of *Archives of Internal Medicine,* the patients with diabetes had a greater prevalence of both upper and lower gastrointestinal symptoms. For example, 26 percent of the diabetic patients had bowel symptoms, compared to about 19 percent of the nondiabetic subjects. In addition, 15.6 percent of the patients with diabetes reported having diarrhea (more than three bowel movements per day, urgency, and loose or watery stools) compared to 10 percent of the nondiabetic patients. The diabetic subjects also reported more problems with dysphagia (5.4 percent versus 1.7 percent for nondiabetics).

The study also showed that patients with good glycemic control (as close to normal blood sugar levels as possible) had a much lower prevalence of gastrointestinal symptoms. For example, 33.3 percent of the diabetic patients with poor glycemic control had abdominal pain. The rate dropped to 15.5 percent for patients with average glycemic control and improved further still to 9.2 percent for patients with good control.

Among the diabetic patients who reported problems with heartburn, those with poor control had a rate of 37.8 percent experiencing this problem. The heartburn rate dropped to 14.0 percent for patients with average glycemic control and further still to 9.3 percent for diabetic patients with good glycemic control. This pattern was observed for nearly all gastrointestinal symptoms, including bloating, nausea, dysphagia, diarrhea, and constipation. Clearly, patients can improve their own health by working to maintain blood sugar levels as close to normal as possible.

Patients with diabetes are at increased risk for nonalcoholic fatty liver disease.

### Types of Diabetes Mellitus and Risk Factors

There are two primary types of diabetes: type 1 diabetes (formerly called juvenile-onset diabetes or insulin-dependent diabetes) and type 2 diabetes (formerly called adult-onset diabetes or non-insulin-dependent diabetes). These terms were changed because adults can be diagnosed with type 1 diabetes and because some people who have long-term type 2 diabetes eventually do need insulin in order to treat the illness.

Type 2 diabetes is the more common form of diabetes, and it represents about 90 to 95 percent of all cases of diabetes in the United States and Canada. The primary risk factors for type 2 diabetes are age (older people have a greater risk, and the risk is greatest among those older than age 65), race (African Americans, Native Americans, and Hispanics have the greatest risk), and health factors; for example, people who are obese have a greater risk for development of type 2 diabetes than people who are of slender or average build. There is also a genetic risk for type 2 diabetes.

Type 1 diabetes, the less common form, is mostly found among whites, and about a million children and adults in the United States have this form of diabetes. Many experts consider type 1 diabetes an autoimmune disorder, in which the immune system mistakenly attacks its own cells for invaders and subsequently harms or destroys them. In the case of type 1 diabetes, the body attacks the beta cells of the pancreas, which make insulin, and ultimately destroys them all.

In some cases, it may be difficult to distinguish between type 1 and type 2 diabetes.

### Background Information

Type 1 diabetes was a fatal disease until the development of insulin in 1921 by Dr. Frederick Banting, a Canadian physician, and Charles Best, a Canadian medical student who assisted him. Many developments have occurred since then to improve the creation and the delivery of insulin, including less painful injection methods and implantable insulin pumps.

In 2000 another medical breakthrough occurred when Dr. Shapiro, another Canadian physician, successfully transplanted pancreatic cells from deceased people into the livers of 11 diabetic patients, through a special catheter. The cells attached to blood vessels in the liver, where the cells began to generate insulin and cured the subjects' diabetes. This procedure became known as the Edmonton Protocol, because it began in Edmonton, Canada.

The reason why this procedure is not now used to cure every person who has type 1 diabetes is that it is experimental and costly, and finding sufficient cadavers (dead people) from whom to excise the pancreas is difficult. As of this writing one pancreas is not sufficient for transplantation and instead, each patient requires two organs, however, there are only about 3,000 cadavers, with one pancreas each.

Research continues on this front, and as of this writing, it still is extremely costly to perform such transplantations and most people who have type 1 diabetes cannot receive them. However, researchers have hope for future improvements and for an actual cure, at some future point.

### Symptoms and Signs of Diabetes

The most common symptoms of diabetes are frequent urination and intense thirst and/or hunger. Other symptoms include the following:

- Excessive fatigue with no apparent cause
- Blurred vision
- Slow healing of cuts or wounds
- Frequent skin or other infections
- Unexplained weight loss (only in type 1 diabetes)

### Key Digestive Problems Associated with Diabetes

Diabetes is often associated with GASTROPARESIS (abnormally slow stomach emptying). It can be very hard for people with diabetes who also have gastroparesis to maintain normal glucose levels. A further problem is that chronic gastroparesis often leads to the development of GASTROESOPHAGEAL REFLUX DISEASE (GERD).

In some cases, the delayed emptying of the stomach is the direct result of nerve damage that was caused by diabetes, which is a condition known as gastroparesis diabeticorum. As many as 25 percent of diabetes patients have gastroparesis.

Many patients with diabetes (about 25 percent) have severe chronic problems with CONSTIPATION and some experience FECAL IMPACTION. People with diabetes may also have DIARRHEA, which is a problem for about 20 percent of patients diagnosed with diabetes. Diarrhea may be due to an abnormal motility or secretions of the intestines, diabetic neuropathy, or small intestinal bacterial overgrowth. Some patients with diabetes have IRRITABLE BOWEL SYNDROME (IBS), although the incidence of IBS among people with diabetes does not appear to be any higher than it is for nondiabetics.

People who have either type 1 and type 2 diabetes are more likely to experience CANDIDA infections of the esophagus, gastrointestinal tract, and mouth.

### Diagnosis of Diabetes

Diabetes is often diagnosed through a fasting blood test, the fasting plasma glucose test. In this test, the patient's blood is drawn within eight to 12 hours after the patient begins fasting. If the fasting glucose level is 126 mg/dl or higher on two different occasions, then diabetes is usually diagnosed. Sometimes in borderline cases, especially if the physician suspects that the patient has type 2 diabetes, the patient is given oral glucose (called an oral glucose tolerance test), and blood glucose levels are then measured. If the blood glucose levels are at or above 200 mg/dl after ingestion of oral glucose, then the person has diabetes.

### Management of Diabetes

Most physicians believe that people who have been diagnosed with diabetes should be treated by a team of medical experts, preferably including an endocrinologist (a physician who specializes in endocrine diseases), a registered dietitian, a certified diabetes educator, and other experts as needed.

The fact remains, however, that individuals diagnosed with diabetes must usually provide most of their own daily care or must receive it from caregivers each day; for example, daily glucose monitoring must be performed, usually at least twice a day, with an evaluation of blood sugar levels. In addition, individuals or their caregivers must act on the information that the blood test supplies, such as eating snacks if the blood sugar level is too low or taking extra insulin or oral medications for diabetes or fluids if glucose levels are too high.

***Common medications taken for diabetes***   Type 1 diabetes is treated with insulin injections, whereas type 2 diabetes is usually treated with a variety of oral medications. Some type 2 diabetes patients may require insulin in addition to oral medications.

Drugs given to people with type 2 diabetes include the following:

- Glyburide (Micronase)
- Repaglinide (Prandin)
- Nateglinide (Starlix)
- Rosiglitazone (Avandia)
- Pioglitazone (Actos)
- Acarbose (Precose)
- Miglitol (Glyset)
- Metformin (Glucophage)

People who have type 1 diabetes must take insulin, which is sold in short-acting, intermediate-acting, and long-acting forms. There are also some fast-acting forms of insulin. Fast-acting insulin, such as insulin lispro, human recombinant deoxyribonucleic acid (rDNA) (Humalog) and Novalog, work within five to 15 minutes of injection, and these drugs can lower a patient's blood sugar level in 45 to 90 minutes.

Short-acting insulin, or regular insulin, starts working within 45 minutes, peaks two to three hours after the patient injects the drug, and can last as long as eight hours. Intermediate insulin (neutral protamine Hagedorn [NPH] or Lente) starts acting about two to four hours after it is injected and peaks about four to 12 hours after injection. Long-acting insulin (ultralente) starts working within four to six hours after injection and peaks about eight to 20 hours from the time of injection. Peakless insulin (glargine) lasts for up to 20 to 24 hours. A combination of short- and long-acting insulin is frequently used to achieve quick and sustained glycemic control for 12 to 24 hours.

***Dietary considerations***   People with diabetes are urged to pay attention to their diet and prevent obesity. Physicians can also check on the patient's glucose levels over a three-month period with a glycosalated hemoglobin level, or hemoglobin A₁C level, test. An elevated A₁C level indicates that blood glucose level has not been adequately controlled.

People who have diabetes may benefit from a high-FIBER diet; however, if they also have GASTRO-PARESIS and a very slow gut, causing megacolon, then a high-fiber diet may create further problems with bowel movements.

*Other lifestyle recommendations* Everyone who has diabetes should stop smoking, because smoking accelerates problems with both diabetes and digestive disorders in addition to worsening diabetes-associated complications, such as heart disease and other medical problems. Physicians also urge people diagnosed with diabetes to obtain regular exercise to improve their health.

For further information about diabetes, contact the following organizations:

American Association of Diabetes Educators
444 North Michigan Avenue
Suite 1240
Chicago, IL 60611
(800) 338-3633, (800) 338-3634 or
    (312) 644-2233

American Diabetes Association (ADA)
1701 North Beauregard Street
Alexandria, VA 22311
(800) 232-3472 (toll free) or (703) 549-1500
http://www.diabetes.org/

Blackwell, D. L., J. G. Collins, and R. Coles. "Summary Health Statistics for U.S. Adults: National Health Interview Survey, 1997." National Center for Health Statistics. *Vital Health Statistics* 10, no. 205 (2002).

Bytzer, Peter, M.D., et al. "Prevalence of Gastrointestinal Symptoms Associated with Diabetes Mellitus: A Population-Based Survey of 15,000 Adults." *Archives of Internal Medicine* 161 (September 10, 2001): 1,989–1,996.

Mesiya, Sikander A., M.D., and Anil Minocha, M.D. "Gastrointestinal Disease in Diabetes Mellitus." *Southern Medical Journal* (winter 1998/1999): 33–38.

National Institute of Diabetes and Digestive and Kidney Diseases. "Conquering Diabetes: Highlights of Program Efforts, Research Advances and Opportunities." U.S. Department of Health and Human Services, NIH Publication no. 02-5137, September 2002.

Pandit, Manjula K., M.D., et al. "Drug-Induced Disorders of Glucose Tolerance." *Annals of Internal Medicine* 118, no. 7 (April 1, 1993): 529–539.

Petit, William, Jr., M.D., and Christine Adamec. *The Encyclopedia of Diabetes*. New York: Facts On File, 2002.

Vinik, Aaron, M.D., et al. "Gastrointestinal, Genitourinary, and Neurovascular Disturbances in Diabetes." *Diabetes Reviews* 7, no. 4 (1996): 346–366.

Wolosin, James D., M.D., and Steven V. Edelman. "Diabetes and the Gastrointestinal Tract." *Clinical Diabetes* 18, no. 4 (fall 2000): 148–151.

**diaphragm** The muscular wall that lies between the abdomen and the chest. This muscle is used for breathing. The hollow gut tube passes through an opening in the diaphragm. Sometimes a hiatal hernia develops, allowing a part of the stomach to protrude into the chest through the esophageal hiatus (opening) in the diaphragm.

See also HERNIA, HIATAL.

**diarrhea** An increase in the frequency and/or fluidity of stools. If diarrhea has lasted for at least four weeks or longer, it is considered chronic. Diarrhea is a symptom caused by many different infections and chronic as well as acute illnesses. In the United States, about eight million people per year see a physician to report diarrhea and of these individuals, about 250,000 are hospitalized. Some individuals experience a chronic problem of having diarrhea that may alternate with constipation, plus experiencing abdominal pain that improves with defecation, a condition that is known as IRRITABLE BOWEL SYNDROME (IBS).

Most cases of acute diarrhea resolve spontaneously. However, if the problem continues and the individual is untreated, diarrhea can sometimes become life-threatening, particularly to infants or to very elderly individuals. Diarrhea can also be dangerous for others who have a compromised immune system, such as people who have human immunodeficiency virus (HIV), cancer, or other serious illnesses.

### Causes of Diarrhea

Diarrhea may be a temporary condition that is caused by a minor or serious illness, indigestion, food-borne illnesses, or contaminated food or water. Diarrhea may be caused by bacteria or viruses or by another agent altogether, such as by a parasitic disease such as amebiasis. Diarrhea may also result from taking some medications; in fact, many different medications produce diarrhea as a side effect, including many antibiotics, antiarrhythmic drugs (for the heart), and anticancer medications and some antidepressants, antihypertensive drugs, and diuretics.

Diarrhea may be a symptom of an acute or chronic disease. Infection with bacteria or parasites in the gastrointestinal tract may also cause diarrhea.

Many people who travel to other countries experience diarrhea, to such an extent that "traveler's diarrhea" is a diagnosis.

### Diagnosis and Treatment

Physicians ask patients with diarrhea how many bowel movements they are having per day, and how long the problem has occurred. Most patients do not require testing; however, laboratory tests, such as the complete blood count (CBC) and stool studies, can also indicate whether an infection is present. Electrolyte tests and tests of renal (kidney) function may be ordered to help the doctor determine the harmful effects of diarrhea, such as dehydration. Physicians may also order a stool sample analysis, to test for infections or other diseases that are causing the problem.

Most cases of acute diarrhea are self-limited and do not require any specific treatment except adequate hydration. Diarrhea is usually treated with over-the-counter (OTC) or prescribed medications. Minor cases of diarrhea may be treated with antidiarrheal medications, rest, and plenty of fluids.

Patients with diarrhea that is associated with bleeding, fever, severe weakness and lethargy, or weight loss should seek medical attention promptly. In addition, replacement of fluids and electrolytes is important to prevent DEHYDRATION. Some individuals may need to be hospitalized so that they can receive intravenous replacement of fluids.

See also COLITIS; CONTAMINATED FOOD OR WATER; DYSENTERY; FOOD-BORNE ILLNESSES; IRRITABLE BOWEL SYNDROME; PARASITIC INFECTIONS.

Bartlett, John G., M.D. "Antibiotic-Associated Diarrhea." *New England Journal of Medicine* 346, no. 5 (January 31, 2002): 334–339.

**diet drugs** Prescribed or over-the-counter medications or herbal remedies that are taken to reduce appetite so that an overweight or obese individual may lose weight more easily. An estimated 5 million people in the United States take prescribed drugs for weight loss, and many millions more take over-the-counter diet drugs. People buy over-the-counter diet remedies in pharmacies and supermarkets as well as through the Internet. There are also print and television advertisements that promote over-the-counter diet drugs.

Medications for weight loss are recommended for some patients who have a BODY MASS INDEX (BMI) of greater than 30 or greater than 27, if there are obesity-related problems that diet and exercise have failed to correct. Diet drugs should not be used by the following individuals:

- Children
- The elderly (older than age 65 years)
- Pregnant or breastfeeding women
- Individuals who have pulmonary hypertension
- Patients who have uncontrolled systemic hypertension
- Patients who have unstable heart disease

In the past, amphetamines were used as diet drugs, but today this category of drugs is not recommended for this use in the United States and in other countries. Some researchers are also looking at the efficacy of some antidepressant drugs, such as bupropion (Wellbutrin) in producing weight loss. Most studies have shown that most diet drugs do not produce massive weight losses and that the weight that is lost is usually regained when the person stops taking the drug.

### Studies on Newer Medications

Researchers are seeking better drugs to control overweight and obesity. Sometimes drugs that have not worked out well in treating other illnesses have had a side effect of causing weight loss, and thus researchers have subsequently performed separate studies to determine whether those medications would help obese people. An antiepileptic drug, zonisamide (Zonegran), has been tested for its efficacy in weight loss by some researchers.

In a study reported in 2003 in the *Journal of the American Medical Association,* the researchers Gadde and colleagues gave obese subjects the drug or a placebo over 16 weeks. All patients were also placed on a hypocaloric (low-calorie) diet, and their compliance was monitored with self-rated food diaries. There were 55 women and five men; of these subjects, 51 completed the protocol. The zonisamide therapy was started at 100 mg orally with a gradual increase to 400 mg. A further increase to 600 mg was made for those patients who had lost less than 5 percent of their body weight after 12 weeks.

The researchers found that zonisamide, combined with a low-calorie diet, was significantly more effective than placebo in producing weight loss. Over the 16-week period, the weight loss in the zonisamide group was an average of 5.9 kg (a 6.0 percent loss), whereas in the placebo group, the average loss was 0.9 kg (a 1.0 percent loss). One reported side effect of zonisamide was fatigue.

In a study reported by Ettinger and colleagues in 2003 in the *Journal of the American Medical Association,* researchers tested the effect of a genetically engineered form of ciliary neurotrophic factor (CNTF) manufactured by Regeneron. This protein had originally been tested as a treatment for amyotrophic lateral sclerosis (ALS) patients, but it had caused significant weight loss in nonobese subjects because it apparently suppresses hunger signals from the hypothalamus.

Researchers decided to test its efficacy on obese patients over 12 weeks. One hundred and twenty-three patients completed the clinical study. Patients taking the protein achieved a significant weight loss when compared to subjects in the placebo group; however, adverse effects were reported, such as nausea as well as pain at the injection site of the medication.

All prescribed diet drugs are offered for short-term use; however, many obesity experts believe that people for whom an antiobesity drug is effective have to continue to use it over the long term, much as patients who have hypertension continue taking hypertension medications once their blood pressure has improved.

### Primary Prescribed Diet Drugs

In the United States, the key prescribed diet drugs are sibutramine (Meridia) and orlistat (Xenical). Orlistat also reduces serum cholesterol level. Phentermine was formerly combined with fenfluramine (Pondimin) or dexfenfluramine (Redux): the phen–fen combination. The combined drug was removed from the consumer market in 1997 in the United States because of an associated problem with a heart valve disease. Phentermine and diethylpriopion are approved only for short-term use (12 weeks).

The side effects of sibutramine are a mild increase in blood pressure, dry mouth, constipation, and headache. It should not be used by those who have a history of heart disease or stroke.

Orlistat's side effects are fecal urgency and incontinence, flatulence, increased frequency of defecation, and oily spotting. An estimated 9 percent of patients discontinue taking orlistat specifically because of these troublesome side effects, although the side effects generally decrease over time. Orlistat decreases the absorption of vitamins A and E, and for this reason, some physicians recommend vitamin supplements to patients who are treated with this drug.

Leptin has been shown to cause a reduction in food intake and to be effective for obese animals and humans; however, its effect is modest and it is not approved for use in the United States.

### An Analysis of the Users of Prescribed Weight Loss Medications

In one analysis of the use of diet drugs, in a 2001 issue of the *Annals of Internal Medicine,* the authors reported that 2.5 percent of adults in the United States used prescription weight loss medications over the period 1996 to 1998. Women were four times more likely to use prescribed diet drugs than men. Hispanic women, at a usage rate of 3.2 percent, were more likely than whites or blacks (both at 2.4 percent) to use these drugs.

The pills were most heavily used by females between the ages of 25 and 44 years. Disturbingly, as many as one-quarter of the individuals taking prescribed weight loss drugs were *not* overweight in terms of their BMI. Hispanic women were most likely to be using these drugs inappropriately. BMI is a measure derived from height and weight that enables physicians to determine whether individuals are overweight or obese. People who are not overweight or obese should not take any diet drugs, whether they are prescribed or over-the-counter medications.

### Use of Over-the-Counter Diet Drugs

In past years, phenylpropanolamine was the primary ingredient in many over-the-counter diet medications; however, because studies showed such drugs increased the risk for heart attack and stroke, these drugs were withdrawn from the market by manufacturers in 2000.

Before 2004, many drugs contained ephedra or ma huang (*Ephedra sinica*), a stimulant combined with caffeine to aid in weight loss. However, ephedra is dangerous for people with hypertension, heart disease, diabetes, and other medical problems. It is also true that some individuals have purportedly died as a result of taking drugs that contain ephedra. Because ephedra is considered an herb under the 1994 Dietary Supplement Health and Education Act, it is not directly under the control of the Food and Drug Administration (FDA) in the United States. However, the Food and Drug Administration after issuing numerous warnings against using ephedra banned the drug in the United States in 2004.

The ingestion of green tea has been shown to produce weight loss. Some use guar gum (derived from the Indian cluster bean) as a weight loss remedy.

In a study reported in a 2001 issue of the *Journal of the American Medical Association*, researchers contacted more than 14,000 individuals in Florida, Iowa, Michigan, West Virginia, and Wisconsin and asked them about their use of over-the-counter diet medications. Ten percent of the consumers reported having used or currently using diet drugs. Most users were obese young women (28 percent), but some users (8 percent) were normal-weight women who apparently wanted to be thinner. There were no ethnic or racial differences among those using over-the-counter diet drugs.

For more information on weight loss, contact the following organization:

Weight-Control Information Network (WIN)
1 WIN Way
Bethesda, MD 20892
(877) 946-4627
Website: www.niddk.nih.gov/health/nutrit/nutrit.htm

See also BARIATRIC SURGERY; OBESITY.

Blanck, Heidi Michels, Laura Kettel Khan, and Mary K. Serdula, M.D. "Use of Nonprescription Weight Loss Products: Results from a Multistate Survey." *Journal of American Medical Association* 286, no. 8 (August 22/29, 2001): 930–935.

Ettinger, Mark P., M.D., et al. "Recombinant Variant of Ciliary Neurotrophic Factor for Weight Loss in Obese Adults: A Randomized, Dose-Ranging Study." *Journal of the American Medical Association* 289, no. 13 (April 9, 2003): 1,826–1,832.

Gadde, Kishore M., M.D., et al. "Zonisamide for Weight Loss in Obese Adults: A Randomized Controlled Trial." *Journal of the American Medical Association* 289, no. 14 (April 9, 2003): 1,820–1,825.

Khan, Laura Kettel, et al. "Use of Prescription Weight Loss Pills among U.S. Adults in 1996–1998." *Annals of Internal Medicine* 134, no. 4 (2001): 282–286.

Wirth, Alfred, M.D., and Jutta Krause. "Long-Term Weight Loss with Sibutramine: A Randomized Controlled Trial." *Journal of the American Medical Association* 286, no. 11 (September 19, 2001): 1,331–1,339.

Yanovski, Susan Z., M.D., and Jack A. Yanovski, M.D. "Obesity." *New England Journal of Medicine* 346, no. 8 (February 21, 2002): 591–602.

**digestion and absorption**  The process by which foods are broken down and nutrients, vitamins, minerals, and other substances are absorbed and used by the body as building blocks and as a source of energy. The process of digestion and absorption is complex and ongoing and is accomplished over several hours.

Food is processed in the stomach and the small intestines for about three hours in each. Thus, digestion does not start with the intake of food and end when a meal is finished. Instead, the food eaten for breakfast and a midmorning snack is still being digested, absorbed, and assimilated while the individual is eating lunch, and digestion and absorption continue continuously until at some point it slows while the individual sleeps for seven or eight hours.

Digestion and absorption normally work very well every day for most people. However, sometimes the digestive system experiences temporary or long-term problems that require treatment.

### Lack of Absorption of Vitamins or Minerals

In some cases, because of disease or medical problems, patients absorb too much or too little of needed nutrients. For example, some people cannot absorb vitamin $B_{12}$ from the food that they eat, so they must take supplemental doses of it. Others suffer from iron deficiency anemia and must take supplemental doses of iron in order for their body to function normally. Others have deficiencies of other substances, such as magnesium or potassium.

Patients with short bowel syndrome have an insufficient length of the small intestines to meet their needs for nutrient absorption and may need to rely upon parenteral nutrition. Patients with hemochromatosis absorb too much iron and suffer from an overload that can lead to liver cirrhosis and heart problems.

### Missing or the Wrong Level of Enzymes Can Be the Problem

In other cases, there is a problem with the specific enzymes that are needed for digestion; for example, patients with chronic pancreatitis cannot produce enough digestive enzymes to digest food. Since these enzymes are needed for digestion, those who have this problem must obtain these enzymes through an external source (pills or capsules) to survive.

### Other Illnesses, Such as Thyroid Disease

Sometimes other systems in the body may cause problems with digestion. For example, if patients have a thyroid disease, they may have sped-up metabolism, caused by hyperthyroidism (high levels of circulating thyroid hormone), or, conversely, they may have very sluggish metabolism, which is caused by hypothyroidism (low levels of thyroid hormone). Both of these conditions can affect the appetite and digestion. Diagnosis and treatment of the underlying thyroid disease usually resolve any digestive problems that the condition has caused.

### Malfunctions of Digestive Organs

Sometimes organs within the digestive system malfunction and may prevent normal digestion and absorption. Organs may have blockages or benign or cancerous tumors that can impede or prevent the normal digestive processes. Organs can also become inflamed and irritated, interfering with the normal digestive process. In addition, slow gut may lead to a small-intestine bacterial overgrowth, causing malabsorption.

### Behavior Can Cause Digestive Problems

The individual can impair normal nutrition, for example, by failing to eat sufficient amounts of food or by eating large quantities of food that lead to obesity and resulting digestive difficulties. Other behavior, such as alcoholism or drug addiction, can cause damage to the digestive system. Depending on how severe the damage is, the digestive system may recover if the abusive behavior ends, or the damage may be irreversible. Examples of the results of abusive behavior are alcoholic liver cirrhosis and narcotic bowel syndrome.

### Infections Impede Digestion

Parasitic or other infectious diseases may make normal digestion difficult or impossible until they are identified and treated. Some infections are spread by contaminated food or water. Many times it is difficult to determine the source of an infection, and the best the doctor can do is to identify the disease and treat it.

### Inherited Defects

Some individuals have hereditary medical problems such as a risk for development of diabetes, that make digestion difficult unless or until they are treated. For this reason, physicians obtain a complete medical history in addition to performing a physical examination when a patient consults them about a medical problem.

### Food Allergies and Food Intolerances

Patients may also have food allergies (in which an immune reaction to a food develops) such as peanut allergy or food intolerances (symptoms that occur in response to eating certain foods, which may be due to the body's lacking a substance that is needed to digest them, such as lactase for the digestion of lactose) of which they are unaware. Some allergies are mild, others are very severe. In addition, food intolerance may also range from mild to severe in scope.

### The Impact of Aging

As individuals age into middle age and then the elderly years (ages 65 and older), the digestive system may become more sluggish, the patient becomes less active, and the risk for development of digestive diseases and/or worsening of existing diseases becomes great. It is also true that older people are much more likely to be using three or more medications than younger individuals. Because many medications can cause digestive difficulties, such as diarrhea or constipation, it is not surprising that many elderly people have difficulties with digestion and problems such as constipation and fecal impaction.

### The Impact of Technology

Diseases and illnesses that physicians could not treat in past years are now treated routinely. Canadian scientists have discovered how to graft cells from the pancreas of deceased individuals into living patients with insulin-dependent diabetes, curing their diabetes. Physicians have found many ways to treat and even cure digestive cancers, through surgery, chemotherapy, and radiation therapy. Nearly every month has new revelations about potential ways physicians can help people of all ages to cope with their digestive problems.

See also ADOLESCENTS; CHILDREN; CANCER; CONSTIPATION; DIABETES MELLITUS; DIARRHEA; DIGESTIVE SYSTEM; ELDERLY; INFANTS.

**digestive enzymes** Substances that are secreted by the body to aid in digesting food. AMYLASE is secreted by the salivary glands as well as the pancreas. Other enzymes are trypsin, chymotrypsin, and carboxypeptidases A and B, all of which are enzymes that transform proteins into amino acids. Lipase is an enzyme that breaks down fats into fatty acids and glycerol. Lactase breaks down milk sugar, which is known as lactose. A deficiency of lactase leads to LACTOSE INTOLERANCE.

Other digestive enzymes include maltase, which breaks down maltose, and sucrase, which digests sucrose.

Some people do not secrete sufficient digestive enzymes, as a result of disease, inflammatory processes, PARASITIC INFECTIONS, and other medical problems. They may need supplemental enzymes; for example, pancreatic enzymes may be needed in cases of chronic pancreatitis. Supplemental pancreatic enzymes are also used to decrease the pain caused by chronic pancreatitis.

**digestive juices** Liquids produced in the stomach and other parts of the gastrointestinal system that help digest and absorb food, for example, hydrochloric acid and pepsin in the stomach. Another organ, the pancreas, secretes pancreatic juice, which contains water; electrolytes such as sodium, potassium, and bicarbonate; as well as enzymes such as trypsin, lipase, and amylase, into the intestines. Another digestive juice is bile, secreted by the liver, stored in the gallbladder, and then delivered into the duodenum at the time of a meal.

See also DIGESTIVE ENZYMES.

**digestive system** The series of interconnected organs that together work to process food, beginning with the mouth, where the salivary glands start processing food that has been ingested. The food then passes into the esophagus, the "food tube" that joins to the stomach, which is the digestive organ where the solid large pieces of food are processed into smaller-sized particles for delivery to the small intestine, where most of digestion and absorption occurs.

Enzymes in the small intestine break down the food further. The liver, pancreas, and gallbladder are also involved in processing food. The pancreas releases special enzymes to break the food down into its elements of carbohydrates, fats, and

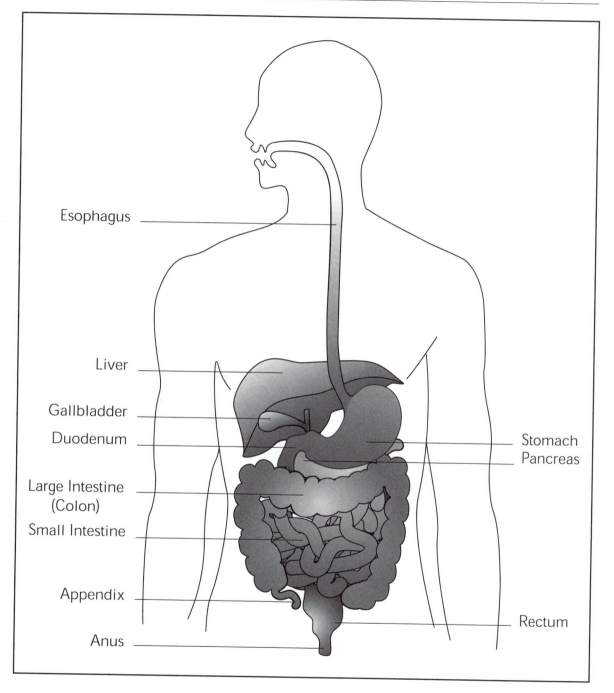

Esophagus

Liver

Gallbladder

Duodenum

Large Intestine
(Colon)

Small Intestine

Appendix

Anus

Stomach
Pancreas

Rectum

proteins. Note: the pancreas is a dual-purpose gland, in that it also secretes the hormone insulin, which helps utilize carbohydrates and maintain a normal blood sugar level. When that function goes awry, diabetes results. However, a person can have diabetes and still have normal pancreatic digestive function, because different parts of the pancreas handle the release of digestive juices and insulin.

The liver produces bile, which is released into the duodenum at meals. Bile juice helps in the processing of the fat. Between meals, the bile that is secreted by the liver is stored and concentrated in the gallbladder, which releases it at mealtime.

The small intestine further breaks down the food and nutrients as fluids and electrolytes that are absorbed into the body. The unused waste products move into the colon, where there is further processing and fluid absorption and conversion of liquid waste matter into solid waste occur. This matter is eliminated in a bowel movement, usually within about a day or two after the food is first consumed.

See also COLON; DIGESTION AND ABSORPTION; ESOPHAGUS; LIVER; PANCREAS; SMALL INTESTINE; STOMACH.

**digital rectal examination (DRE)**    The physician's gloved manual examination using a finger. It involves insertion of a finger into and examination of the rectum and (in men) also of the prostate gland, for the purpose of identifying cancer, hemorrhoids, polyps, or other serious medical conditions or problems.

The rectal examination generally takes about 30 seconds. The digit is the lubricated finger of the physician; the examination is usually performed during a routine physical examination. Most physicians recommend that the rectal examination be a standard part of the annual physical examination. This is particularly true for men, because the DRE may sometimes detect abnormalities of the prostate gland, and indicator of prostate disease or prostate cancer.

Most men and women detest having a rectal examination and may consider it the worst part of the physical examination. They may try to deter the physician from performing the rectal examination or even refuse to have one. They may not realize the importance of the examination and the major findings that may result from it, which sometimes may save their life.

See also CANCER, ANAL; CANCER, COLORECTAL.

**diverticulitis**    An inflammatory infective condition that is a complication of chronic diverticulosis, which is the presence of pouches (diverticula), usually in the colon. Many people have diverticulosis (although most of them do not realize this and it is undiagnosed) but do not have diverticulitis. If the diverticulitis is acute, however, it is a painful condition that may produce mild to severe pain. Patients with diverticulitis may experience constipation or loose stools. In some cases, diverticulitis can become very severe and even life-threatening.

The conditions of diverticulosis and diverticulitis are frequently confused by many patients because of the similarity of the terms. To distinguish them, keep in mind that diverticulosis is the cause of the problem, and diverticulitis, when it occurs, is the complication of diverticulosis.

Diverticulitis results from a tiny perforation in the diverticular pouches, which causes the pouch and the surrounding area to become infected and inflamed. Diverticulitis usually involves a diverticulum on the left side of the colon, although it can occur anywhere along the colon.

### Risk of Diverticulitis

About 5 to 10 percent of people in the United States and Canada who are older than 45 years old may have an attack of acute diverticulitis. Diverticulitis is less of a problem in such places as Asia and Africa, where fewer people have diverticulosis.

Some patients with diverticulitis are younger individuals, and an estimated 10 to 20 percent of patients with diverticulitis are younger than 50 years. It is also possible, although it is not common, for children and adolescents to experience diverticulitis.

### Symptoms and Signs

Some symptoms of diverticulitis are fever, abdominal pain that is usually in the left lower abdomen, constipation or diarrhea, indigestion, gas, and bloating. Patients also have a belly that is sore to the touch, especially on the left side. Blood test results may suggest the presence of an infection.

### Diagnosis and Treatment of Diverticulitis

The diagnosis of diverticulitis is based on clinical grounds. An ultrasound and computed tomography (CT) scan are also helpful. When physicians suspect diverticulitis, they do not perform a colonoscopy because this procedure can exacerbate the problem by causing the inflamed pouch to burst and spill its contents. Patients with diverticulitis are prescribed a liquid diet and a course of ANTIBIOTICS. Patients with severe cases of diverticulitis may need to be hospitalized and may, rarely, require surgery.

When the condition has resolved, physicians may then order a colonoscopy to rule out the presence of cancer that is masquerading as diverticulitis. Patients with recurrent bouts of diverticulitis need surgery for an excision of the involved segment.

See also DIVERTICULOSIS.

Ferzoco, L. B., M.D., V. Raptopoulos, M.D., and W. Silen, M.D. "Acute Diverticulitis." *New England Journal of Medicine* 338, no. 21 (May 21, 1998): 1,521–1,526.

**diverticulosis**    A condition in which small pouches (diverticula) occur, usually in the colon. It usually causes no symptoms. Diverticulosis is common in the United States, Canada, and Western European countries, perhaps because of the low fiber in the diet of most citizens. Diverticulosis is rare in Asian and African populations.

Most people older than the age of 60 years have diverticulosis, but the majority of them have no symptoms of or problem with this condition. Many people do not even know that they have diverticulosis unless they are informed by their doctor of the presence of the condition, for example, after they undergo a barium enema or COLONOSCOPY. Diverticuli may also occur in the small intestine, often as a result of a disease such as SCLERODERMA.

Diverticulosis may lead to DIVERTICULITIS, which is a condition in which the pouches become inflamed and infected. Diverticulosis and diverticulitis are frequently confused because of the similarity of the names. However, diverticulosis is the cause and diverticulitis, when it occurs, is the result.

### Symptoms

Many people with diverticulosis have no symptoms; however, some individuals have vague symptoms, such as abdominal cramping. This is called painful diverticular disease. Patients who also have diverticulitis (inflammation of the diverticuli) experience left lower abdominal pain with fever and a belly that is sore to the touch. Blood test results may also suggest the presence of an infection. Diverticula are a common cause of lower gastrointestinal bleeding, which is usually painless and massive, often requiring a blood transfusion.

### Diagnosis

The diagnosis of diverticulosis is often made incidentally, when a colonoscopy, sigmoidoscopy, or barium enema is performed. The diagnosis of diverticulitis, on the other hand, is made on clinical grounds with or without noninvasive imaging studies, and a colonoscopy or barium enema is not performed in such circumstances, since the inflamed pouch may actually burst and worsen the patient's condition, even becoming life-threatening.

A colonoscopy would be performed within a few weeks after the diverticulitis was resolved, to make sure there was no other medical problem such as cancer, which could mimic a bout of diverticulitis. Diverticulitis and diverticular bleeding usually do not occur simultaneously. Patients who have lower gastrointestinal bleeding require a colonoscopy to look for the cause of the bleeding, including diverticulosis, and to allow the physician to treat the bleeding lesion as appropriate.

### Treatment: Lifestyle Recommendations

People who have diverticulosis are advised to drink plenty of water and to eat fruits and vegetables each day so that they have sufficient fiber to help move fecal material through thecolon. Some physicians routinely advise patients who have diverticulosis to avoid eating popcorn or nuts, which may get trapped into the diverticular pouches and cause diverticulitis. This dietary modification recommendation is considered controversial.

See also MECKEL'S DIVERTICULUM.

**dumping syndrome**    A condition in which after a person eats food it travels very rapidly (within 30 minutes) directly from the stomach into the jejunum of the small intestine.

Dumping syndrome may sometimes be a result of surgery, such as elective BARIATRIC SURGERY. Some obese individuals have this surgery to lose large amounts of weight or other forms of gastric surgery (for example, surgery for a peptic ulcer).

### Early and Late Dumping Syndromes

There are two types of dumping syndrome: early and late. Early dumping syndrome is caused by the rapid and uncontrolled entry of food into the small intestine. Late dumping syndrome involves the release of an increased quantity of insulin, which results in reactive hypoglycemia (low blood sugar level).

### Symptoms and Signs of Dumping Syndrome

The symptoms and signs differ in early dumping syndrome and late dumping syndrome. The key symptoms of early dumping syndrome, which occur shortly after eating, are sweating, heart palpitations, weakness, abdominal pain, and nausea that may be accompanied by vomiting and even by syncope (fainting). In late dumping syndrome, the symptoms occur a few hours after eating, and they may include anxiety, restlessness, tremors, a rapid and pounding heartbeat, and even mental confusion.

### Diagnosis and Treatment

Doctors diagnose the illness on the basis of the symptoms and a careful medical history, particularly noting past surgeries. The recommended treatment for dumping syndrome is that the patient eat small and frequent meals that are high in fat and proteins and low in carbohydrates. Solids and liquids are generally separated, and patients are advised to drink their liquids *between* meals, rather than with them, as is the usual custom. Octreotide is used for patients who still have problems despite complying with these recommendations. Sometimes anticholinergic drugs may

be taken before meals to decrease the effect of dumping syndrome.

**dysentery**    An infectious disease that is often caused by CONTAMINATED FOOD OR WATER, and that causes severe bloody DIARRHEA and stomach upset. People who are living in poor countries, especially children, can die of dysentery. Some forms of dysentery, such as bacillary dysentery, are caused by SHIGELLA bacteria. AMEBIASIS also causes dysentery.

See also FOOD-BORNE ILLNESSES.

**dyspepsia**    Abdominal pain or discomfort in the upper abdomen that is presumed to have originated in the upper gastrointestinal system. Pain is exacerbated by food intake, and there may be accompanying nausea, vomiting, and bloating. Dyspepsia may indicate a minor or a more serious condition. The main causes of dyspepsia are gastroduodenal ulcer, atypical GASTROESOPHAGEAL REFLUX, and GASTROPARESIS; occasionally gastric cancer may cause dyspepsia.

### Other Digestive Causes

Dyspepsia may have a variety of other causes. HELICOBACTER PYLORI may be the culprit that causes chronic dyspepsia as a result of ulcer disease. However, whether *Helicobacter pylori* alone, without the presence of an ulcer, can cause dyspepsia is a controversial issue among experts. Excessive gastric acid may be seen in as many as 20 percent of all patients with dyspepsia. Other patients may have problems with GASTROPARESIS, very slow emptying of the stomach contents into the intestines. In some cases, dyspepsia may be a symptom of gastrointestinal cancer.

Most of the time, however, despite investigations, no specific cause of the dyspepsia can be found, and consequently, the diagnosis is nonulcer dyspepsia (dyspepsia with no ulcer).

### Nondigestive Causes of Dyspepsia

Other causes, some of which may emanate from outside the gut which are also considered in the diagnosis of dyspepsia include the following:

- Angina pectoris of the heart (atypical angina)
- Abdominal aortic aneurysm
- Intestinal angina
- Biliary colic
- Pancreatic cancer
- Pancreatitis

### Diagnosis of the Cause of Dyspepsia

Physicians determine the cause of the dyspepsia by taking a careful medical history, performing a physical examination of the patient, and ordering appropriate tests. The major causes of dyspepsia can be best evaluated by an upper gastrointestinal endoscopy. An alternate option is for the physician to order upper gastrointestinal X rays. In the case of young and healthy patients without alarming symptoms such as weight loss or bleeding, the physician may elect simply to test the patient for the presence of *Helicobacter pylori,* and if the finding is positive, treat the patient as if he or she has an ulcer without specifically testing for ulcer.

See also CANCER, PANCREATIC; ENDOSCOPY; PANCREATITIS; ULCER, PEPTIC.

Bytzer, Peter, M.D., and Nicholas J. Talley, M.D. "Dyspepsia." *Annals of Internal Medicine* 134, no. 9, part 2 (2001): 815–822.

Fisher, Richard S., M.D., and Henry P. Parkman, M.D. "Management of Nonulcer Dyspepsia." *New England Journal of Medicine* 339, no. 19 (November 5, 1998): 1,376–1,381.

Minocha, A., et al. "Helicobacter Pylori Is Associated with Alterations in Intestinal Gas Profile Among Patients with Non-ulcer Dyspepsia." *Digestive Disease Sciences* 39, no. 8 (1994): 1,613–1,617.

Minocha, Anil, et al. "Alterations in Upper Gastrointestinal Motility in Helicobacter Pylori Positive Non Ulcer Dyspepsia." *American Journal of Gastroenterology* 89, no. 10 (1994): 1,797–1,800.

**dysphagia** Difficulty and sometimes choking with swallowing. Dysphagia may be due to an inability to transfer food from the throat to the esophagus, which is called transfer dysphagia. This problem may be seen in patients with stroke, DIABETES MELLITUS, Parkinson's disease, and other medical problems. Another type of dysphagia is esophageal dysphagia, wherein the transfer occurs normally, but the transit through the esophagus is impaired, as is found with chronic GASTROESOPHAGEAL REFLUX DISEASE (GERD). The esophagus (food tube) in GERD can become constricted, often as a result of years of untreated disease.

In severe dysphagia, even tiny pieces of food may be blocked, and then if the condition worsens, even fluids cannot pass through. Such blockages need to be treated before normal feeding can resume. Benign strictures can be dilated by using dilators. In the case of a stricture due to cancer, an esophageal stent can be placed to maintain the patency of the esophageal lumen. Treatment of ACHALASIA involves pneumatic dilation, surgery, and sometimes botulinum toxin (Botox). GERD is not the only cause of dysphagia; patients may have SCLERODERMA, an enlarged heart, CANCER, or other medical problems. Those who experience dysphagia should have a medical evaluation.

See also BARRETT'S ESOPHAGUS; BOTULINUM TOXIN.

Havu, Kalyana, M.D., Thomas Matthew, and Anil Minocha. "Effectiveness of Esophageal Dilation in Relieving Non-Obstructive Esophageal Dysphagia and Improving Quality of Life." *Southern Medical Journal* 97, no. 2 (February 2004): 137–140.

**eating disorders**  Medical and psychological problems that lead to either excessive undereating or extreme overeating. The three most common eating disorders are ANOREXIA NERVOSA, BULIMIA NERVOSA, and OBESITY. Some experts also consider periodic binge eating to be an eating disorder as well, especially if the binges occur in the evening and the patient avoids eating during the daytime. People with eating disorders are in danger of becoming either underweight, if they are not eating enough, or becoming overweight or obese if their food consumption is greater than their body needs. Physicians use the concept of BODY MASS INDEX to determine whether individuals are underweight, normal weight, overweight, or obese.

Whether they are too thin or obese, individuals who have eating disorders are all obsessed with food and consider it paramount to their self-image.

### Risk Factors

People of all ages may suffer from eating disorders, although obesity is by far the most common form of eating disorder. In general, women are more likely to be diagnosed with eating disorders, with the exception of binge eating, which is different from bulimia nervosa because there is no purging. Binge eating is a disorder that is more common among men. Sometimes elderly people fail to eat, either because they have a lack of appetite or depression or because they are unable to prepare their own food. (Sometimes all three conditions are present.)

### Symptoms of Eating Disorders

An extreme preoccupation with food is a key indicator of an eating disorder. Both the anorexic and the obese person, despite the disparities in their weight and appearance, constantly think about food. In the case of the obese person, when food is desired, it is usually consumed. Conversely, the anorexic is also obsessed with food, but primarily with thoughts of avoiding food, to maintain the current body weight. (Some anorexics also want to lose more weight.)

### Diagnosis and Treatment

The diagnosis of an eating disorder is based on information provided by the patient as well as the physician's observations during a physical examination. Often patients deny that they have an eating disorder and insist that they are healthy and it is others who truly have a problem.

If the eating disorder causes severe health problems, as in extreme cases of anorexia nervosa or bulimia nervosa, then the patient may need to be hospitalized and treated. In severe cases of obesity in which the patient has been unable to gain control over eating habits, sometimes medicines may help, and some patients may succeed with bariatric surgery.

See also BARIATRIC SURGERY; DIET DRUGS.

Becker, Anne E., M.D., et al. "Eating Disorders." *New England Journal of Medicine* 340, no. 14 (April 8, 1999): 1,092–1,098.

Cassell, Dana K., and David H. Gleaves. *Obesity and Eating Disorders*. 2d ed. New York: Facts On File, 2000.

***E. coli***  See ESCHERICHIA COLI.

**elderly people and digestive diseases**  Senior citizens (ages 65 and older) who have ailments or medical problems of the digestive tracts. Older individuals have many of the same digestive diseases and disorders experienced by the general population. However, aging creates additional risks of development of digestive diseases and disorders, and people age 65 and older are more likely to have such problems as CONSTIPATION, GASTROE-SOPHAGEAL REFLUX DISEASE, and forms of cancer of the digestive tract, particularly PANCREATIC CANCER, COLORECTAL CANCER, GALLBLADDER CANCER, LIVER CANCER, and STOMACH CANCER. HIATAL HERNIA is also a common diagnosis among older people, as are DIVERTICULITIS and DIVERTICULOSIS.

Older people are also more likely to have type 2 DIABETES MELLITUS, which is often undiagnosed. Long-term diabetes leads to serious digestive problems. According to Doctors Mesiya and Minocha in their 1998/1999 article for *Southern Medical Journal:* "Acute problems include acute stress gastritis during ketoacidosis, acute pancreatitis and acute cholecystitis [gallbladder inflammation]. Most problems are, however chronic, and may manifest with remissions and relapses."

Older people may have digestive diseases such as GASTROPARESIS (significant slowing of stomach emptying) that stem from other illnesses that they have, such as diabetes, as well as from medications that they may take. Motility (the movement of food through the gastrointestinal system) is also often slowed among people diagnosed with Parkinson's disease (which is primarily seen among the elderly), and sometimes it can be very difficult for Parkinson's patients to maintain their usual weight because of the digestive problems due to the disease. Parkinson's disease patients may need to consume liquid nutritional supplements to increase their calorie count.

Elderly individuals may also have EATING DISORDERS, primarily disorders in which they fail to eat, such as anorexia, but OBESITY as well. Older people may not eat because of problems with depression or mental confusion or because of inability to shop, prepare food, or feed themselves. They may also become obese as a result of eating a poor diet and failing to exercise sufficiently (or at all).

### Effects of Medications on Older People

Many older individuals take medications for a variety of chronic and serious diseases, such as DIABETES MELLITUS, HYPERTENSION, arthritis, and heart trouble, and these medications may cause or contribute to the development of digestive disorders.

For example, GASTRITIS is a common side effect of nonsteroidal anti-inflammatory drugs (NSAIDs) that are used to treat arthritis. The use of NSAIDs may lead to the development of ULCERS.

Another problem is that many older people experience GASTROESOPHAGEAL REFLUX DISEASE (GERD), but large numbers of them rely upon over-the-counter antacids to resolve the problem and do not consult a physician about the condition (or they do not report this problem when they do see a physician). Over-the-counter drugs such as antacids usually cannot provide enough protection to the esophagus when a person has chronic GERD; nor can these drugs resolve the problem as can prescription medications, such as proton pump inhibitor medications. As a result, older people are more likely to have BARRETT'S ESOPHAGUS, a precancerous condition, which in some people causes the development of esophageal cancer.

In the case of older individuals, the physician usually takes an extremely careful history of all the current prescribed, over-the-counter, and supplemental (such as herbal remedies) medications that the individual is taking. The reason for this is that many older individuals see more than one physician and consequently may be taking many different medications. Abdominal distress and pain, diarrhea, and constipation are all very common side effects of many drugs.

It is also possible that digestive problems that older people experience may result from an interaction of the many medications that the individual takes. Sometimes lowering the dosage or decreasing the number of medications can resolve a digestive problem that is experienced by an older person.

Sometimes people do not realize that medications can affect older people differently than younger people; for example, the body water content of older people is generally lower than that of younger people. As a result of physiological differences between older and younger individuals, older adults may need lower dosages or different medications. For example, a dosage of digoxin for the heart that is considered normal for the average person can sometimes induce side effects such as nausea, vomiting, and confusion, in an elderly person that the same dosage would not cause in younger people. One key reason for this particular difference is that older people have a lower body fluid–to–body weight ratio than younger individuals.

### Lack of Physical Activity

Physical inactivity can lead to serious digestive problems. Older people who live a very sedentary life or are bedridden are the most likely individuals to have some digestive problems, such as constipation or FECAL IMPACTION (in which case the individual is unable to have a bowel movement because the stool is dry and hard and is stuck like a rock, not allowing any movement). Further, it is often difficult for older individuals to eat a healthy diet because of the following problems:

- Inability to prepare food
- Lack of transportation to shopping facilities because of inability to drive and lack of mass transportation
- Difficulty with eating and swallowing, because of ill-fitting dentures or other dental or oral problems
- Inability to feed themselves, caused by weakness

### Diagnosis and Treatment

Older individuals are screened for digestive diseases by their physicians with the same type of laboratory tests that are used for younger people, such as blood tests and imaging tests such as computed tomography (CT) scans or magnetic resonance imaging (MRI) scans. They may have procedures such as colonoscopy, upper endoscopy, or sigmoidoscopy, as well as barium enemas and other tests that the physician may order.

Treatment depends on the underlying medical problem and may be as simple as changing a dosage of a medication or as complicated as performing major surgery.

Most physicians recommend lifestyle changes whenever possible; for example, all patients who smoke should stop smoking because smoking is very harmful to the digestive system and worsens existing medical problems. Doctors also recommend regular exercise, and even patients in wheelchairs can do some simple exercises as recommended by their physicians or physical therapists.

It is also important to be wary of drug interactions in elderly people. For example, patients who use NSAIDs, including baby aspirin, should take additional protective medications (such as misoprostol or lansoprazole) to protect against the development of an NSAID-induced ulcer.

See also CANCER; CONSTIPATION; NONSTEROIDAL ANTI-INFLAMMATORY MEDICATIONS; ULCER, PEPTIC.

Aparasu, Rajender R., and Jane R. Mort. "Inappropriate Prescribing for the Elderly: Beers Criteria-Based Review." *The Annals of Pharmacotherapy* 34 (2000): 338–346.

Kandel, Joseph, M.D., and Christine Adamec. *The Encyclopedia of Senior Health and Well-Being.* New York: Facts On File, 2003.

Mesiya, Sikander A., M.D., and Anil Minocha, M.D. "Gastrointestinal Disease in Diabetes Mellitus." *Southern Medical Journal* (Winter 1998/1999): 33–38.

**electrocoagulation** The use of an electrical current to cauterize during surgery as well as during such procedures as ENDOSCOPY. Electrocoagulation may also be used to stop gastrointestinal bleeding or to remove a polyp during an endoscopy.

**electrogastrogram** A procedure that measures gastric electrical activities. Just as electrocardiograms (ECGs or EKG) study the rhythms of the heart, the electrogastrogram can detect abnormally fast, irregular, or slow rhythms of the stomach. The electrogastrogram can be useful in diagnosing the cause of GASTROPARESIS (slow stomach emptying). The test can be performed while patients are fasting, or after a meal is consumed. Patients with DIABETES MELLITUS have a high risk for gastroparesis, and thus physicians may use the electrogastrogram as an adjunctive test for such patients to help with diagnosis.

**electrolytes** Essential chemical substances in the body, both within the cells and in the body fluids, including the blood. Electrolyte levels can become low when an individual has DEHYDRATION, fever, vomiting, and DIARRHEA, as a result of infection or disease. Electrolytes can be replaced with oral hydration solutions or by intravenous feeding in the hospital.

In a matter of hours, illnesses such as cholera can cause massive fluid loss and electrolyte imbalance which can be fatal. Ironically, intravenous potassium is given as part of the three-drug "cocktail" (very high dosages are given) that is used in a lethal injection to execute convicted prisoners.

Mild electrolyte imbalances can be resolved with preparations available at most pharmacies. For example, for children who have mild electrolyte imbalance the electrolyte Pedialyte may be recommended.

See also CHOLERA; FOOD-BORNE ILLNESSES.

**encopresis** Accidental bowel movement, a problem that usually occurs in small children. Technically, *encopresis* may be defined as a repeated passage of feces in inappropriate places for at least once a month for three months. This frequency and duration criteria are appropriate for patients who are older than four years: younger children may not be fully toilet trained. The possibility of physical abuse should be excluded in small children with encopresis. Some patients with encopresis may have CONSTIPATION with FECAL IMPACTION.

**endoscopic retrograde cholangiopancreatography (ERCP)** An endoscopic procedure in which the pancreatic and biliary ducts can be examined by the physician, who is usually a gastroenterologist. The ERCP is usually an outpatient procedure, although sometimes a patient may be observed overnight in the hospital after the procedure, depending on the interventions that are undertaken during the procedure. The ERCP is used to diagnose suspected disorders of the bile ducts and the pancreas. Some conditions that may be diagnosed with an ERCP are bile duct stones, strictures (narrowing), and cancerous tumors.

Preoperative antibiotics are administered in cases of suspected bile duct obstruction before ERCP. The patient is given local anesthetic medication to numb the throat before the ERCP, as well as intravenous sedatives to calm him or her during the procedure. Sometimes general anesthesia is used. The physician places the endoscope down the throat. The scope is propelled downward to the duodenum until the doctor reaches the ampulla, where the openings of both the biliary and the pancreatic ducts lie. The doctor then inserts a catheter through the endoscope and penetrates the opening, passing the catheter into the ducts, and then injects radiocontrast dye. Examination under fluoroscopy is performed, and X rays of the area are taken.

The ERCP not only is a diagnostic procedure but can also be used for therapeutic purposes. For example, a physician who notes a stone in the bile duct can make a cut in the ampulla to widen the opening and can remove the stone with instruments that are inserted through the scope. Similarly, a stricture of the duct can be dilated. The doctor also may take a biopsy sample to test for cancer.

The aftereffects of ERCP may be a sore throat and feeling of bloating or abdominal pain. In about 5 to 10 percent of patients who have this procedure, pancreatitis may develop. This is an inflammation of the pancreas that may require hospitalization. Death is a rare complication.

See also ENDOSCOPY.

**endoscopic ultrasound (EUS)** A procedure involving both the endoscope and an ultrasound. The ultrasound is attached to the tip of the endoscope, which is passed into the gut, and ultrasound images are then taken from within the gut. The endoscopic ultrasound is useful in diagnosing and assessing the severity of many cancers, such as cancer of the esophagus, pancreas, and rectum. Biopsies can also be undertaken during the procedure, as guided by the ultrasound images. Endoscopic ultrasound is also useful for detecting stones in the bile ducts.

**endoscopy** A procedure that is performed usually by a physician who is also frequently a GASTROENTEROLOGIST in which a device (the endoscope) is inserted into the gut to visualize the inside of the digestive system. Surgeons and physicians in other specialties may also perform endoscopies. The endoscopy may be an upper endoscopy or a colonoscopy of the colon. Biliary endoscopy is another form of endoscopy. The ENTEROSCOPY procedure examines the small intestine.

In an upper endoscopy or esophagogastroduodenoscopy (EGD), the endoscope is inserted through the throat and into the stomach of the patient for the purpose of detecting the presence of any diseases and disorders of the esophagus, stomach, and duodenum: cancer of the esophagus or stomach, GASTROESOPHAGEAL REFLUX DISEASE, hiatal hernia, peptic ulcer, or a variety of other digestive ailments. The cause of upper gastrointestinal bleeding can be identified and treated as needed.

In biliary endoscopy, or endoscopic retrograde cholangiopancreatography (ERCP), physicians can observe the bile and pancreatic ducts and see any obstructions that may be present such as stones, stricture, or cancer. Occasionally, specialized endoscopes with an ultrasound transducer attached may be used to take sonographic pictures from inside the gut.

In most cases, mild sedation (also known as conscious sedation or twilight sleep) is administered to the patient; however, some physicians believe that the procedure is actually safer when it is performed without sedation, and it is also less expensive to perform the procedure without sedation. Most endoscopies in the United States are undertaken with patient sedation. In addition, newer and narrower ultrathin endoscopes make sedation less necessary because these endoscopes can be introduced either transnasally (through the nose) or transorally (through the throat) with much less discomfort to the patient.

### Reasons Why Gastroenterologists Order Endoscopies

Physicians perform at least 10 million endoscopic procedures each year. In a survey of 276 gastroenterologists nationwide in the United States on the reasons why they performed endoscopies, reported in a 2000 issue of *Gastroenterology* by David A. Lieberman and his colleagues, the researchers found that upper endoscopies (EGD) were most frequently performed to evaluate the cause of abdominal pain or dyspepsia (23.7 percent). Other reasons for performing endoscopies included dysphagia, or difficulty in swallowing (20 percent); acid reflux symptoms (17 percent); suspicion of gastrointestinal bleeding (16.1 percent); and nausea/vomiting (10.9 percent). Other primary reasons for performing endoscopy were checking a patient who had Barrett's esophagus and evaluating chest pain.

### Association of Endoscopies with Other Diseases

In an interesting study to determine whether the appendix may play a role in immune-modulation of the gut, Minocha and colleagues studied 524 patients, 55 who had previously had appendectomy and 469 in the control group who had not had this surgery. These findings were reported in a 1999 issue of the *Southern Medical Journal.*

The researchers did find a significant association in individuals who had an appendectomy and needed an endoscopy after the appendectomy (if one was performed). The previous appendectomy group had a rate of 33.46 percent of endoscopies versus the rate of 20.55 of the patients who had not had an appendectomy.

### Advances in Endoscopy

In 2000 an endoscope that is actually a tiny camera the size of a capsule that could be swallowed was introduced. This device transmits images remotely and eliminates the need for endoscopy or for sedation. No preparation is needed before the special endoscope is swallowed. It is useful for examining the small intestine, most of which is not within easy reach of the endoscope. A disadvantage of the device is that the physician has no control over its speed or the region that it covers; nor can the doctor perform a biopsy or any procedures if a problem is identified.

CHROMOENDOSCOPY, currently an experimental technique, is another 21st-century advance of the endoscope. This procedure uses special color sprays that highlight body tissues and any areas of abnormalities. Other devices, such as the EndoCinch suturing system made by Bard and approved by the Food and Drug Administration (FDA) in 2000, allow physicians to perform surgery on patients who have gastroesophageal reflux disease. The cost of the surgery with the Bard EndoCinch is markedly lower than the cost of surgery performed in the traditional manner.

### The Virtual Endoscopy

Recent developments with the endoscope have enabled some physicians to image the lower gastrointestinal system, thus avoiding the invasive COLONOSCOPY. If the virtual colonoscopy detects a possible medical problem, it is followed with an actual colonoscopy. Some physicians are also performing virtual colonoscopy to screen for colorectal cancer. However, as of this writing, virtual colonoscopy has not been endorsed by gastroenterology organizations as an acceptable method of screening for colon cancer.

For further information on endoscopies, contact the following organization:

American Society for Gastrointestinal Endoscopy (ASGE)
13 Elm Street
Manchester, NH 01944
(978) 526-8330
http://www.asge.org

See also CANCER, COLORECTAL; COLONOSCOPY; CONSCIOUS SEDATION; ENDOSCOPIC ULTRASOUND; ENTEROSCOPY; SIGMOIDOSCOPY.

Brugge, William R., M.D., and Van Dam, Jacques, M.D. "Pancreatic and Biliary Endoscopy." *New England Journal of Medicine* 341, no. 24 (December 9, 1999): 1,808–1,818.

Lieberman, David A., et al. "Patterns of Endoscopy Use in the United States." *Gastroenterology* 118, no. 3 (2000): 619–624.

Minocha, Anil, M.D., and Radhika Srinivasan, M.D. "Conscious Sedation: Pearls and Perils." *Digestive Diseases and Sciences* 43, no. 8 (August 1998): 1835–1,844.

Minocha, Anil, M.D., et al. "Prevalence of Previous Appendectomy among Patients Needing Gastrointestinal Endoscopy." *Southern Medical Journal* 92, no. 1 (January 1999): 41–43.

Newman, Julliana. "Radiographic and Endoscopic Evaluation of the Upper GI Tract." *Radiologic Technology* 69, no. 3 (January/February 1998): 213–227.

Van Dam, Jacques, M.D., and Brugge, William R., M.D. "Endoscopy of the Upper Gastrointestinal Tract." *New England Journal of Medicine* 341, no. 23 (December 2, 1999): 1,738–1,748.

Wood, Bradford J., and Razavi, Pouneh. "Virtual Endoscopy: A Promising New Technology." *American Family Physician* 66, no. 66 (July 1, 2002): 107–112.

**enema** Procedure in which the colon is evacuated (emptied) through the external introduction of water and chemicals into the rectum, thus inducing a bowel movement. Enemas can be self-performed or may be given by other individuals. They are usually used for severe constipation or for emptying of the colon of waste before medical procedures, such as the sigmoidoscopy or COLONOSCOPY. Enemas may be self-administered through insertable packaged chemicals that can be purchased at pharmacies or supermarkets or may be administered by medical personnel in the home or hospital. Fleet enemas are the most popular brand used; however, different medications are found in different forms of Fleet enemas.

An enema is not the same as a barium enema, which is a procedure performed by a doctor in which barium is inserted into the rectum so that the colon is highlighted and shows up well on X rays.

**enteral nutrition** Food that is provided to a patient through a tube that is placed into the stomach or small intestine and is also called tube feeding. Enteral nutrition may be provided in a long tube that is inserted into the nose and travels to the stomach or the small intestine. Alternatively, it may be provided via a small tube that is inserted directly through the abdominal wall into the stomach or intestine, which can be placed by a physician during an endoscopy or surgery. Radiologists can also place such tubes.

Enteral nutrition is provided to individuals who are unable to eat normally because of illness and/or incapacity but have a functional gut. On the other hand, patients for whom enteral feeding cannot be administered into the gut, such as those who have bowel obstruction, require parenteral nutrition.

See also FEEDING TUBE; PARENTERAL NUTRITION.

**enteric nervous system** Network of nerves in the gastrointestinal system that are the "brains" of the gastrointestinal system and that control numerous functions, including movement of food through the system, intestinal secretions, as well as inflammatory and immune processes.

Goyal, Raj K., M.D., and Hirano, Ikuo, M.D. "The Enteric Nervous System." *New England Journal of Medicine* 334, no. 17 (April 25, 1996): 1,106–1,115.

**enteroscopy** The endoscopic examination of the small intestine through a scope that is inserted through the mouth and into the stomach and then passed into the small intestine. Biopsy specimens can be taken during the procedure if any suspicious areas are seen by the physician. The enteroscopy examines the region of the small bowel that is beyond the reach of the esophagogastroduodenoscopy. Occasionally during a colonoscopy, the scope inserted through the rectum and into the colon can move farther into the last part of the small intestine called the ileum, in a procedure known as ileoscopy.

See also COLONOSCOPY; ENDOSCOPY; SIGMOIDOSCOPY.

**enterovirus** A common virus in the picornavirus family that is found worldwide. The virus generally multiplies within the intestinal tract. The coxsackievirus is an example of an enterovirus, as are the poliovirus and echovirus. To identify them better, since 1970 enteroviruses that have been identified have been given numbers, starting with enterovirus 68.

Some enteroviruses can trigger severe diseases, such as encephalitis and meningitis. Older people, small children, and people who have a weakened immune system are usually affected more severely by enteroviruses than other people; for example, enterovirus 71 has been associated with some deaths among children age five and younger.

### Transmission of Enteroviruses
Medical researchers believe that enteroviruses are spread by fecal–oral contamination (as occurs after a person does not wash his or her hands after using a toilet and then touches others or touches items that others touch, such as food), and they may be spread through respiration as well (by an infected person's breathing on someone and transmitting the disease).

### Symptoms
The symptoms caused by enterovirus vary; they often include nausea, vomiting, and diarrhea, as well as abdominal pain.

### Diagnosis and Treatment
Physicians suspect and clinically diagnose an enterovirus illness on the basis of symptoms. Laboratory diagnosis is based on the identification of the virus in the cell culture. Other methods include detection of enterovirus RNA by polymerase chain reaction (PCR) or retrospectively by serologic methods. Cell culture is cumbersome and expensive and is not commonly performed except in cases of mass infections. A blood test for serology may be helpful in select cases.

Patients are treated with antiemetics (to control vomiting) and antidiarrheal drugs (to limit diarrhea). Dehydrated patients may need to be hospitalized, particularly if they are infants, elderly people, or individuals who have a weakened immune system.

See also ANTIDIARRHEALS; ANTIEMETICS; CONTAMINATED FOOD OR WATER; DIARRHEA; NAUSEA AND VOMITING.

Raphael Dolin, M.D. "Enterovirus 71—Emerging Infections and Emerging Questions." *New England Journal of Medicine* 341, no. 13 (September 23, 1999): 984–985.

**enzyme** See DIGESTIVE ENZYMES.

**enzyme-linked immunosorbent assay (ELISA)** A blood test that detects a range of antibodies, allowing the identification of various forms of diseases, infections, and organisms, such as *HELICOBACTER PYLORI,* viral HEPATITIS, human immunodeficiency virus, tumors, PARASITIC INFECTIONS, and other medical problems, such as CELIAC SPRUE.

**eosinophilic gastroenteritis (EG)**   A rare disease that is often misdiagnosed as IRRITABLE BOWEL SYNDROME. In EG, any part of the gastrointestinal tract, from the esophagus to the colon and including the bile ducts, can be affected.

EG may be caused by intestinal parasites; often the cause cannot be determined. Approximately 50 percent of patients who have EG have other allergic disorders, such as asthma, eczema, or rhinitis.

### Signs and Symptoms

Common symptoms of EG include nausea and vomiting, abdominal pain, and diarrhea. Some patients experienced weight loss; others have problems with malabsorption. The gut may become rigid and lead to intestinal obstruction. Patients may also have a fluid-filled abdomen (ASCITES).

### Diagnosis of EG

Eosinophilic gastroenteritis can be confirmed with a biopsy of the affected region of the stomach and small intestine or colon, taken during an ENDOSCOPY. In addition, some laboratory tests may provide abnormal results for patients with EG with malabsorption, such as reduced serum iron concentration and a prolonged prothrombin time. Peripheral eosinophil counts are frequently elevated, although they are normal in about 20 percent of patients with EG.

### Treatment of EG

Mild cases of EG can be treated symptomatically; for example, antidiarrheals are given to patients for diarrhea and iron supplementation is given in cases of an iron deficiency. If patients are symptomatic, the treatment also usually includes the administration of a steroid, such as prednisone. The steroid is administered to patients for two weeks; then the dosage is tapered over two more weeks. A few patients may require prolonged treatment. EG patients may experience flares of the disease months or years later, requiring short-term dosages of prednisone, which are tapered off. Some patients have also been treated with oral cromolyn.

See also PARASITIC INFECTIONS.

**erythema nodosum**   Reddish purple sores in the lower legs that are painful and that occur in a variety of diseases. Erythema nodosum can accompany a streptococcal throat infection, TUBERCULOSIS, and other infections. In digestive diseases, erythema nodosum may accompany a flare-up of CROHN'S DISEASE or ULCERATIVE COLITIS. The treatment for erythema nodosum is symptomatic. These lesions are self-limited and usually disappear when the disease goes into remission and when the underlying disease is successfully treated.

See also SCLERODERMA.

***Escherichia coli* (*E. coli*)**   Common bacteria normally found in the colon of humans and animals, some strains acquire certain genetic material and they can become pathogenic to cause infection. *E. coli* may also be found in contaminated foods, such as meat or other foods that are prepared under unsanitary conditions.

Sometimes swimmers contract *E. coli* from swimming in water or swimming pools that are contaminated with feces and are inadequately chlorinated.

### Types of E. coli

There are several forms of harmful *E. coli,* such as enterohemorrhagic *E. coli* (EHEC). This bacterium causes bloody diarrhea, and it may also lead to kidney failure in adults and children who have weakened immune systems. The most common harmful form of EHEC that is found in the United States as of this writing is O157:H7, which can severely harm the intestinal lining as well as cause hemolytic uremic syndrome (HUS), which can be fatal. Antibiotics are not useful against *E. coli* 0157:H7, and treatment is symptomatic. Other harmful types of *E. coli* are also found in the United States.

### Foods in Which E. coli is Most Commonly Found

Although any food can theoretically be contaminated by *E. coli,* this bacterium has been found most frequently in the following types of foods:

- Raw or undercooked hamburger
- Lettuce
- Salami

- Unpasteurized milk, apple cider, and apple juice
- Contaminated well water

### Symptoms of E. coli O157:H7 Infection

Common symptoms of the most frequently found strain of *E. coli* (0157:H7) are as follows:

- Watery or bloody diarrhea
- Nausea
- Painful abdominal cramps

Some patients also have low-grade fever and may experience vomiting. If the disease is caused by contaminated food, the patient's symptoms usually start within two to five days of the time the food is ingested. Symptoms may last up to eight days.

### Other Types of E. coli Infection

Enterotoxigenic *E. coli* (ETEC) is usually the cause of "traveler's diarrhea," an infection that develops when tourists consume contaminated food or water.

Another form of *E. coli* is enteropathogenic *E. coli* (EPEC). This form causes diarrhea that lasts two weeks or longer. It is transmitted through contaminated water or infected animals.

### Diagnosis and Treatment

The physician diagnoses patients with *E. coli* infections on the basis of symptoms as well as results from laboratory stool sample tests. Generally, patients are advised to rest and to drink plenty of water to prevent dehydration. Antibiotics are not effective for diarrheal illness in most cases, and they are usually not prescribed. However, antibiotics may be helpful in selected cases of traveler's diarrhea.

### Preventing E. coli Infections

To prevent the food-borne transmission of *E. coli*, experts recommend that individuals take the following actions:

- Avoiding raw and undercooked beef products
- Drinking no unpasteurized milk or juices
- Washing fresh fruits and vegetables, whether they are to be eaten raw or cooked

See also CONTAMINATED FOOD OR WATER; DIARRHEA; FOOD-BORNE ILLNESSES; TRAVEL.

**esophageal cancer**   See CANCER, ESOPHAGUS.

**esophagitis**   An inflammation of the esophagus (the upper food tube). The esophagus may also be ulcerated, in the condition called ulcerative esophagitis. Esophagitis may be caused by a disease, such as GASTROESOPHAGEAL REFLUX DISEASE, or other factors, such as use of medications (such as tetracycline). It may also be caused by infections.

### Infectious Esophagitis

Esophagitis may also be induced by infections, such as *Candida* infection (particularly by *Candida albicans*), CYTOMEGALOVIRUS, and herpes. Patients who have a weakened immune system, such as those who have human immunodeficiency virus (HIV) or cancer, are more prone to development of such infection.

People in the following categories are more likely to have infectious esophagitis than others:

- Patients with diabetes
- Patients who are alcoholics
- Patients who are on chemotherapy drugs
- Patients who have had organ transplantation and are taking immunosuppressive drugs

Some patients have had ulcers in the esophagus as a consequence of an infection with viruses.

### Pill Esophagitis

Sometimes esophagitis is caused by medications; the disorder is called pill esophagitis. The key drugs that induce this form of esophagitis contain tetracycline antibiotics, iron, ascorbic acid, and potassium chloride. Tetracycline used for acne in adolescents and alendronate (Fosamax) used to treat osteoporosis in the elderly are both common culprits in causing pill esophagitis. The form of the drug is also significant; for example, doxycycline capsules are more likely to cause damage than doxycycline tablets are, primarily because gelatin

**PERCENTAGE OF ADULTS 18 YEARS OF AGE AND OLDER WHO WERE PHYSICALLY INACTIVE DURING THEIR LEISURE TIME AND PERCENTAGE OF ADULTS WHO ENGAGED IN SOME LEISURE-TIME PHYSICAL ACTIVITY FOR AT LEAST 10 MINUTES, BY SELECTED CHARACTERISTICS: UNITED STATES, AVERAGE ANNUAL, 1997–1998**

| Selected Characteristic | Physically Inactive[1] | | | At Least Some Physical Activity[2] | | |
|---|---|---|---|---|---|---|
| | Both Sexes | Men | Women | Both Sexes | Men | Women |
| Ages 18 years and over (age-adjusted)[3,4] | 38.3 | 35.4 | 40.9 | 61.7 | 64.6 | 59.1 |
| Ages 18 years and over (crude)[3] | 38.0 | 34.7 | 41.1 | 62.0 | 65.3 | 58.9 |
| Age | | | | | | |
| 18–24 years | 30.4 | 25.0 | 35.7 | 69.6 | 75.0 | 64.3 |
| 25–44 years | 33.3 | 31.1 | 35.3 | 66.7 | 68.9 | 64.7 |
| 45–64 years | 39.5 | 37.9 | 40.9 | 60.5 | 62.1 | 59.1 |
| 65–74 years | 47.9 | 44.2 | 51.0 | 52.1 | 55.8 | 49.0 |
| 75 years and over | 61.3 | 53.9 | 66.0 | 38.7 | 46.1 | 34.0 |
| Race-ethnicity[4] | | | | | | |
| Hispanic | 53.2 | 48.9 | 57.4 | 46.8 | 51.1 | 42.6 |
| White non-Hispanic | 34.5 | 32.5 | 36.2 | 65.5 | 67.5 | 63.8 |
| Black non-Hispanic | 50.2 | 44.1 | 55.2 | 49.8 | 55.9 | 44.8 |
| Asian/Pacific Islander non-Hispanic | 38.2 | 30.9 | 45.5 | 61.8 | 69.1 | 54.5 |
| Education[4] | | | | | | |
| Less than high school graduate | 60.1 | 57.1 | 63.1 | 39.9 | 42.9 | 36.9 |
| GED diploma[5] | 45.6 | 43.0 | 48.7 | 54.4 | 57.0 | 51.3 |
| High school graduate | 43.3 | 41.1 | 45.2 | 56.7 | 58.9 | 54.8 |
| Some college—no degree | 32.2 | 29.3 | 34.9 | 67.8 | 70.7 | 65.1 |
| Associate of Arts degree | 30.8 | 28.0 | 33.3 | 69.2 | 72.0 | 66.7 |
| Bachelor of Arts, Science degree | 22.7 | 19.6 | 25.9 | 77.3 | 80.4 | 74.1 |
| Master's, doctorate, medical degree | 21.8 | 21.5 | 22.8 | 78.2 | 78.5 | 77.2 |
| Poverty status[4,6] | | | | | | |
| Below poverty level | 56.9 | 54.2 | 58.8 | 43.1 | 45.8 | 41.2 |
| 1.00–1.99 times poverty level | 48.9 | 47.2 | 50.3 | 51.1 | 52.8 | 49.7 |
| 2.00–3.99 times poverty level | 36.2 | 34.3 | 38.0 | 63.8 | 65.7 | 62.0 |
| 4.00 times poverty level or more | 24.3 | 22.6 | 26.3 | 75.7 | 77.4 | 73.7 |

capsules tend to stick to the wall of the esophagus easily instead of moving down as they should.

According to Drs. Minocha and Greenbaum in a 1991 article in the *American Journal of Gastroenterology,* gelatin capsules are more adhesive in nature and thus more likely to stick to the tissue in the esophagus. An additional problem occurs if patients take medicine at bedtime while lying down.

The authors say:

Sometimes even large quantities of water may fail to dislodge the tablet stuck in the esophagus. Similarly, swallowing in supine position delays esophageal transit. Esophageal clearance of pills taken at bedtime is also delayed by marked decreases in salivation and swallowing that occur during sleep.

Ingestion of alcohol may worsen pill esophagitis, especially when alcohol is taken with aspirin.

### Symptoms of Esophagitis

Individuals who have esophagitis may have chest pain and experience painful swallowing of foods or even liquids. Other symptoms of esophagitis include nausea and vomiting. Fever may be seen in infectious esophagitis.

### Diagnosis and Treatment

Physicians take a complete medical history and examine the throat. An endoscopy is frequently indi-

| Selected Characteristic | Physically Inactive[1] | | | At Least Some Physical Activity[2] | | |
|---|---|---|---|---|---|---|
| | Both Sexes | Men | Women | Both Sexes | Men | Women |
| Marital status[4] | | | | | | |
| Never married | 38.8 | 34.5 | 43.1 | 61.2 | 65.5 | 56.9 |
| Married | 37.5 | 35.5 | 39.3 | 62.5 | 64.5 | 60.7 |
| Cohabiting | 41.1 | 38.6 | 47.0 | 58.9 | 61.4 | 53.0 |
| Divorced or separated | 44.0 | 41.1 | 45.9 | 56.0 | 58.9 | 54.1 |
| Widowed | 51.9 | 54.2 | 47.2 | 48.1 | 45.8 | 52.8 |
| Geographic region[4] | | | | | | |
| Northeast | 37.7 | 34.3 | 40.7 | 62.3 | 65.7 | 59.3 |
| Midwest | 35.0 | 32.8 | 36.9 | 65.0 | 67.2 | 63.1 |
| South | 44.2 | 41.3 | 46.9 | 55.8 | 58.7 | 53.1 |
| West | 32.2 | 28.8 | 35.4 | 67.8 | 71.2 | 64.6 |
| Place of residence[4] | | | | | | |
| MSA, central city[7] | 41.1 | 37.0 | 44.6 | 58.9 | 63.0 | 55.4 |
| MSA, not central city[7] | 35.2 | 32.2 | 38.0 | 64.8 | 67.8 | 62.0 |
| Not MSA [7] | 41.8 | 40.7 | 42.9 | 58.2 | 59.3 | 57.1 |

[1]Engaged in no light-moderate or vigorous leisure-time physical activity lasting 10 minutes or longer. Persons classified as physically inactive may include individuals who engaged in strengthening activities but no other type of physical activity.

[2]Includes engaging in vigorous leisure-time physical activities, lasting 10 minutes or longer, that cause heavy sweating or large increases in breathing or heart rate and/or engaging in light-moderate leisure-time physical activities, lasting 10 minutes or longer, that cause only light sweating or a slight to moderate increase in breathing or heart rate.

[3]Persons of other races and unknown race and ethnicity, unknown education, unknown poverty status, and unknown marital status are included in the total but not shown separately.

[4]Age adjusted to the 2000 projected U.S. population using age groups 18–24 years, 25–44 years, 45–64 years, 65–74 years, and 75 years and over.

[5]GED is General Educational Development high school equivalency diploma.

[6]Poverty status is based on family income and family size using the U.S. Census Bureau poverty thresholds.

[7]MSA is metropolitan statistical area.

Source: Department of Health and Human Services. *Advance Data from Vital and Health Statistics* no. 325 (April 7, 2002). National Institutes of Health. "The Practical Guide: Identification, Evaluation, and Treatment of Overweight and Obesity in Adults." National Heart, Lung and Blood Institute, NIH Publication no. 00-4084, October 2000.

cated in many cases of esophagitis, especially of suspected infectious esophagitis. If the physician finds that the patient is infected with *Candida* organisms or a viral infection, then appropriate medications can be prescribed. If the doctor believes that other illnesses, such as diabetes, are predisposing the patient to esophagitis, in addition to fighting the infection, he or she urges the patient to work hard to reach a blood glucose level that is as close to normal as possible.

If the patient's esophagitis is caused by medications, doctors should consider another medication as well as advise the patient to take the drug while in an upright position with at least a glass of water. Sometimes changing from a capsule to a table form of the medication can help resolve much of the problem.

See also BARRETT'S ESOPHAGUS; CANCER, ESOPHAGEAL; DYSPHAGIA.

Davis, Dirk R., M.D. "Esophageal Infections." *GI/Liver Secrets.* 2d ed. Philadelphia: Hanley & Belfus, 2001.

Minocha, Anil, M.D., and David S. Greenbaum, M.D. "Pill-Esophagitis Caused by Nonsteroidal Antiinflammatory Drugs." *American Journal of Gastroenterology* 86, no. 8 (1991): 1,086–1,089.

**esophagus**    The food tube that connects the throat to the stomach. The esophagus is a part of the digestive system. If problems arise, the esophagus may become inflamed (ESOPHAGITIS). If an individual has chronic GASTROESOPHAGEAL REFLUX

DISEASE, in which some food that has already been acidified by the stomach travels backward up the esophagus, this condition can cause esophagitis. Chronic acid reflux may also cause BARRETT'S ESOPH-AGUS, a precancerous condition. Infections caused by viruses or fungi may occur in the esophagus of patients who have a compromised immune system, such as patients who have acquired immunodeficiency syndrome (AIDS). The incidence of cancer of the esophagus is rising in the United States.

See also ACID REFLUX; CANCER, ESOPHAGEAL.

**exercise**   Physical activity that achieves the goals of improving digestion, maintaining a healthy weight, and improving an individual's overall physical and emotional health. Physicians believe that at least some form of exercise is advisable for most people. Exercise reduces the risk of medical problems such as constipation. It can also decrease the risk of some diseases; for example, a study reported in 1999 in the *New England Journal of Medicine* found that physical activity (or inactivity) is an independent risk factor for decreasing (or increasing) the risk of need for a cholecystectomy among women.

Many experts believe that walking, one of the simplest exercises that can be performed, is recommended for most ambulatory people. Even elderly individuals who are wheelchair bound may be able to perform some simple exercises. Exercise reduces not only the risk of heart disease, but also the risk

for development of many cancers, including cancers of the digestive system.

### Tailoring Exercise

Exercise should be tailored to the individual's health and abilities, and any medical problems that are present should also be considered. For example, individuals who have GASTROESOPHAGEAL REFLUX DISEASE should avoid exercises that cause abdominal strain, such as weightlifting.

### National Problems with Physical Inactivity in the United States

A lack of physical activity and exercise can lead to problems such as overweight and obesity. Many people in the United States are physically inactive, and that is one reason for the high rate of obesity. According to the National Center for Health Statistics in their 2002 Advance Data report, 35.4 percent of men and 40.9 percent of women ages 18 and older were physically inactive in 1997–98. The percentages of people who are physically inactive increase with age: nearly half (47.9 percent) of people 65 to 74 years are physically inactive.

In looking at exercise and race and ethnicity, whites (34.5 percent) and Asians (38.2 percent) have the lowest rates of physical inactivity; more than half of blacks (50.2 percent) and Hispanics (53.2 percent) are physically inactive. (See table on page 110.)

Physical activity is clearly correlated with education. Among people with less than a high school

---

### EXAMPLES OF MODERATE AMOUNTS OF PHYSICAL ACTIVITY*

| Common Chores | Sporting Activities |
|---|---|
| Washing and waxing a car for 45–60 minutes | Playing volleyball for 45–60 minutes |
| Washing windows or floors for 45–60 minutes | Playing touch football for 45 minutes |
| Gardening for 30–45 minutes | Walking 1 3/4 miles in 35 minutes (20 min/mile) |
| Wheeling self in wheelchair for 30–40 minutes | Basketball (shooting baskets) for 30 minutes |
| Pushing a stroller 1 ½ miles in 30 minutes | Bicycling 5 miles in 30 minutes |
| Raking leaves for 30 minutes | Dancing fast (social) for 30 minutes |
| Walking 2 miles in 30 minutes (15 min/mile) | Water aerobics for 30 minutes |
| Shoveling snow for 15 minutes | Swimming laps for 20 minutes |
| Stairwalking for 15 minutes | Basketball (playing a game) for 15–20 minutes |
| | Jumping rope for 15 minutes |
| | Running 1 1/2 miles in 15 minutes (15 min/mile) |

*A moderate amount of physical activity is roughly equivalent to physical activity that uses approximately 150 calories of energy per day, or 1,000 calories per week. Some activities can be performed at various intensities; the suggested durations correspond to expected intensity of effort.

education, 60.1 percent are physically inactive. Of people who have a high school diploma in the United States, 43.3 percent are inactive. The least inactive group (which, turning it around, means the most physically active group) were people who have a master's degree or higher level of education: only 21.8 percent were physically inactive.

In considering the geographic region of the country, the most inactive people are found in the South (44.2 percent) and the least inactive people in the West (32.2 percent). See table on page 111 for further information.

See also ANOREXIA NERVOSA; BULIMIA NERVOSA; CHOLECYSTECTOMY; EATING DISORDERS; OBESITY; WALKING.

Leitzmann, Michael F., M.D., et al. "Recreational Physical Activity and the Risk of Cholecystectomy in Women." *New England Journal of Medicine* 341, no. 11 (September 9, 1999): 777–784.

National Institutes of Health. "The Practical Guide: Identification, Evaluation, and Treatment of Overweight and Obesity in Adults." National Heart, Lung and Blood Institute, NIH Publication no. 00-4084, October 2000.

**failure to thrive (FTT)** Condition in which an infant or a small child up to the age of two years old does not eat adequately and shows markedly abnormal growth (or no growth) as well as development that is much slower than is normally expected for a child in this age group. Rather than growing and increasing proportionately in weight, as is normal for healthy children, some children who have failure to thrive (FTT) are actually losing weight, causing concern or alarm.

For about 1 to 5 percent of children younger than age two who are admitted to the hospital failure to thrive is diagnosed. Children in orphanages may experience failure to thrive, particularly when they receive minimal care and caregivers vary from day to day.

Studies of children who have FTT have shown that about half are below the 5th percentile in terms of growth and weight—that means that 95 percent of all other children are taller and weigh more. Some people also use the term *failure to thrive* to describe elderly patients who are losing weight and declining in health, but not as a result of any apparent medical problem. However, most experts use the term exclusively to describe severely undernourished and late-developing infants and children.

The failure to thrive is a cause for concern for both parents and pediatrician, because the condition can lead to (or can indicate already-existing) developmental delays and/or emotional problems. Some experts believe that FTT may indicate a neuroendocrine disturbance resulting from emotional deprivation; however, one should not assume that children with FTT have uncaring parents unless there is clear evidence of child abuse or neglect.

There are two classifications of failure to thrive: organic and nonorganic. Organic failure to thrive may be caused by a chronic severe medical prob-lem; it may also be an indicator of a genetic disorder with an early onset. Organic causes of FTT include the following medical problems:

- Gastroesophageal reflux disease (GERD)
- Postnatal infections
- Cystic fibrosis
- Milk protein intolerance
- Human immunodeficiency virus (HIV) infection
- Intestinal parasites
- Congenital heart disease

In contrast, nonorganic failure to thrive may result from social disruption, an emotional disorder, starvation, maternal drug addiction, or other causes. Severe abuse and neglect are also causes of nonorganic failure to thrive among some children.

### Risk Factors
Mothers in poor neighborhoods and who are drug abusers are more likely to have children who are diagnosed with FTT. Malnourished mothers are also more likely to have infants who fail to thrive. There appears to be an increased incidence of FTT among children who are receiving Medicaid, as well as among those who are homeless or living in rural areas.

### Symptoms of Failure to Thrive
Infants with failure to thrive usually appear listless, apathetic, and weak. They may appear malnourished and exhibit poor muscular development. Some babies with FTT exhibit behavior that is characteristic of this condition; for example, according to *The Encyclopedia of Child Abuse*, "Infants suffering from the sensory deprivation associated with FTT often maintain a posture in which the arms are

held out, flexed at the elbow with the hands up and legs drawn in. This position of apparent surrender is held for long periods of time."

### Diagnosis and Treatment

Laboratory tests cannot diagnose the presence of failure to thrive, but they are a useful adjunct. Thus, tests, including a complete blood count (CBC) and a complete metabolic profile, should be done judiciously. Laboratory tests to search for a cause should be ordered on the basis of clues obtained from the medical history and the physical examination.

Tests can only screen out other medical problems, such as infections, low thyroid level, vitamin deficiencies, or other medical illnesses. Physicians base a diagnosis of failure to thrive on a comparison of the child's past height and weight to his or her current height and weight as well as to those of children who are of the same age. If the child is not growing or is actually losing weight, then the physician actively seeks to identify the problem and resolve it.

The physician is in close contact with the family, assisting them with ways to help the child improve. If the doctor thinks that the family is in some way causing the child's failure to thrive, he or she must report the family to the authorities who oversee and investigate child abuse and neglect accusations. Some physicians may worry that placing the child in foster care could cause further harm; however, if the underlying problem is abuse or neglect, then remaining with the family could cause further deterioration of the child's health or even the death of the child.

See also MALNUTRITION.

Clark, Robin E., Judith Freeman Clark, with Christine Adamec. *The Encyclopedia of Child Abuse.* 2d ed. New York: Facts On File, 2000.

**familial juvenile polyposis (FJP)**   A hereditary condition with an onset in childhood in which a patient has at least 10 polyps (abnormal growths of tissue) of the juvenile type. This condition occurs in one in 100,000 live births. These polyps can lead to the development of colorectal cancer. Children with a family history of this condition should be screened for familial juvenile polyposis. Familial

juvenile polyposis is different from familial adenomatous polyposis (FAP): up to 20 percent of patients with FJP develop cancer, whereas in FAP, the long-term risk of cancer is 100 percent.

In late childhood or early adolescence, patients with this condition have rectal bleeding. In most cases, the polyps are located in the colon, but sometimes they may also be seen throughout the digestive tract. Rarely, they may be found only in the stomach. The polyps usually range in size from five millimeters to five centimeters.

### Symptoms and Signs

Although many patients with this condition have no symptoms, especially in the early stages, if symptoms do occur, they may include the following:

- Visible blood in the stool
- Diarrhea or an extended period of constipation
- Abdominal pain
- Rectal prolapse of the polyp
- Intestinal obstruction
- Fatigue due to anemia

Familial juvenile polyposis patients are also at increased risk for development of cancer of the colon, which may occur at an average age of 37 years.

### Diagnosis and Treatment

Polyposis can be diagnosed with a colonoscopy, barium enema, or sigmoidoscopy; colonoscopy gives the most comprehensive results. If polyps are present and they are few in number, they are removed by the physician, usually during a colonoscopy. A biopsy can help distinguish juvenile polyps from other kinds of polyps.

Colonoscopic polypectomy with regular periodic surveillance colonoscopy is probably adequate therapy when only a small number of polyps are present. Prophylactic surgery may be used for patients who have a large number of polyps, as well as those who have large polyps that cannot be removed by an endoscopy or patients with a strong family history of colon cancer. An upper endoscopy or an upper gastrointestinal X ray with a small bowel X ray is also recommended as part of the surveillance of patients with familial juvenile polyposis, starting at the age of 25 years.

See also CANCER, COLORECTAL; COLONOSCOPY; ENDOSCOPY; MULTIPLE LYMPHOMATOUS POLYPOSIS; POLYPS.

Altman, Roberta, and Michael J. Sarg. *The Cancer Dictionary*. Rev. ed. New York: Facts On File, 2000.

**fasting**  Purposely avoiding consuming food and sometimes fluids as well for a given period. Fasting may be done for a religious purpose or because of a belief that fasting somehow "cleans out" the body. Fasting may be perceived as therapeutic, but it can become dangerous if it extends beyond the duration that an individual's body can handle. Individuals who are also avoiding fluids may experience severe DEHYDRATION.

Fasting may be undertaken on physician orders, for example, before ENDOSCOPY or an ultrasound test for the gallbladder. Prolonged fasting may also be appropriate in situations in which food intake may worsen a condition, as in acute PANCREATITIS. However, if fasting is continued for more than several days, PARENTERAL NUTRITION is administered.

See also ANOREXIA NERVOSA; DIET DRUGS.

**fecal impaction**  A condition of severe constipation in which the person's stools become stuck and cannot be moved normally through a bowel movement, often because they are very hard and solid, and bowel movements are too sluggish. In most cases, the person has not had a bowel movement for at least two or three days, and possibly for a much longer period. On occasion, the person who has fecal impaction may have loose stools, which are liquefied stools that are trying to pass around the blockage that is being caused by the impacted stool.

### Risk Factors

The problem of fecal impaction is most commonly found among elderly individuals in nursing homes, as well as among those who have severe physical and/or mental and/or developmental disabilities. Sometimes use of medications that strongly slow action of the gut can lead to fecal impaction, particularly prolonged use of narcotic painkillers, which can lead to narcotic bowel syndrome.

### Treatment of Fecal Impaction

If the person who has fecal impaction cannot cause the removal of the feces with the use of laxatives or enemas, he or she must be disimpacted manually by medical personnel or others to resolve the blockage created by the stool and allow bowel movements to occur. Over the long term, individuals who have been diagnosed with fecal impaction are often advised to take stool softeners and/or laxatives on a regular basis, along with drinking plenty of fluid, to prevent a recurrence of the problem. The treatment for fecal impaction is individualized by the physician, on the basis of the patient's clinical situation and on the cause that precipitated the impaction.

See also CONSTIPATION; NARCOTIC BOWEL SYNDROME.

**feeding tube**  A flexible cylindrical tube into which nutrition formula is placed when a person is unable to eat and swallow food normally, such as after a severe accident or serious medical procedure, or during a severe chronic illness. In addition, some very weak older people or younger individuals who are permanently disabled may need to receive nutrition through a feeding tube on a regular basis. The feeding tube may be inserted through the nose down through the throat and threaded directly into the stomach. A patient's nutritional and fluid needs are calculated on the basis of his or her height and weight and then delivered through the tube.

Patients requiring long-term feeding may have a feeding tube placed directly into the stomach (gastrostomy) or the small intestine (jejunostomy) through the abdominal wall, bypassing both the nose and the throat. These tubes can be placed by gastroenterologists, surgeons, and radiologists, using different techniques.

See also ENTERAL NUTRITION; PARENTERAL NUTRITION.

**fiber**  Vegetable matter from plant cell walls, which is often included in the diet as an aid to bowel function and helps to protect against the development of cancer. Fiber is found in such items as wheat bran and some fruits and vegetables, as well as in oats, beans, peas, and other vegetables. A high-fiber diet may also help to lower high CHOLESTEROL levels. It can also often prevent problems with constipation. Commercial forms of fiber that are available in the United States include Metamucil, Citrucil, and Fibercon, as well as many other brands.

Some experts believe that the risk of development of colorectal cancer can be reduced by increasing the amount of dietary fiber. In a study reported in a 2003 issue of the *Lancet,* the researchers described their study of dietary fiber intake and the subsequent development of colorectal cancer in more than a half-million individuals ages 25 to 70 years old in 10 European countries who participated in the European Prospective Investigation into Cancer and Nutrition (EPIC). According to the researchers, fiber reduced the risk of colorectal cancer development in some individuals: "In populations with low average intake of dietary fibre, an approximate doubling of total fibre intake from foods could reduce the risk of colorectal cancer by 40 percent."

A high-fiber diet is not always advisable; for example, it is not recommended when a person has severe GASTROPARESIS or megacolon, because it can worsen both conditions. Often people who have DIABETES MELLITUS have gastroparesis.

See also CANCER, COLORECTAL; CONSTIPATION.

Bingham, Sheila A., et al. "Dietary Fibre in Food and Protection against Colorectal Cancer in the European Prospective Investigation into Cancer and Nutrition (EPIC): An Observational Study." *Lancet* 361, no. 9368 (May 3, 2003): 1,496–1,501.

**fibromyalgia syndrome (FMS)** A chronic and widespread muscle pain disorder that is also often associated with the ACID REFLUX that occurs in people who are diagnosed with GASTROESOPHAGEAL REFLUX DISEASE. In addition, many people who are diagnosed with fibromyalgia also have arthritis and IRRITABLE BOWEL SYNDROME as well as several other chronic pain disorders, such as migraines and irritable bladder. An estimated six million people in the United States have fibromyalgia. It is unknown how many people have this medical problem worldwide.

### Risk Factors

Fibromyalgia is a condition that is more commonly diagnosed among women than men (although men can have fibromyalgia, too, as can children), and it is also diagnosed most frequently among females of childbearing age, although it is not known whether this group most often has a diagnosis of FMS because physicians assume that older or younger individuals (or men) never have fibromyalgia.

### Causes of FMS

The cause of fibromyalgia is unknown; there is much speculation about possible causes. Some experts have suggested that physical trauma (such as being in a car crash or experiencing physical or sexual abuse, as a child or as an adult) can cause the problem. Other experts point to prior severe infections or illnesses or to autoimmune reactions as among the possible causes of this medical problem. There may also be a genetic predisposition to the development of fibromyalgia, since the illness appears to "run in" families, particularly among related females, and a genetic linkage is under investigation by medical researchers.

### Symptoms of Fibromyalgia

Rheumatologists have identified 18 specific "tender points" throughout the body that people with fibromyalgia may have, and if an individual experiences pain when at least 11 of these points are gently pressed, then the physician may diagnose fibromyalgia. These tender points may be very painful to the touch, although the physician cannot feel any bumps or other differences from other areas. (Tender points are not the same as trigger points, which are painful areas that the physician can actually feel when touching them.)

Other symptoms of fibromyalgia include overall muscle stiffness (particularly stiffness that is experienced in the morning, when the patient first wakes up) and extreme fatigue. Some patients also experience a mild form of mental confusion that some experts have labeled "fibro fog," in which they forget appointments and lose items, symptoms that are also common to adults who have attention deficit disorder. Most people with fibromyalgia also have chronic sleep problems, including difficulty in falling asleep and/or frequent wakening. These sleep problems may be part of the reason for the confusion.

*A Valid Medical Problem*

Researchers such as Roland Staud, M.D., at the University of Florida in Gainesville, have found in clinical studies that people who have fibromyalgia are more pain-sensitive than others and that their pain lasts longer. Despite this research finding, there are still many medical doctors and other experts who persist in believing that fibromyalgia is not a "real" medical problem, and that people exhibiting such symptoms should be referred to psychiatrists for treatment, rather than to rheumatologists or pain management centers.

*Diagnosis and Treatment*

In addition to palpating the tender points that are commonly associated with fibromyalgia, physicians usually order laboratory tests (such as blood and urine tests) to rule out other medical problems. There are no specific medical tests that detect fibromyalgia. It is also possible—and indeed it is common—for patients to have both fibromyalgia and other illnesses. Generally, physicians diagnose fibromyalgia on the basis of physical examination, medical history, and results of laboratory tests.

Fibromyalgia is treated by some experts with recommended lifestyle changes, such as the avoidance of foods and drinks that contain caffeine, including soft drinks and chocolate. Some individuals who have fibromyalgia improve by avoiding citrus fruits and foods that contain monosodium glutamate (MSG), a flavor enhancer that is added to many canned and frozen foods. Weight loss among individuals with FMS who are obese may also help to improve the condition, and exercise is also recommended; however, exercise should not be overly vigorous, since some fibromyalgia patients may tire rapidly and may be injured more readily than others.

Individuals with fibromyalgia may need medications such as nonsteroidal anti-inflammatory medications or painkilling drugs. Some doctors believe that guaifenesin, a cough medicine, may be helpful in treating fibromyalgia. Guaifenesin is a mild analgesic and a mild muscle relaxant, and it may make some individuals feel better, although it is not a cure for fibromyalgia. Mild doses of antidepressants may help some patients, even when they are not depressed. Such drugs can also help improve problems with sleep.

Massage therapy and/or meditation may be helpful. Patients should avoid vigorous and painful massages, which can exacerbate overall pain. Some patients improve with hypnotherapy.

Some physicians also treat the pain of fibromyalgia with BOTULINUM TOXIN (Botox) injections into several painful areas. (Botox is also used by cosmetic surgeons to rid the face of facial wrinkles temporarily.) Botox treatment for fibromyalgia is controversial, and it is also very expensive. Beyond some anecdotal reports from some physicians of success with their patients, it is still unknown as of this writing whether Botox injections are a good treatment for fibromyalgia.

See also PAIN.

Staud, Roland, M.D., and Christine Adamec. *Fibromyalgia for Dummies.* New York: John Wiley & Sons, 2002.

**fish oil**  Generally capsules that contain oil extracted from fish. Fish oil has anti-inflammatory qualities, but it can cause digestive problems such as abdominal discomfort, heartburn, or diarrhea. However, when it is enteric-coated, fish oil can be tolerated by most people.

In one small study of 78 patients with Crohn's disease who were in remission, reported in a 1996 issue of the *New England Journal of Medicine,* the researchers found that the group who took fish oil had significantly fewer relapses of Crohn's disease symptoms (28 percent in the fish oil group versus 69 percent in the placebo group). Fish oil may be helpful for patients with ULCERATIVE COLITIS. It can also lower triglyceride levels in the body.

See also ALTERNATIVE MEDICINE; CROHN'S DISEASE; ULCERATIVE COLITIS.

Belluzzi, Andrea, M.D., et al. "Effect of an Enteric-Coated Fish-Oil Preparation on Relapses in Crohn's Disease." *New England Journal of Medicine* 334, no. 24 (June 13, 1996): 1,557–1,560.

**fissure**  A small crack or tear in the anal opening. It may be caused by straining to have a bowel movement or passing a very hard stool. Fissures may also be caused by TUBERCULOSIS, herpes infection, ACQUIRED IMMUNODEFICIENCY SYNDROME, CAN-

CER, INFLAMMATORY BOWEL DISEASE, and other disorders that should be considered.

The patient who has a fissure experiences severe pain that worsens during defecation as well as during a routine digital rectal examination by a physician. There may also be some bleeding associated with a fissure. Physicians treat most patients with fissures with sitz baths, rectal suppositories, or creams containing corticosteroids and local anesthetics. Patients are also advised to eat a high-fiber diet to keep their stools soft so that the fissure has an opportunity to heal. Some patients are given nitroglycerin ointments. BOTULINUM TOXIN injection is also useful. Chronic fissures may require surgery.

Pfenninger, John L. "Common Anorectal Conditions. Part III. Lesions." *American Family Physician,* July 1, 2001.

**fistula**   An artificially created passage between two hollow organs or between an organ and an external part of the body. Fistulas usually develop as a result of damaged tissues' contacting with each other and uniting during healing. If the fistula causes harm, it requires medical treatment or surgery. Examples of different types of fistulas are gastrocolic (the stomach and the colon), rectovaginal (the rectum and the vagina), colovesical (the colon and the urinary bladder), and enterocutaneous (the intestines and the skin).

Conditions that can cause fistula formation include CROHN'S DISEASE, DIVERTICULITIS, and CANCER. A fistula can also occur as a complication of abdominal surgery.

**fluid and electrolyte balance**   Levels of fluids and electrolytes in the body. To retain normal health, the body needs to maintain a healthy level of fluids and electrolytes. Sometimes, the fluid and electrolyte levels can become unbalanced as a result of disease, such as gastroenteritis, excessive vomiting, sweating, or severe infections.

Some medications can also cause fluid losses. In such cases, patients need fluid and electrolyte replacement. In acute cases of imbalances, some patients may even require hospitalization so that they can receive intravenous fluid and electrolyte replacements. When a patient's condition is stabilized, he or she can usually drink sufficient fluids to maintain a normal level of fluids and electrolytes.

Most individuals who have diarrhea can replenish their fluid and electrolyte levels by drinking fluids. People who exercise heavily often drink the commercial product Gatorade, which was developed by researchers at the University of Florida. Patients who have low potassium levels caused by some diuretic drugs such as furosemide (Lasix) often routinely take potassium supplements.

See also DEHYDRATION; DIARRHEA; ELECTROLYTES.

**food-borne illnesses**   Disorders caused by organisms, often bacteria, viruses, molds, or parasitic infections, that are carried and transmitted in food. The food is unknowingly ingested by others, who may become infected and then ill. (Some people become more ill than others do, depending on their general health, their immune system, and other factors.)

According to the Centers for Disease Control and Prevention (CDC) in the United States, an estimated 76 million people have food-borne illnesses each year, and of this number, 325,000 people are hospitalized and 5,000 people die. Food-borne illnesses are an even greater problem in many areas throughout the globe, especially in developing countries, often because of diseases that are transmitted through the consumption of contaminated food and water.

In addition to the pain, suffering, and, in some cases, even deaths that are caused by food-borne illnesses, the economic cost is also high, and experts estimate the annual cost in the United States alone at about $6 billion in medical expenses and loss of productivity when workers are too ill to work. Of this estimated $6 billion cost, *Salmonella* bacteria cause the largest single expense. An estimated 1.4 million people in the United States are infected by *Salmonella* organisms each year, usually as a result of eating contaminated food, such as beef, poultry, pork, eggs, or milk.

*Primary Bacterial Causes of Food-Borne Diseases*
There are about 250 different identified food-borne diseases; however, bacteria cause most food-borne diseases, followed in number by viruses and then

parasites, such as those that cause AMEBIASIS. In addition, manufactured or natural chemicals make some people ill. Others become sick from toxins that are produced by the food-borne agent, and it is that toxin rather than the food-borne agent itself that causes illness; for example, BOTULINUM TOXIN causes botulism.

Although there are many different types of bacteria that may cause food-borne illnesses, five create most problems: SALMONELLA, CLOSTRIDIUM, CAMPYLOBACTER, ESCHERICHIA COLI, and SHIGELLA. The symptoms caused by these diseases vary, but in general, they cause diarrhea (which may be severe and bloody, depending on the bacterium and the severity of the infection), nausea, vomiting, and abdominal pain. (For a detailed list of bacteria that cause food-borne illnesses, see table.)

### How Food-Borne Illnesses Are Transmitted

Frequently the cause of food-borne illnesses is fecal contamination spread by food preparation workers who have not washed their hands after using the toilet and have unknowingly transferred bacteria from their own feces to food to be ingested by others. This is a key reason why employee bathrooms in restaurants frequently have signs reminding employees to wash their hands with soap before returning to work. Unfortunately, sometimes these warnings are unheeded.

Other causes of food-borne illnesses are as follows:

- Preparing food on dirty and contaminated countertops or tables that have not been wiped clean ahead of time

### BACTERIA THAT CAUSE FOOD-BORNE ILLNESS

| Bacteria | Found | Transmission | Symptoms |
| --- | --- | --- | --- |
| *Campylobacter jejuni* | Intestinal tracts of animals and birds, raw milk, untreated water, and sewage sludge. | Contaminated water, raw milk, and raw or under-cooked meat, poultry, or shellfish. | Fever, headache, and muscle pain followed by diarrhea (sometimes bloody), abdominal pain, and nausea that appear 2 to 5 days after eating; may last 7 to 10 days. |
| *Clostridium botulinum* | Widely distributed in nature, soil, water, on plants, and in intestinal tract of animals including fish. Grows only in little or no oxygen. | Bacteria produce a toxin that causes illness. Improperly canned foods, garlic in oil, vacuum-packaged and tightly wrapped food. | Toxin affects the nervous system. Symptoms usually appear in 18 to 36 hours but can sometimes appear as few as 4 hours or as many as 8 days after eating; double vision, droopy eyelids, trouble with speaking and swallowing, and difficulty with breathing. Fatal in 3 to 10 days if not treated. |
| *Clostridium perfringens* | Soil, dust, sewage, and intestinal tract of animals and humans. Grows only in little or no oxygen. | Called "the cafeteria germ" because many outbreaks result from food left for long periods in steam tables or at room temperature. Bacteria destroyed by cooking, but some toxin-producing spores may survive. | Diarrhea and gas pains may appear 8 to 24 hours after eating; usually last about 1 day, but less severe symptoms may persist for 1 to 2 weeks. |
| *Escherichia coli* O157:H7 | Intestinal tract of some mammals, raw milk, unchlorinated water, one of several strains of *E. coli* that can cause human illness. | Contaminated water, raw milk, raw or rare ground beef, unpasteurized apple juice or cider, uncooked fruits and vegetables; person to person. | Diarrhea or bloody diarrhea, abdominal cramps, nausea, and malaise; can begin 2 to 5 days after food is eaten, lasting about 8 days. Some, especially the very young, have hemolytic-uremic syndrome (HUS) that causes acute kidney failure. A similar illness, thrombotic thrombocytopenic purpura (TTP), may occur in adults. |

*(continues)*

**BACTERIA THAT CAUSE FOOD-BORNE ILLNESS** *(continued)*

| Bacteria | Found | Transmission | Symptoms |
|---|---|---|---|
| *Listeria monocytogenes* | Intestinal tract of humans and animals, milk, soil, leaf vegetables; can grow slowly at refrigerator temperatures. | Ready-to-eat foods such as hot dogs, luncheon meats, cold cuts, fermented or dry sausage, and other deli-style meat and poultry; soft cheeses and unpasteurized milk. | Fever, chills, headache, backache, sometimes upset stomach, abdominal pain, and diarrhea; may take up to 3 weeks to become ill; more serious illness may later develop in at-risk patients (pregnant women and newborns, older adults, and people with weakened immune system). |
| *Salmonella* (more than 2,300 types) | Intestinal tract and feces of animals; *Salmonella* enteritidis in eggs. | Raw or undercooked eggs, poultry, and meat, raw milk and dairy products; seafood; and food handlers. | Stomach pain, diarrhea, nausea, chills, fever, and headache usually appear 8 to 72 hours after eating; may last 1 to 2 days. |
| *Shigella* (more than 30 types) | Human intestinal tract; rarely found in other animals. | Person to person by fecal–oral route; fecal contamination of food and water. Most outbreaks result from food, especially salads, prepared and handled by workers with poor personal hygiene. | Disease referred to as shigellosis or bacillary dysentery. Diarrhea containing blood and mucus, fever, abdominal cramps, chills, and vomiting; 12 to 50 hours from ingestion of bacteria; can last a few days to 2 weeks. |
| *Staphylococcus aureus* | On humans (skin, infected cuts, pimples, nose, and throat). | Person to person through food from improper food handling. Multiply rapidly at room temperature to produce a toxin that causes illness. | Severe nausea, abdominal cramps, vomiting, and diarrhea occur 1 to 6 hours after eating; recovery within 2 to 3 days—longer if severe dehydration occurs. |

Source: Food Safety and Inspection Service, United States Department of Agriculture. "Foodborne Illness: What Consumers Need to Know." Undated.

- Leaving food that should be refrigerated out of the refrigerator, causing it to spoil
- Eating food from a common container and with the hands

### *Diagnosing and Treating Food-Borne Illnesses*

Physicians may suspect a food-borne illness, particularly if multiple people who ate at the same restaurant or who attended the same function and consumed common food or water also became ill with similar symptoms of nausea and vomiting, and sometimes diarrhea as well. Most food-borne illnesses are short-lived and resolve on their own.

Sometimes antibiotics improve the condition, especially if the food-borne illness is bacterial. In severe cases of food-borne illnesses, individuals need to be hospitalized to treat dehydration and electrolyte depletion that can result from severe vomiting and diarrhea. Individuals who are elderly or are in a weakened condition due to cancer or a compromised immune system are likely to have more severe symptoms than others exposed to the same germs.

### *Preventing Food-Borne Illnesses*

It is not possible to eradicate all food-borne illnesses, but certain precautions can limit the risks for consumers. Such basic precautions include taking the following actions:

- Washing hands before food preparation
- Washing hands and food preparation surfaces after raw meat or poultry has been touched
- Washing hands every time after using the toilet

- Cooking meats, particularly beef, chicken, and eggs, thoroughly

- Washing fruits and vegetables before eating, particularly if they are to be eaten raw

- Preventing cross-contamination of foods by preparing poultry, beef, chicken, or eggs separately from other foods

- Drinking only pasteurized milk and juices

- Refrigerating leftover food within two hours of cooking

For further information, contact the following organizations:

Centers for Disease Control and Prevention
National Center for Infectious Diseases
Division of Bacterial and Mycotic Diseases
1600 Clifton Road NE
Atlanta, GA 30333
(888) 232-3228 (toll-free)
http://www.cdc.gov

United States Department of Agriculture
Food Safety and Inspection Service
1400 Independence Avenue SW, Room 2932-S
Washington, DC 20250
(800) 256-7072 (toll-free)
http://www.fsis.usda.gov

United States Food and Drug Administration
Center for Food Safety and Applied Nutrition
5100 Paint Branch Parkway
College Park, MD 20740
(888) SAFEFOOD (toll-free)
http://vm.cfsan.fda.gove/list.html

See also CONTAMINATED FOOD OR WATER; PASTEURIZATION; TRAVEL.

**functional bowel disorders**  Disorders of the functioning of nerves and muscles of the gastrointestinal system that cause diarrhea, constipation, and pain, such as in IRRITABLE BOWEL SYNDROME. There is no grossly apparent (visible to the naked eye) structural damage to the organ involved in a functional bowel disorder; thus, irritable bowel syndrome causes no visible damage to the colon.

Thus, the diagnosis is primarily or solely made by taking the patient's medical history and performing a physical examination, as well as by excluding other mimicking diseases by ordering tests such as blood tests, X rays, and ENDOSCOPY.

In addition to irritable bowel syndrome, other functional bowel disorders include functional dyspepsia, noncardiac chest pain, and functional heartburn, for which the causes are unknown. Visceral hypersensitivity or a lowered pain threshold is seen in these patients. Treatments include use of antidepressants to increase the patient's pain threshold.

See also CONSTIPATION; DIARRHEA.

**fundoplication**  A surgical treatment for GASTROESOPHAGEAL REFLUX DISEASE, which is also called Nissen's fundoplication. The procedure may be performed laparoscopically, or it may be accomplished through a large open incision in the abdomen. A part of the stomach is wrapped around the junction of the esophagus and the stomach in order to tighten the junction and to prevent the reflux of gastric contents back into the esophagus. In a modification of the Nissen's fundoplication procedure the surgeon creates a partial wrap (270 degrees) rather than a 360-degree wrap around the esophagus; this modified procedure is used for patients with impaired esophageal motility.

See also ACID REFLUX.

**fungi**  Yeast or mold that cause infection, such as *Candidiasis* species or THRUSH. In addition to infection in other organs, fungal infection occurs in the digestive organs among patients whose immune function is suppressed or suboptimal, such as patients who have acquired immunodeficiency syndrome (AIDS). Sometimes diabetes patients experience a fungal infection in the esophagus, leading to pain during swallowing of food. Oral medications can be administered to treat fungi. If the fungus is external, antifungal creams are recommended by physicians. Sometimes intravenous medications are needed to eradicate the fungus, especially if it has spread to the bloodstream.

See also *CANDIDA; LACTOBACILLUS;* THRUSH.

**gag reflex**   The natural tendency of the throat to prevent swallowing that may occur if a noxious substance, fluids, or foods touches the back of the tongue and the throat (the back of the pharynx, or soft palate). This reflex does not have any relation to the swallowing process.

### Testing the Gag Reflex

The gag reflex can be checked by touching or stroking the posterior pharynx on one side with a cotton swab and then comparing this response to the response elicited by touching the other side. About 15 to 30 percent of normal individuals do not have a gag reflex response to this test. The test result is most informative when the responses are asymmetric (differing from one side to the other).

### Gag Reflex and Endoscopy

Many people worry that because of the gag reflex they cannot endure endoscopy, a procedure in which a tube is inserted down the throat so that the physician can inspect both the esophagus and the stomach. However, most people have little or no problem with this procedure, and the gag reflex does not prevent the doctor from performing the endoscopy.

### Abnormal Gag Reflexes

An abnormal gag reflex may be elicited in patients who have swallowing problems after a stroke or who are in a coma. However, the absence of the gag reflex does not mean that this absence is the cause of dysphagia.

The gag reflex is abnormal and asymmetric in diseases involving cranial nerves IX and X.

An abnormal gag reflex is not protective and does not occur when food falls into the back of the throat in an uncontrolled way.

**gallbladder**   The digestive organ that stores bile that is manufactured by the liver. When the gallbladder malfunctions, stones and infection may develop. GALLSTONES usually do not cause symptoms, but they can block the flow of bile to the duodenum, causing CHOLECYSTITIS, CHOLANGITIS, or PANCREATITIS, which can be extremely painful and sometimes even life-threatening. If the gallbladder must be surgically removed, patients can continue to digest their food and function without it. Most cases of cholecystectomy are currently undertaken laparoscopically.

See also CANCER, GALLBLADDER; CHOLECYSTECTOMY.

**gallbladder cancer**   See CANCER, GALLBLADDER.

**gallstones**   Yellow, black, or brown stonelike material that can cause severe pain when they become lodged in the ducts carrying bile from the liver or the gallbladder to the small intestine. Individuals may have one gallstone or many of them.

The presence of stones in the gallbladder, called cholelithiasis, may lead to a chronic inflammation of the gallbladder known as chronic cholecystitis. If gallstones are lodged in the bile ducts, this condition is known as choledocholithiasis. About 15 to 20 percent of gallstone patients have choledocholithiasis, which can lead to inflammation of the bile ducts as well as to pancreatitis. When impacted in the cystic duct, gallstones cause acute cholecystitis.

Most gallstones (about 90 percent) comprise cholesterol; others may comprise many different materials. Cholesterol gallstones are yellow. Noncholesterol gallstones are either black or brown. People who have some blood diseases (such as thalassemia and sickle cell anemia) are more likely to have noncholesterol gallstones. Individuals who have liver cirrhosis may also have black or brown gallstones. Brown stones are often related to parasitic or bacterial infections. Coffee, aspirin, and vitamin C appear to protect against gallstones.

Gallstones can be as small as one grain of sand or as large as a golf ball.

### Risk Factors

An estimated 15 to 20 percent of the population in the United States have gallstones at some point in their life. About one million cases of gallstone disease are diagnosed each year in the United States. Native Americans in the United States have the highest risk of development of gallstones. Worldwide, people in Scandinavian countries are at high risk for gallstones, and as many as half the population in these countries have gallstones by the age of 50.

Although almost anyone can have gallstones, there are some key risk factors among patients that doctors look for:

- Obesity is a major risk factor, especially among women.
- High levels of estrogen caused by pregnancy, birth control pills, or hormone replacement estrogen that is given to menopausal women increase risk.
- Race and ethnicity: Native Americans, particularly the Pima of Arizona, have the highest risk of development of gallstones. An estimated 70 to 80 percent of all Pima women have gallstones by the age of 30. Native Americans are followed by Mexican Americans in high risk of development of gallstones.
- Gender: Women who are between the ages of 20 and 60 have double to triple the risk of development of gallstones of men.
- Age: People age 60 and older have a higher risk than younger individuals.
- Medications: People taking cholesterol-lowering drugs like clofibrate or antibiotics like ceftriaxone have a higher risk.

- Patients who have had bariatric surgery as a treatment for severe obesity, have a risk of development of gallstones after surgery of about 30 percent.
- Presence of diabetes raises risk.
- Presence of Crohn's disease increases risk.
- Very rapid weight loss.

### Symptoms and Signs of Gallstones

In general, the following symptoms and signs may indicate the presence of gallstones, although only a physician can confirm the diagnosis. It is important to keep in mind that in most patients gallstones produce no symptoms, and health problems related to them never develop. When patients are symptomatic, the symptoms that indicate gallstones may also be indicators of other serious problems, such as a heart attack, appendicitis, ulcers, or pancreatitis.

Pain characteristics of biliary colic gallstones may include the following:

- Pain in the upper and right abdomen that has lasted for at least 30 minutes to several hours. Pain lasting longer than six hours suggests acute cholecystitis (inflammation of the gallbladder). The term biliary *colic* is a misnomer, since the pain is not colicky but constant.
- Pain may be preceded by a heavy meal.
- Pain may radiate to the center, between the patient's shoulder blades.
- Pain may radiate to the tip of the right shoulder.
- Pain may be accompanied by nausea and vomiting.
- Pain may be accompanied by restlessness.

Symptoms such as bloating, vague abdominal discomfort, and gas occur with the same frequency as in other conditions such as ulcers.

### Diagnosis

Unless the patient has emergency symptoms, in many cases, doctors identify gallstones during routine tests for other medical problems, with tests such as ultrasound. Ultrasound is considered the best test for identifying gallstones; however, it is possible that gallstones will not be identified by an ultrasound examination, especially when the stones are in the bile duct.

Other tests that doctors may order include blood tests to identify infection, jaundice, or pancreatitis as well as magnetic resonance imaging (MRI) tests to check for blocked bile ducts or computed tomography (CT) tests to check for gallstones in the ducts as well as for inflammation of the gallbladder and the pancreas. Blood test results that show elevated levels of liver enzymes and bilirubin may indicate biliary duct stones (choledocholithias). Elevated blood levels of amylase and lipase may indicate the presence of bile duct stones and/or pancreatitis.

One older diagnostic test is oral cholecystography, in which patients took one dose of a contrast dye, and the gallbladder was imaged in plain X rays. This test is not usually chosen today, because it is cumbersome and takes several hours. In addition, this test is no more accurate than the ultrasound test.

### Treatment of Gallstones

If gallstones are identified, and the physician believes that the patient's problems are related to the gallstones, usually the physician recommends surgery to remove the entire gallbladder. This surgery not only removes existing gallstones but ensures that additional gallstones will not develop. Rarely, stones may develop in the bile duct after the removal of the gallbladder.

Surgery to remove the gallbladder is called CHOLECYSTECTOMY; an estimated 500,000 patients in the United States have cholecystectomy every year. In most cases, the surgery is performed laparoscopically: it is done through multiple small incisions in the abdomen. A cholecystectomy is not performed if gallstones are not causing symptoms except in cases when a condition carries a high risk for disease or cancer, such as calcified gallbladder or a large gallbladder polyp.

If surgery is not considered advisable for some reason, because the patient is a poor surgical risk or the patient declines surgery, then doctors may prescribe nonsurgical therapy. A functioning gallbladder as assessed by oral cholecystography is an essential prerequisite to nonsurgical therapy. Ursodiol (Actigall) is a medication to help dissolve the gallstone. The drug works only on cholesterol gallstones, but since this form of gallstone is the more common, most patients have the potential to benefit from this therapy. This drug is not very effective for large, multiple, or calcified stones. The drug may take months or longer to dissolve existing stones and may cause some diarrhea as a side effect.

Contact dissolution is a method whereby a needle is inserted into the gallbladder and a solvent such as methyl tert-butyl ether (MRBE) is injected to dissolve the stone. Complete stone dissolution may be achieved in 65 percent of the cases, and selected patients are subsequently recommended oral dissolution therapy to prevent recurrence of stones. This method is not widely available as of this writing.

Another treatment for gallstones is extracorporeal shockwave lithotripsy (ESWL). In this treatment, the gallstones are broken up by shock waves that are administered; however, patients may have severe pain after their treatment. The best candidates for this treatment are patients who have only one gallstone with a diameter of less than two centimeters that is radiolucent. Some physicians use the procedure when there are multiple stones with an aggregate size of three centimeters.

Lithotripsy is followed by administration of ursodiol, as described earlier. ESWL is not a very popular method because of its poor efficacy, and it is used only for patients at poor surgical risk.

See also CHOLELITHIASIS; GALLBLADDER; PANCREATITIS.

Agrawal, Sangeeta, M.D., and Sreenivasa Jonnalagadda, M.D. "Gallstones, from Gallbladder to Gut." *Postgraduate Medicine* 108, no. 3 (September 1, 2000).

Cox, Cheryl A., and Stephen J. Bickston. "Right Upper Quadrant Pain: Gallbladder Disease and Its Complications." In *20 Common Problems in Gastroenterology.* New York: McGraw-Hill Medical Publishing Division, 2002.

**gas**  Air that is produced as a normal part of the digestive process. When gas is expressed through the mouth, the process is called burping, and when it is expressed through the rectum, it is called farting or flatulence. The gas that is belched is usually the air that is swallowed and does not stem from the colon. On the other hand, the gas of flatus is produced in the colon as a result of bacterial fermentations of the unabsorbed carbohydrates.

Gas production in the colon is normal; there is always some gas in the gut. There is a wide range in the number of flatulent expulsions that people may have. Elderly subjects expel small amounts but more frequently than younger individuals.

A variety of measures are used by patients who have "excessive gas," such as avoiding gas-producing foods and taking over-the-counter medications such as alpha-D-galactosidase enzyme (Beano), simethicone, and activated charcoal. However frequently, treatment is unsatisfactory.

If the gas problem is a severe one, individuals should see their physician to determine whether there is another underlying problem.

See also BELCHING; GAS-BLOAT SYNDROME.

**gas-bloat syndrome**   A rare medical problem that results from an inability to belch (burp), causing the patient to experience a buildup of gases in the stomach. Gas-bloat syndrome is sometimes seen after fundoplication surgery for GASTROESOPHAGEAL REFLUX DISEASE (GERD).

Patients who have gas-bloat syndrome should avoid foods that lead to production of excessive gas, including carbonated beverages. Prokinetic medications may help. In very severe cases, patients may require surgery to correct gas-bloat syndrome.

See also GAS.

**gastrectomy**   The surgical excision of all or part of the stomach, usually performed because of the diagnosis of cancer, especially stomach cancer. The gastrectomy may also be performed as part of surgery for ulcers as well as for cancer of the pancreas. The gastrectomy can also lead to other medical problems and conditions, such as dumping syndrome.

See also CANCER, PANCREATIC; CANCER, STOMACH; DUMPING SYNDROME; STOMACH; ULCERS, PEPTIC.

**gastric emptying**   Part of the normal digestive process, in which the contents of the stomach are

emptied and delivered into the duodenum. During this process in a fed state, only small particles of food measuring one to two millimeters are allowed to pass through. The gastric emptying test is used to determine whether the patient has abnormal gastric emptying. Delayed gastric emptying is called GASTROPARESIS.

See also DIGESTION AND ABSORPTION.

**gastrin**   A digestive hormone that directs the stomach to release hydrochloric acid to help with the digestion of food as well as to kill many of the foreign infectious organisms that are ingested with food. Gastrin also helps maintain the normal growth of the stomach lining.

See also HORMONES.

**gastritis**   Inflammation of the stomach. The problem may be temporary, due to food or other substances that have irritated the stomach, such as alcohol. Some individuals, however, suffer from chronic gastritis, which may be caused by infection with *Helicobacter pylori*. The use of drugs that damage the stomach, such as NONSTEROIDAL ANTI-INFLAMMATORY DRUGS (NSAIDs), also causes gastritis. Chronic gastritis may lead to the development of ulcers and, rarely, may lead to cancer.

See also ALCOHOL ABUSE AND DEPENDENCE/ALCOHOLISM; CANCER, STOMACH; *HELICOBACTER PYLORI*; ULCERS, PEPTIC.

**gastroenterologist**   A medical doctor who specializes in diagnosing and treating diseases and disorders of the digestive system. The gastroenterologist also performs a variety of diagnostic procedures, such as esophagogastroduodenoscopy (upper gastrointestinal endoscopy), COLONOSCOPY, SIGMOIDOSCOPY, and ENDOSCOPIC RETROGRADE CHOLANGIOPANCREATOGRAPHY (ERCP).

See also PEDIATRIC GASTROENTEROLOGIST.

**gastroesophageal reflux disease (GERD)**   A chronic digestive disease whose primary characteristic is a chronic backflow (reflux) of food and digestive juices from the stomach into the esophagus and sometimes into the mouth as well. About 55 million people in the United States, six million people in Canada, and millions of people in other countries worldwide suffer from GERD. Many people with GERD are untreated (other than by taking over-the-counter antacids) because they do not realize that they have the illness or they do not know about the seriousness of this chronic illness over time.

Chronic GERD can lead to damage of the food tube called the ESOPHAGUS (the condition of ESOPHAGITIS), and it may also cause a narrowing (stricture) of the esophageal passage so that the individual has difficulty in swallowing (DYSPHAGIA). GERD that has been untreated for many years may also lead to BARRETT'S ESOPHAGUS, a precancerous condition of the esophagus that can ultimately lead to cancer.

### Causes of GERD

The cause of GERD is usually not excessive acid level but acid that is in the wrong place. There are a variety of different potential factors contributing to GERD, and the physician may have difficulty determining a specific cause; for example, GERD may be related to a genetic factor; it may also be caused or exacerbated by obesity. However, most of the time there is no clear cause, and most reflux occurs during transient lower esophageal relaxations. GASTROPARESIS (slow stomach emptying) and gastroduodenal surgery each predispose patients to development of GERD.

Another common risk factor for GERD and esophagitis is the regular use of nonsteroidal anti-inflammatory drugs (NSAIDs), which are medications that are usually prescribed for arthritis and related illnesses. Medications such as calcium channel blocker medications that are taken to treat hypertension or heart disease can also cause or contribute to the development of GERD. A variety of other medications may cause GERD, including estrogen or progesterone preparations taken by menopausal women and sumatriptan (Imitrex) taken for migraine headaches, antidepressants such as amitriptyline (Elavil), doxepin (Sinequan), and nortriptyline (Pamelor).

### Risk Factors

Certain categories of people are more prone to development of GERD than others, such as people who

- Have diabetes
- Have hypothyroidism (low level of thyroid hormone)
- Have a hiatal hernia
- Have chronic constipation and straining to move the bowels
- Smoke
- Have asthma
- Are pregnant
- Have decreased production of saliva (caused by medications and/or aging)
- Are overweight
- Have gastroparesis

### Symptoms

The key symptoms of chronic GERD are frequent heartburn and entry of a sour (acid)-tasting fluid into the mouth. Many other atypical symptoms may occur; they may include

- Asthma
- Chronic throat clearing
- Hoarseness and cough
- Possible difficulty in swallowing
- Frequent episodes of bronchitis and recurrent pneumonia
- Frequent ear, nose, and throat infections

Some people who have GERD may also experience severe chest pains that even physicians may confuse with heart attack; a heart attack should always be ruled out by a physician before GERD is considered as a possibility. It is also possible to have both heart disease and GERD.

### Diagnosis of GERD

GERD is often diagnosed on the basis of the presence of a clinical history of chronic heartburn alone. In general, the physician takes a full medical history and performs a complete physical examination of the patient.

In some cases, the patient may have an upper endoscopy, in which a special instrument is inserted down the throat and into the esophagus and then into the stomach. Besides detecting damage to the esophagus due to GERD, this test can detect other medical problems, such as hiatal hernias, ulcers, or STOMACH CANCER. The endoscopy results are normal in about half of the cases of patients with GERD; in those cases it is known as nonerosive reflux disease (NERD).

### Treatment

People diagnosed with GERD may be treated with medications, lifestyle recommendations, and even surgery, although surgery is not the usual treatment. However, some surgeons believe that almost every patient who has GERD requires surgery. Many patients can improve their medical status by taking simple actions such as giving up smoking or avoiding certain types of foods.

*Recommended medications*  Many patients are treated with a drug in the PROTON PUMP INHIBITOR (PPI) class, such as omeprazole (Prilosec), pantoprazole (Protonix), rabeprazole (Aciphex), lansoprazole (Prevacid), or esomeprazole (Nexium). Generic versions of omeprazole are available. Some patients are treated with a drug in the histamine-2 inhibitor class (also known as H-2 blockers) such as cimetidine (Tagamet) or ranitidine (Zantac), which are effective in about half of the cases. PPIs are superior to H-2 blockers and are effective in about 90 percent of patients. There are many other possible medications that may be administered and new ones are continually in development by pharmaceutical companies.

*Drugs to be avoided*  Some medications should be avoided whenever possible by people who have GERD, because they may further aggravate the condition. Examples of drugs that patients should try to avoid are

• Progesterone

• Calcium channel blockers

• Nonsteroidal anti-inflammatory drugs

• Tricyclic antidepressants

Some experts also believe that herbal remedies such as goldenseal and peppermint may worsen the condition, although good studies to address this issue are lacking.

*Lifestyle changes*  Most doctors strongly advise GERD patients to make changes in their lifestyle, such as raising the head of their bed, so they are less likely to experience acid reflux at night. Patients with GERD should not go to bed for at least two to three hours after eating a meal.

Patients who are overweight are urged to lose weight, because obesity may worsen the symptoms of GERD. Patients are also urged to exercise but should avoid weightlifting and other strenuous exercises, instead concentrating on walking and riding a stationary bicycle or participating in other forms of low-impact aerobic activity.

Dietary changes may improve symptoms; for example, patients should forgo consuming large fatty meals, alcohol, chocolate, onions, orange juice, and carbonated beverages.

Patients who smoke should stop smoking immediately. Smoking aggravates many medical conditions, including GERD.

See also ACID REFLUX; CHEST PAIN, NONCARDIAC; HISTAMINE-2 INHIBITORS.

Minocha, Anil, M.D., and Christine Adamec. *How to Stop Heartburn: Simple Ways to Heal Heartburn and Acid Reflux.* New York: John Wiley & Sons, 2001.

**gastrointestinal bleeding**  See BLEEDING, GASTROINTESTINAL; OCCULT GASTROINTESTINAL BLEEDING.

**gastroparesis**  A delayed emptying of the stomach. In the early stages of gastroparesis, the patient's main problem is the stomach's delaying of the emptying of solids. If the condition worsens further, there is also a delay in the emptying of liquids from the stomach to the small intestine. This condition makes a normal three-meal-a-day schedule difficult, because the food from breakfast may still be in the stomach when food from lunch is consumed and has to be processed.

### Risk Factors

Gastroparesis may be caused by or linked to diseases such as DIABETES MELLITUS, neurological disorders, thyroid disease, or peptic ulcer. Older people (ages 65 and older) are more likely to experience gastroparesis.

Gastroparesis may also be caused by medications, which can have the side effect of slowing the process of digestion. Examples of types of drugs that can have that effect are antidepressants, tranquilizers, and calcium blocker medications. In many cases, no cause of the gastroparesis can be found, and it is often believed to be triggered by a viral illness.

SMOKING is also known to exacerbate gastroparesis, and smokers are urged to stop smoking immediately to prevent the problem from worsening. (Even if the smoker does not yet have a problem with gastroparesis, it is advisable to quit smoking before the condition develops.)

### Symptoms of Gastroparesis

Some people have no symptoms of gastroparesis, others have symptoms or signs, which include

- Nausea and vomiting
- Anorexia (lack of appetite)
- Early satiety (feeling of fullness that occurs soon after eating)
- Bloating
- Abdominal pain and distention
- Acid reflux

### Diagnosis and Treatment

Physicians generally suspect that their patients have gastroparesis on the basis of their symptoms, and they confirm the diagnosis with a gastric emptying test, after first excluding the presence of a gastric obstruction with either the upper gastrointestinal X ray or an endoscopy.

A *low-fiber* diet is usually recommended for people who are diagnosed with gastroparesis (because fiber may exacerbate the condition), as is eating five or six small meals per day rather than three large meals. Some patients are placed on a liquid diet. A person who has diabetes and gastroparesis should try to maintain a blood sugar level that is as close to normal as possible in order to improve gastric emptying.

There are several medications used for treating gastroparesis, and in the United States, metoclopramide (Reglan) is frequently prescribed. However, metoclopramide can cause tremors and parkinsonian effects. Another drug, domperidone, works as metoclopramide does but without causing the same parkinsonian side effects; however, it has to be made in pharmacies on a special order. Some physicians have also used erythromycin to treat gastroparesis, but it is effective only for short periods.

Some conditions improve with a special device that is implanted to treat gastroparesis. The Food and Drug Administration (FDA) has approved the implantation of a gastric electrical stimulator or stomach pacemaker (Enterra Therapy), which is similar to the pacemaker of the heart. However, this treatment is only used in severe cases. Injection of botulinum toxin (Botox) into the pylorus helps improve gastric emptying of people who have diabetic gastroparesis.

In patients who are unable to eat, an endoscopic insertion of a percutaneous endoscopic jejunostomy (PEJ) or a surgical jejunostomy may be done. In this procedure, a tube is placed through an incision in the abdominal wall into the small bowel, bypassing the stomach. As a result, food is directly fed into the intestine rather than into the stomach through the mouth. Some patients need to be fed via long-term intravenous nutritional methods.

See also BOTULINUM TOXIN; DIABETES MELLITUS; FIBER.

**gastrostomy** A procedure that creates an artificial hole in the abdominal wall and connected to the stomach, through which a feeding tube can be inserted and the patient can be supplied with ENTERAL NUTRITION. In the case of severe GASTROPARESIS, a venting gastrostomy may be done to suction gas from the stomach in order to prevent distention, whereas feeding is done through a tube in the small intestine. Feeding into the small intestine is accomplished through a jejunostomy tube that is placed farther down in the jejunum.

**ghrelin**   A hormone that was discovered in 1999. Ghrelin is released by the stomach and appears to affect appetite and satiety (a feeling of fullness after eating) directly. Preliminary studies indicate that suppression of ghrelin may become a treatment for OBESITY. Comparisons of patients that have lost weight by dieting or by gastric bypass surgery have demonstrated that the gastric bypass patients experienced significant drops in their blood level of ghrelin after the surgery.

Because obesity is a major problem in the United States, Canada, and many other developed countries, the finding that blood levels of ghrelin apparently can increase or decrease an individual's appetite appears to be a major breakthrough. Some researchers anticipate that ghrelin antagonist medications will be developed to create a new diet drug that will help many patients who are overweight or obese.

See also BARIATRIC SURGERY; DIET DRUGS.

**Giardia/giardiasis**   *Giardia* is the protozoon that causes the infection giardiasis. In the United States, most infections are caused by *Giardia lamblia,* which harbors in the human intestinal tract and is also found in human feces. Giardiasis is generally a nonfatal and common infection of the small intestine. Giardiasis is transmitted through contaminated food or water. Periodic outbreaks occur in institutions, especially those that cater to small children, and at functions such as large picnics.

### Symptoms

Most people with giardiasis (as many as two-thirds) have no symptoms. When symptoms do occur, they generally appear within one to three weeks or longer after infection and may include the following

- Diarrhea
- Bad-smelling and oily feces
- Abdominal pains
- Loss of appetite
- Gas
- Nausea and vomiting

### Diagnosis and Treatment

Doctors may particularly suspect giardiasis if others in the same environment (such as a day care center) have already been diagnosed. But the only way to confirm giardiasis is with an analysis of a stool sample or duodenal aspirate. Generally, three samples are required because *Giardia* organisms may be missed otherwise.

Medications help most patients and prevent further transmission. The medication that is most commonly used is metronidazole. Other medications that may be used include quinacrine, furazolidone, and paromomycin.

### Preventing Giardiasis

There is no medication or vaccine to protect against *Giardia* organisms; however, simple precautions can and should be taken by people to limit the incidence of infection, including the following actions:

- Washing hands after using the toilet
- Avoiding unwashed fruits or vegetables unless the surface of the food can be peeled away
- Keeping children who attend a day care center who have severe diarrhea at home, to prevent infecting other children
- Boiling drinking water if *Giardia* organisms may be present

See also CONTAMINATED FOOD OR WATER; DIARRHEA; FOOD-BORNE ILLNESSES; PARASITIC INFECTIONS.

**Gilbert's disease**   An inherited liver disorder that is not dangerous but may sometimes be confused with serious liver diseases. If such confusion occurs, patients may receive unnecessary investigations for HEPATITIS or other serious liver ailments that they do not have. Gilbert's disease is estimated to be present in about 3 to 7 percent of adults, and usually is diagnosed in adolescence or early adulthood. The disease was first identified in 1901 by the French physician Nicolas A. Gilbert.

### Diagnosis

The diagnosis is made on the basis of laboratory tests. The primary characteristic of Gilbert's disease is a changing level of serum bilirubin, which may appear to the physician to indicate JAUNDICE. The subtype pattern of the bilirubin level that is elevated is indirect or unconjugated, which is different from the predominantly direct or conjugated bilirubin level elevation that is seen in liver disease.

The increases in bilirubin level that are characteristic of Gilbert's disease occur during periods of physical stress, such as when the patient is fasting, is feverish, or has an acute illness; however, the individual's liver functions continue to be normal and no treatment is required. When the period of fasting or acute illness subsides, the bilirubin level returns to normal again.

For further information on Gilbert's disease, contact the following organization:

American Liver Foundation
75 Maiden Lane
New York, NY 10038
(212) 668-1000 or (800) 465-4837 (toll-free)
http://www.liverfoundation.org

See also BILIRUBIN.

Wynbrandt, James, and Mark D. Ludman. "Gilbert disease." *The Encyclopedia of Genetic Disorders and Birth Defects.* 2d ed. New York: Facts On File, 2000, p. 146.

**glucose**    Blood sugar. Normal levels of glucose are essential to good health. High levels constitute hyperglycemia and are characteristic of DIABETES MELLITUS, in which low insulin levels occur. In diabetic patients, insulin may have to be taken every day in injections in order to maintain the blood glucose level. Patients who have type 2 diabetes may be treated with oral medications and not need insulin.

Low levels of blood glucose are known as hypoglycemia. Sometimes people who have diabetes may take insulin but eat inadequate amounts of food; they may then experience unusually low glucose levels. Low glucose level can lead to mild symptoms, or, in extreme cases, even to coma. Because of this problem, diabetes patients frequently carry candy, fruit, or another form of sugar for use in an emergency.

Certain tissues in the body, such as the brain, red blood cells, bone marrow, parts of the eyes, and kidneys, can utilize only glucose as an energy source.

**guaiac**    A substance that is used in fecal occult blood testing to screen patients for colorectal cancer. Guaiac is a gumlike or resinous substance that is obtained from two tree species: *Guaiacum officinale* and *Guaiacum sanctum.* The test was discovered by Van Deen in 1864, who found that guaiac changes color when it is applied to stool that contains blood.

Various tests that are based on guaiac are used. Guaiac tests do produce some false positive results, such as those caused by the patient's eating red meat, turnip, or horseradish before having the test or ingesting stomach-irritant drugs that cause gastritis, such as aspirin. On the other hand, the ingestion of vitamin C before testing can cause a false negative test result.

See also CANCER, COLORECTAL; OCCULT BLEEDING.

**halitosis** Unpleasant breath, which may be caused by poor oral and dental hygiene or by a digestive illness, such as GASTROESOPHAGEAL REFLUX DISEASE or ZENKER'S DIVERTICULUM, or by another medical problem.

**heartburn** Occasional or chronic acidic feeling behind the chest that is usually caused by acid reflux. Chronic heartburn is also known as GASTROESOPHAGEAL REFLUX DISEASE; however, sometimes even a heart attack may produce a burning pain in the chest, and distinguishing between acid reflux and heart attack can be difficult.

See also ACID REFLUX.

**Helicobacter pylori** (*H. pylori* or **HP**) Common bacteria that are found in the stomach of many people in the United States and other countries and that are the primary cause of peptic ulcers. In addition, sometimes an infection with *Helicobacter pylori* (HP) precedes certain forms of stomach cancer. In the past, HP was also associated with other medical problems, such as heart disease and short stature, but these links have been scientifically refuted.

One association based on scientific data was found by researchers who looked at studies of people infected with HP in Japan; their findings were reported in the *New England Journal of Medicine* in 2001. The research showed that infected people had a higher risk of development of gastric cancer when they were compared to those patients who were not infected with HP. In one study 1,526 Japanese patients who had duodenal or gastric ulcer or other serious gastric problems were evaluated for an infection with HP. Of these patients, 280 individuals were infected. The patients were then followed up for about eight years. The researchers found that about 3 percent of the patients who had been diagnosed with HP developed gastric cancer, whereas cancer developed in none of the uninfected patients.

### Some Historical Background

Until the late 20th century, most physicians worldwide believed that ulcers were caused by stress, diet, or acid; however, in 1982, the Australian physicians Marshall and Warren theorized that ulcers are actually caused by bacteria. In fact, Dr. Marshall actually consumed some HP bacteria and caused the development of an infection. He contracted gastritis, had antibiotic treatment, and was cured of both gastritis and HP.

Despite this research, for a while, most physicians worldwide refused to believe that bacteria could cause gastritis or ulcers, believing instead that the primary causes were diet and/or stress, and consequently they ridiculed Marshall and Warren. It was not until 1994, when the National Institutes of Health (NIH) in the United States confirmed the association between HP and ulcers and the NIH then recommended that antibiotics be used to prevent recurrence of HP-induced ulcers, that most physicians began to accept that *Helicobacter pylori* is the true culprit in the majority of ulcers. This was a dramatic paradigm shift for physicians worldwide.

### Risk Factors for Contracting HP

Although HP is more commonly found in poor countries, the bacteria are ubiquitously present in every society. Researchers report that the incidence of infection in developed countries is 20 to 50 percent, whereas it is greater than 80 percent in poor countries. Generally, the bacteria are contracted by children and harbored in the stomach unless or until they are eradicated by antibiotics.

### Risk of Development of an Ulcer Caused by HP

People infected with HP have a much higher risk of development of ulcers, although not everyone who has had HP infection has an ulcer. Researchers report that the risk of development of a peptic ulcer among people who are infected with HP is about 15 percent.

Interestingly, Dr. Minocha and his colleagues have found that patients who have a prior history of having a tonsillectomy have a significantly reduced risk of being infected with HP, possibly because patients with bad tonsils are more likely to have used antibiotics in the past, thus eradicating the HP infection in the stomach. The same patients are also likely to undergo subsequent tonsillectomy. Thus, the possible linkage between HP and tonsillectomy may be merely an association and not a cause-and-effect relationship.

Another possibility is that the tonsils serve as a kind of collecting place for bacteria, although researchers are not sure whether this is true. Minocha's findings were reported in 1997 in the *Journal of Clinical Gastroenterology.*

### Symptoms and Signs

Most individuals who are infected with HP have no symptoms. Most have chronic gastritis and a few patients develop ulcers. Symptoms of indigestion in the presence of HP but without an overt ulcer are usually not relieved by eradicating the HP.

### Diagnosis of HP

If physicians suspect that HP is the underlying cause of the patient's problem, they can confirm the diagnosis with the urea breath test, or with blood tests or stool antigen tests. In addition, if an endoscopy is performed, the physician can take a biopsy of extracted tissue to determine whether it is infected with HP. Physicians usually do not test patients who have endoscopy for HP unless they also suspect that they may have a problem related to HP *and* they intend to treat the HP. If the patient has no symptoms, then it is not considered necessary to confirm or refute the presence of HP. Therefore, patients who are receiving long-term

treatment for GASTROESOPHAGEAL REFLUX DISEASE (GERD) are usually not tested for HP. Interestingly, HP may be protective against GERD.

In the breath test, the patient ingests a urea-laden meal that is laced with minute amounts of radioactivity. The patient then merely breathes into a device that measures the presence of radioactivity, and a high level of radioactivity or radio labeled carbon dioxide indicates infection with HP. This test is highly reliable for adults and children older than age six but may not be available at some clinics. Blood testing for HP is considered relatively inexpensive and thus is used by many physicians; however, it is only a screening test, as it tests for antibodies. The blood test cannot be used for testing whether bacteria have been eradicated after treatment because antibodies may persist for years even after HP has been eradicated.

The stool test for HP is also highly reliable and can be used to confirm after treatment that HP has been eradicated.

### Treating **Helicobacter pylori**

HP is a very resistant bacterium. Single-drug regimens are ineffective. Once HP has been diagnosed, physicians usually treat patients with combination therapy, with at least two and usually three or more antibiotics for about two weeks. Some doctors confirm that HP is truly eradicated from their patients after the treatment is complete by examining for HP with a stool antigen test or a breath test. A 2002 article in the *Annals of Internal Medicine* revealed that the stool antigen test successfully identifies patients who continue to be infected.

See also ANTIBIOTICS; BREATH TESTS; CANCER, STOMACH; DYSPEPSIA; ENZYME-LINKED IMMUNOSORBENT ASSAY; GASTRITIS; ULCERS, PEPTIC.

Minocha, Anil, M.D., et al. "Alterations in Upper Gastrointestinal Motility in *Helicobacter pylori*-Positive Nonulcer Dyspepsia." *American Journal of Gastroenterology* 89, no. 10 (1994): 1,797–1,800.

Minocha, Anil, M.D., et al. "*Helicobacter pylori* Is Associated with Alternations in Intestinal Gas Profile among Patients with Nonulcer Dyspepsia." *Digestive Diseases and Sciences* 39, no. 8 (August 1994): 1,613–1,617.

Minocha, Anil, M.D., C. A. Racakowski, M.D., and
    Robert J. Richards, M.D. "Is a History of Tonsillectomy
    Associated with a Decreased Risk of *Helicobacter pylori*
    Infection?" *Journal of Clinical Gastroenterology* 25, no. 4
    (1997): 580–582.
Uemura, Naomi, M.D., et al. "*Helicobacter Pylori* Infection
    and the Development of Gastric Cancer." *New England
    Journal of Medicine* 345, no. 11 (September 13, 2001):
    784–789.
Vaira, Dino, M.D., et al. "The Stool Antigen Test for
    Detection of Helicobacter pylori after Eradication
    Therapy." *Annals of Internal Medicine* 136, no. 4
    (February 19, 2002): 280–287.

**hemochromatosis**  A disease that is caused by
excessive absorption of iron from food with prefer-
ential deposition of the iron into the liver, pancreas,
heart, and other organs. If untreated, this disease
causes damage to these organs and others in the
body. In most cases, hemochromatosis is a hereditary
disease that is caused by a defect in the *HFE* gene. In
a few cases, the disease is not linked to this gene and
may or may not be hereditary. Hemochromatosis
increases the risk for development of cirrhosis
(liver inflammation) and liver cancer.

A secondary iron overload may be caused by
increased absorption of iron that is related to the
inability of the body to produce red blood cells adequately. It may also be related to chronic liver disease and sometimes to excessive use of iron
supplements. In some cases, an increased iron level
may be caused by repeated and multiple blood
transfusions or the administration of intravenous
iron. In cases of hereditary hemochromatosis,
symptoms do not appear until adulthood; non-
hereditary hemochromatosis may appear in infancy or childhood.

Neonatal hemochromatosis (NH), also called
neonatal iron storage disease, was first noted in
1957, but only about 100 cases have been identified since then. This medical problem is believed to
be related to an intrauterine infection that causes
babies to be born with excessive levels of iron in
their liver.

Babies who have NH are usually small for gesta-
tional age or premature. The pregnancy of their
mothers was often complicated by intrauterine
growth retardation, placental edema, or other serious problems. The baby's distress is usually noted
shortly after birth. Infants have liver failure,
hypoalbuminemia, hypoglycemia (low blood sugar
level). Usually ascites (fluid in the abdomen) and
hyperbilirubinemia develop. The prognosis of the
babies is poor and they usually die without liver
transplantation.

Another form of hemochromatosis is called
African iron overload, or bantu hemosiderosis,
which was once believed to be caused by an
increased level of iron that was absorbed through
the alcohol in iron drums. It is now believed
instead that this form of hemochromatosis is a
genetic disorder, but it is different from the disease
related to the *HFE* gene.

### Risk Factors for Hemochromatosis

Most people with hereditary hemochromatosis are
whites of Northern European descent. An estimated one in 200 whites carries the hemochromatosis
gene and is at risk for development of the disease.

Men have a five times greater risk of developing
hemochromatosis than women.

In general, the symptoms of hemochromatosis
do not appear until the age of 30 to 50 years for
men and after age 50 for women. In many cases,
people who are diagnosed with the disease have no
symptoms at the time of diagnosis. Some physicians see neonatal hemochromatosis (diagnosed in
some newborn babies) as distinct from the
hemochromatosis that is experienced by children
and adults.

### A Systemic Effect on the Body

When hemochromatosis continues untreated, it
affects the major organs of the body by causing
deposits of iron in the body tissues. As a result, the
following diseases may develop:

- Liver disease (cirrhosis, liver cancer, and liver
  failure)
- Pancreatic damage (which may cause diabetes)
- Low thyroid level
- Adrenal gland damage
- Cardiac problems, such as congestive heart
  failure or heart arrhythmias

- Impotence
- Early menopause
- Arthritis

### Diagnosis and Treatment

Diagnosis is usually delayed since symptoms do not develop until the late stages of hemochromatosis. When physicians observe that a patient has a constellation of abnormal blood tests or diseases that are commonly caused by hemochromatosis, they screen for the disease by ordering blood testing.

Physicians generally order the following tests to screen their patients for hemochromatosis: serum iron, serum transferrin, and serum ferritin. If tests show an abnormally high level of iron, doctors may then order a blood test that checks for the *HFE* genetic mutations. A positive test result confirms the presence of hemochromatosis, whereas a negative test result does not exclude hemochromatosis but does make it less likely. In addition, doctors may also order a liver biopsy to test for iron in the liver, to determine whether the liver is damaged, and, if it is, to evaluate the extent of damage.

The treatment for hemochromatosis sounds to many people like a throwback to medieval times: removing blood from the patient. Hemochromatosis is one of the few diseases in which patients actually benefit from bloodletting, which is technically called phlebotomy. In general, physicians order a pint of blood to be removed from adults once or twice a week for a few months or for as long as a year, depending on how severe the iron overload is in the body. Iron overload is monitored by serum ferritin levels. By decreasing the quantity of blood, and consequently blood and body iron, the body function stabilizes and in many cases returns to normal, although after the condition is stabilized, periodic phlebotomy every one to two months is required for life because the basic problem of excessive iron absorption is still present.

If the disease is treated in time, and before the development of liver cirrhosis, patients have a normal life expectancy. Patients start to feel better and have an increased energy level shortly after phlebotomy; however, patients with already damaged joints and hypogonadism do not revert to the predamaged condition.

Hemochromatosis patients should *never* take iron supplements, since their body is already naturally overloaded with iron. If patients have liver damage, they should also avoid alcohol so that the liver does not become overtaxed.

Most infants who have neonatal hemochromatosis die of the disease, although some infants have survived with liver transplantation. In one study of five infants who had liver transplantation, three survived a year later.

### Testing Siblings and Other Relatives

When one family member is diagnosed with hemochromatosis, his or her siblings should also be tested, since they are at high risk for the disease. In addition, the parents of the hemochromatosis patient as well as other genetic relatives should consult doctors about testing.

In one study of 214 homozygous relatives (test positive for hemochromatosis) of people diagnosed with hemochromatosis, primarily siblings, researchers found that 85 percent of the men and 68 percent of the women had iron overload and that a substantial number of them had conditions related to hemochromatosis that had yet to be detected clinically.

For further information, contact the following organizations:

American Hemochromatosis Society
777 East Atlantic Avenue
Suite Z-363
Delray Beach, FL 33484
(888) 665-IRON (toll-free) or (561) 266-9037
http://www.americanhs.org

American Liver Foundation
75 Maiden Lane
Suite 603
New York, NY 10038
(800) 465-4837 (toll-free) or (888) 443-7222
http://www.liverfoundation.org

Hemochromatosis Foundation, Inc.
P.O. Box 8569
Albany, NY 12208
(518) 489-0972
http://www.hemochromatosis.org

National Organization for Rare Disorders (NORD)
55 Kenosia Avenue
P.O. Box 1968
Danbury, CT 06813
(800) 999-6673 (toll-free) or (203) 744-0100
http://www.rarediseases.org

See also ANEMIA; CANCER, LIVER; CIRRHOSIS; DIGESTION AND ABSORPTION; IRON; VITAMIN DEFICIENCIES/EXCESSES.

Bulaj, Zaneta J., M.D., et al. "Disease-Related Conditions in Relatives of Patients with Hemochromatosis." *New England Journal of Medicine* 343, no. 21 (November 23, 2000): 1,529–1,535.

Murray, Karen F., M.D., and Kris V. Kowdley, M.D. "Neonatal Hemochromatosis." *Pediatrics* 108, no. 4 (October 2001): 960–964.

**hemorrhoids/hemorrhoidal disease**   Hemorrhoids are normal in the human body and present at birth. Hemorrhoids are a cushion of widened blood vessels called the hemorrhoidal plexus. However, when the term *hemorrhoids* is used, physicians and others are referring to hemorrhoidal disease, as when hemorrhoids are causing problems by becoming enlarged or irritated causing bleeding or when a blood clot forms within them.

Hemorrhoids are said to be internal when they are located inside the lower rectum, whereas hemorrhoids that are located around the anus are called external hemorrhoids. Both internal and external hemorrhoidal problems may coexist in the same patient.

Hemorrhoids cause few or no problems in most individuals. In some cases, however, they cause minor or severe painless bleeding, as well as pain and itching. Other features may include the protrusion of an internal hemorrhoid through the anus and pain resulting from the blood clots that lie within the hemorrhoids. Fecal soiling may also occur. The true incidence of hemorrhoidal problems is not known; it is believed that at least 4 percent of the adults in the United States experience such problems. Hemorrhoids occur in both sexes and are seen most commonly in people who are between 45 and 65 years old.

### Causes of Hemorrhoids

The exact cause of hemorrhoidal disease remains to be established. Some key risk factors include straining during defecation, chronic constipation or diarrhea, prolonged sitting, advancing age, pregnancy, and abdominal or pelvic tumors. Medications may indirectly cause hemorrhoids by drying out the stool and making passing it difficult.

### Diagnosis and Treatment

Hemorrhoidal disease is often diagnosed by a physician by taking a complete history of the patient and performing a physical examination, including a routine rectal examination. Anoscopy (examination of the anal canal) can be performed in the office.

Rectal bleeding, either overt or invisible, should not be automatically attributed to hemorrhoids, unless other causes such as cancer have been excluded since the two can coexist. Hemorrhoids can also be diagnosed during a routine sigmoidoscopy or colonoscopy, and such a procedure is usually performed not just to diagnose hemorrhoids but to exclude the presence of any other disease that might cause hemorrhoidal symptoms.

In many cases, patients can manage and improve their own hemorrhoids symptoms by taking specific actions, such as increasing the level of fiber in their diet as well as the quantity of water that they drink so that having bowel movements becomes easier. Some patients may also take laxatives or stool softener medications, if they are advised to do so by their physician.

Patients who are experiencing pain and itching from hemorrhoids may gain benefit from taking sitz baths (shallow soaking baths). Small tubs that fit over the toilet can be used for this purpose, or the patient may soak in the bathtub. Cold packs over the anal area may help, if they are recommended by the patient's doctor. Medicated over-the-counter (nonprescribed) suppositories can be purchased at pharmacies or prescribed. Because of the risk of side effects, creams and suppositories, especially those containing hydrocortisone, should not be used by patients longer than one week, unless recommended by a physician.

Patients are also advised to avoid sitting on the toilet for a long period. In addition, constipation should be prevented whenever possible, and regular exercise such as walking can often help with this problem.

Minimally invasive procedures for hemorrhoids include rubber band ligation, laser therapy, sclerotherapy (injection of chemicals into hemorrhoids to obliterate them), and cryosurgery.

Sometimes surgical removal of the hemorrhoids is needed, especially if the patient is experiencing severe and protruding hemorrhoids with frequent bleeding and pain and medical treatments are not relieving the symptoms. However, complications can follow surgery, and the physician weighs the risks versus the benefits of surgery before embarking on the surgical course.

See also CONSTIPATION; FECAL IMPACTION.

**hepatitis A, B, C, D, and E**    Inflammation of the liver that is caused by an infectious virus. Other viruses can also cause hepatitis; however, the five primary forms of viral hepatitis are hepatitis A, B, C, D, and E. (There are also causes of liver inflammation other than viruses, such as alcohol abuse and alcoholism and use of some drugs.) Chronic hepatitis B and C can lead to cirrhosis (inflammation of the liver), which, in turn, can cause liver cancer of the HEPATOCELLULAR CARCINOMA type.

### Hepatitis A

Hepatitis A is a common form. It is contracted through consuming food or water contaminated with the virus. Some outbreaks are attributed to the consumption of raw or half-cooked shellfish that are contaminated. Transmission of hepatitis A through blood and blood products is rare.

*Risk factors*    People who are at most risk for contracting hepatitis are those who fit one or more of the following categories. They are individuals who

- Reside with someone who has the disease
- Are children who attend day care
- Are adults who work in a day care center
- Are men who have sex with other men

- Travel to countries where hepatitis A is a common problem, particularly to poor countries where there is inadequate sanitation

*Symptoms of hepatitis A*    There are a range of symptoms that may be experienced by a person with hepatitis A. These symptoms are common to other illnesses, and only a physician can properly diagnose the presence of hepatitis, with appropriate laboratory tests. The common symptoms of hepatitis A include the following symptoms (not everyone has these symptoms, and most people with hepatitis A have no symptoms at all):

- Fatigue
- Nausea
- Lack of appetite
- Abdominal pain
- Diarrhea
- Easy bruising
- Headache
- Light-colored stools
- Fever
- Darkened urine
- Jaundice (yellowed eyes and skin)

*Diagnosis and treatment*    Hepatitis A can be diagnosed with a blood test to check for antibodies to hepatitis A. Levels of liver enzymes such as serum alanine aminotransferase (ALT) are typically elevated in individuals who have any form of viral hepatitis.

Treatment for acute hepatitis is supportive, and most patients do not require hospitalization unless the hepatitis is severe. Hepatitis patients must avoid all alcohol. This is because the liver metabolizes alcohol, and alcohol injures the liver by causing alcoholic hepatitis. As a result, since people with viral hepatitis have a liver that is already in a weakened condition, alcohol can further exacerbate the problem. Hepatitis A does not progress to chronic hepatitis.

*Prevention of hepatitis A*    Children and adults can be vaccinated against hepatitis. Children must be at least age two before they can receive the vaccine. Adults generally have a vaccination for hepatitis only if they are in a high-risk category: travelers going to an endemic area where hepatitis is known to be prevalent, children and adults living in endemic areas, and chronic liver disease patients.

Passive immunity can be quickly achieved by giving patients pooled immunoglobulin after an acute exposure to hepatitis A. Pooled immunoglobulin already includes the antibodies; it is used *after* the person has had a potential exposure, in order to provide immunity quickly against the virus that has already entered the system quickly. It is also given in cases when there is potential to be exposed soon (travel to endemic area).

Basic good hygiene can also protect against contracting hepatitis A, such as washing the hands before eating or before preparing food or after using the toilet. If a person travels to another country, it is best to drink only bottled water or soft drinks while there and to avoid using ice. Any fruits or vegetables should be thoroughly washed before they are eaten. It is best to eat fruits or vegetables that can be peeled, such as oranges or carrots.

### Hepatitis B

Another common form of hepatitis is hepatitis B, which is caused by the hepatitis B virus. Unlike hepatitis A, hepatitis B is caused by contact with body fluids of an infected person, such as the blood or the semen. Worldwide, there are an estimated 300 million persons infected with hepatitis B, or about 5 percent of the global population.

*Risk factors*   Individuals who are at risk for contracting hepatitis B are those who

- Have sex with an infected person without a condom
- Are men who have sex with other men
- Share a needle used by an infected person
- Have body piercing or a tattoo performed by a facility that reuses needles or tools used on an infected person
- Are born to a mother who has hepatitis B
- Have kidney dialysis

- Get a needle stick with infected blood (a problem for some health care workers)
- Are medical personnel
- Share a toothbrush with an infected person

*Symptoms*   The symptoms of hepatitis B are virtually identical to those of any other form of hepatitis, such as hepatitis A. Most patients with hepatitis B have no symptoms when they acquire the infection. Acute hepatitis can progress to chronic hepatitis and even cancer.

*Diagnosis and treatment*   A doctor who suspects hepatitis B may order blood tests to confirm the diagnosis. These tests check the blood for hepatitis B virus and/or antibodies against the virus. In some cases, the doctor also orders a liver biopsy, which is the removal of a small amount of tissue from the liver. The biopsy can show whether the virus is affecting the liver and, if so, how severely.

Hepatitis B patients are treated with injections of interferon or with oral medications such as lamivudine or adefovir. Some patients experience total liver failure and must have liver transplantation in order to stay alive. Hepatitis B also increases the risk for development of liver cancer.

*Prevention of hepatitis B*   Vaccines for hepatitis B can protect individuals from the disease. These vaccines are given to newborn infants, as well as to older children and adults. Universal vaccination of all newborns is the rule. Catch-up vaccination implies vaccination of children who were born before universal neonatal vaccination was implemented amd most of these children are schoolage. The vaccine is given in three injections spread over about six months. All three shots must be received for protection against hepatitis B.

Behavioral ways to protect against contracting hepatitis B include the following:

- Using a condom when having sex
- Avoiding using needles that have been used by others to self-inject drugs
- Avoiding using the personal items of another person, such as a toothbrush, razor, or any item that could have any blood on its surface

- Not having body piercing or tattooing, or, if they are done, making sure that the person doing the piercing or tattooing uses clean tools by observing that they are removed from sterile packaging

### Hepatitis C

A very common viral infection of the liver, hepatitis C is caused by the hepatitis C virus. It is transmitted through body fluids, such as blood. The sexual transmission of hepatitis C is uncommon. There are an estimated four million people in the United States who are infected with hepatitis C. About 28,000 new infections of hepatitis C are estimated to occur each year.

Chronic hepatitis develops in about 60 to 85 percent of the cases of hepatitis C. In about 10 to 20 percent of hepatitis C patients cirrhosis of the liver develops over time (about 20 years). This risk is accelerated if patients are diagnosed when they are older than age 50, and the risk is further exacerbated if they consume alcohol or have concurrent hepatitis or a human immunodeficiency virus (HIV) infection.

According to Zamani and Herrine in their chapter in *20 Common Problems in Gastroenterology,* "Chronic hepatitis C, accompanied by cirrhosis and hepatic [liver] failure, is the leading indication for liver transplantation in adults in the United States, accounting for 30 to 40 percent of cases at most transplant centers."

**Risk factors**   Individuals who are at risk for contracting hepatitis C include the following groups:

- Those who have injected drugs with needles that were used by others
- People who have experienced a prick from a needle that has infected blood (a problem faced by some health care workers)
- Infants born to a woman who has hepatitis C
- People who have had tattoos or body piercings performed by people using equipment infected with hepatitis C (new needles and sterilized equipment should be used for each person)
- Individuals who had blood transfusions or organ transplantation before 1990 in the United

States or Canada or in the present in poor countries
- People who use intranasal cocaine
- People who have kidney dialysis
- Rarely, those who have had sexual contact, especially if one or both partners have other sexually transmitted diseases (however, the risk is minimal to nonexistent if a couple have been in a monogamous relationship for more than five years and the infected person has not yet transmitted the hepatitis to the partner)

There are several different forms of hepatitis C. Genotype 1 is the predominant form found in the United States. It causes more severe disease and is more refractory to medical treatment. Genotypes 2 and 3 cause less severe disease among infected individuals, and these forms of hepatitis C also respond to treatment better.

**Symptoms and signs**   Most people who have hepatitis C have no symptoms or signs until the advanced stages of liver disease. Those who do have symptoms experience the same nonspecific flulike symptoms experienced by hepatitis A or B patients: fatigue, abdominal pain, fever, lack of appetite, and diarrhea

**Diagnosis and treatment**   Physicians usually detect hepatitis C through a blood test. If hepatitis C is found, the physician may order a liver biopsy to determine how severe the hepatitis is and whether the liver has sustained damage.

Hepatitis C is usually treated with two medications, interferon and ribavarin, unless the case is very mild. In that instance, physicians may postpone treatment while they continue to monitor the patient. If the liver is very damaged, the patient may need liver transplantation.

**Prevention of hepatitis C**   There is no vaccine that is available against hepatitis C as of this writing. Actions that an individual can take to limit the risks of contracting hepatitis C are as follows:

- Never share drug needles
- Wear surgical gloves if the blood of another person must be touched
- Avoid using another person's toothbrush or other item that may have blood on it

- Avoid body piercing or tattooing or make sure that the equipment used is sterile
- If having sex with multiple partners, make sure that males use condoms

### Hepatitis D

Hepatitis D is a rare form that is mostly found in Southern Italy, some areas of the former Soviet Union, and Romania. Hepatitis D is primarily spread through the sharing of contaminated needles for drug use. It is also known as the delta virus. It does not occur independently, but only as a coinfection in patients who also have hepatitis B. Hepatitis D may infect the subject at the same time that he or she is infected with hepatitis B, or chronic hepatitis B patients may be infected later with hepatitis D. Worldwide, 5 percent of hepatitis B carriers also have hepatitis D.

*Symptoms*   The symptoms of acute hepatitis D are the same as those of all other forms of hepatitis.

*Diagnosis and treatment*   Diagnosis can be made with blood tests for the virus. Interferon alfa is used for treatment of patients who are candidates for this therapy such as patients with chronic hepatitis D and active liver disease as evidenced by abnormal liver enzymes and/or chronic hepatitis on liver biopsy. This is because chronic hepatitis D can be a severe liver disease, and interferon treatment is more likely to be effective in patients with a short duration of infection. Asymptomatic hepatitis D carriers with normal liver enzyme levels do not require therapy, but should be observed to see if more active liver disease develops. The role of foscarnet (Foscavir) in treatment appears promising.

Prevention of hepatitis D involves the same measures used to prevent hepatitis B.

### Hepatitis E

A form of hepatitis that is rare in the United States and Canada, hepatitis E is transmitted through contaminated water or food.

*Risk factors*   Person-to-person transmission of hepatitis E is uncommon. International travelers and people living in areas where there is an outbreak of hepatitis E are at risk for contracting hepatitis E.

*Symptoms and signs*   The symptoms of hepatitis E infection are the same as those of hepatitis A,

B, and C. Often there are no symptoms. Fulminant liver failure may occur, especially among pregnant females.

*Diagnosis and treatment*   Doctors can diagnose the presence of hepatitis E with blood tests. There is no specific treatment for the illness, and generally supportive care is provided. Most patients improve within days to weeks. No chronic hepatitis is caused by hepatitis E.

*Prevention of hepatitis E*   There is no vaccine for hepatitis E. International travelers should avoid drinking tap water while in other countries and should wash their hands before eating or preparing food and after using the toilet.

For more information, contact the following organizations:

American Liver Foundation
75 Maiden Lane
Suite 603
New York, NY 10038
(800) 465-4837 (toll-free)
http://www.liverfoundation.org

Centers for Disease Control and Prevention (CDC)
National Center for Infectious Diseases
Hepatitis Branch
1600 Clifton Road
Atlanta, GA 30333
(888) 443-7232 (toll-free)

Hepatitis B Foundation
700 East Butler Avenue
Doylestown, PA 18901
http://www.hepb.org

Hepatitis Foundation International
504 Blick Drive
Silver Spring, MD 20904
(800-891) 0707 (toll-free) or (301) 622-4200
http://www.hepfi.org

National Digestive Diseases Information
    Clearinghouse
2 Information Way
Bethesda, MD 20892
(800) 891-5389 (toll-free)

See also CIRRHOSIS; LIVER; LIVER FAILURE; LIVER TRANSPLANTATION.

Farci, Patrizia, et al. "Treatment of Chronic Hepatitis D with Interferon Alfa-2a." *New England Journal of Medicine* 330, no. 2 (January 13, 1994): 88–94.

Herrine, Steven K., M.D. "Approach to the Patient with Chronic Hepatitis C Virus Infection," *Annals of Internal Medicine* 136, no. 10 (May 21, 2002): 747–757.

Charles S. Lieber, M.D. "Alcohol and Hepatitis C." *Alcohol Research & Health* 25, no. 4 (2001): 245–254.

Zamani, Saeed, and Steven K. Herrine. "Viral Hepatitis." In *20 Common Problems in Gastroenterology.* New York: McGraw-Hill Medical Publishing Division, 2002.

**hepatocellular carcinoma (HCC)**  The most prominent form of liver cancer, representing about 70 percent of all liver cancers. It is also known as malignant hepatoma or simply hepatoma and as primary liver cancer. Hepatocellular carcinoma (HCC) is usually associated with cirrhosis of the liver that stems from infection with chronic HEPATITIS B and C or from chronic alcoholism or diseases such as HEMOCHROMATOSIS. In addition, infection with hepatitis B increases the risk for hepatocellular carcinoma even if the liver has no evidence of cirrhosis. HCC occurs more frequently among men.

The researchers El-Sarag and Mason studied risk factors for an increase in the rate of hepatocellular cancer between 1993 and 1998 and reported their findings in *Archives of Internal Medicine* in 2000. They considered the increase from an incidence of 36.4 patients per 100,000 between 1993 and 1995 to 47.5 patients per 100,000 between 1996 and 1998. The researchers found that hepatitis C represented most of the cause of the increase. They found that the rates for liver cancer patients who also had either alcoholic cirrhosis or hepatitis B infection stayed about the same.

In this study, of 1,605 patients in the Veterans Administration (VA) Medical Center patient files in the United States who were diagnosed with primary liver cancer, nearly all (99.5 percent) were men. Note: because of the specific population that VA hospitals serve (military veterans), most of their patients are males. The average age of the patients was 64 years. Most of the patients were white (65 percent), followed by blacks (21 percent) and Hispanics (10 percent). Only 1 percent of the patients were Native American and 1 percent were Asians. In 2 percent of the cases, the race of the patient was unknown.

The researchers found that half of the patients had hepatitis C. The major risk factors for other patients with hepatocellular carcinoma were cirrhosis, autoimmune hepatitis, and hepatitis B infection. According to the researchers, in about a third of hepatitis C patients cirrhosis develops, and the interval from contracting of hepatitis C to development of cirrhosis is about 20 years. When a patient has cirrhosis, the annual risk of development of hepatocellular cancer is about 1 to 4 percent.

Another study, of patients in Taiwan, including 111 male patients who had recently been diagnosed with hepatocellular cancer, was described in a 2002 issue of the *New England Journal of Medicine.* The researchers found a higher risk for development of hepatocellular carcinoma among patients who had a positive finding of infection with hepatitis B e antigen (HBeAg). In addition, if patients had positive findings for both hepatitis B e antigen and hepatitis B surface antigen (HBsAg), the risk escalated markedly. The blood can be tested for hepatitis BeAg and hepatitis B surface antigen, as well as for antibodies against them. The presence of such antibodies indicates that immunity is present.

Among the patients who had a negative result for either hepatitis B e antigen or hepatitis B surface antigen, the incidence of hepatocellular carcinoma was 39.1 per 100,000 people. Among those with a positive result for HBsAg but a negative result for HBeAg, the incidence increased dramatically to 324.4 per 100,000. When patients had positive results for *both* HBsAg and HBeAg, the risk rose greatly: to 1,169.4 per 100,000 patients. Thus, the researchers concluded that both HBeAg and HBsAg may be important risk markers of those in whom hepatocellular carcinoma develops. Selected patients with this form of cancer may be candidates for liver transplantation.

See also CANCER; CANCER, LIVER; CIRRHOSIS; LIVER; LIVER FAILURE; LIVER TRANSPLANTATION.

El-Sarag, Hashem B., M.D., and Andrew C. Mason, M.D. "Risk Factors for the Rising Rates of Primary Liver Cancer in the United States." *Archives of Internal Medicine* 160 (November 27, 2000): 3,227–3,230.

Yang, Hwai-I, et al. "Hepatitis B e Antigen and the Risk of Hepatocellular Carcinoma." *New England Journal of Medicine* 347, no. 3 (July 18, 2002): 168–174.

**hereditary pancreatitis**  An inherited condition that causes inflammation of the pancreas. Cases of hereditary pancreatitis constitute only a small fraction of all cases of pancreatitis. The condition usually appears before the 20th birthday (usually around age 10) and in some cases may appear before the age of five years. The condition may be mild at first, with increasingly severe occurrences of attacks.

Computed tomography (CT) and ultrasound scans help doctors to diagnose pancreatitis, but these imaging tests do not indicate that the illness is hereditary. An ENDOSCOPIC RETROGRADE CHOLANGIOPANCREATOGRAPHY (ERCP) may be needed in some cases, especially to determine whether surgery is indicated. Genetic testing for hereditary pancreatitis may be undertaken after obtaining full informed consent from a child's parents or guardian.

See also PANCREAS; PANCREATITIS.

**hernia, hiatal**  A medical condition that is caused by the sliding of a section of the upper part of the stomach into the chest through an opening in the diaphragm (esophageal hiatus). It may be a very dangerous condition, but in most cases, hiatal hernias are not symptomatic, and they remain undiagnosed and are not a problem for most people who have them.

The hiatal hernia may be a sliding hernia or a paraesophageal hiatal hernia. In sliding hiatal hernia, part of the stomach along with the junction of the stomach and the esophagus slide up into the chest. In the case of paraesophageal hiatal hernia, the junction stays at the level of the DIAPHRAGM, whereas part of the stomach moves into the chest cavity.

### *Risk Factors*

People who are obese have a greater risk of development of hiatal hernia than others. The presence of GASTROESOPHAGEAL REFLUX DISEASE (GERD) worsens a hiatal hernia.

### *Symptoms*

As mentioned, in most cases, there are no symptoms or signs of a hiatal hernia. A few patients may have ulcers in the hernia and may experience gastrointestinal bleeding as well as ANEMIA. The paraesophageal hernia can become twisted in a life-threatening fashion, and the patient may enter an emergency room with severe upper abdominal pain.

### *Diagnosis and Treatment*

If hiatal hernias cause severe symptoms, they can be surgically repaired. In many cases, the surgery can be performed laparoscopically, through small incisions that are made in the abdomen. In many cases, however, the treatment for the hiatal hernia is the same as for GERD; for example, physicians recommend lifestyle changes, such as advising obese patients to lose weight, which may result in the reduction of the hiatal hernia, along with recommending acid blocking drugs.

For further information on hiatal hernias, contact the following organizations:

American College of Gastroenterology
4900-B South 31st Street
Arlington, VA 22206
(703) 820-7400
http://www.acg.gi.org

American Gastroenterological Association
7910 Woodmont Avenue
Suite 700
Bethesda, MD 20814
(301) 654-2055
http://www.gastro.org

Minocha, Anil, M.D., and Christine Adamec. *How to Stop Heartburn: Simple Ways to Heal Heartburn and Acid Reflux.* New York: John Wiley & Sons, 2001.

**Hirschsprung's disease (HD)**   A severe disease of the colon that causes a loss of nerve cells in part of the colon/rectum and is usually diagnosed for the first time in infants or small children and occasionally in adults. The disease was named after Harald Hirschsprung, a Danish pediatrician who wrote about the condition in 1888. In the case of infants and children who have the disease, a PEDIATRIC GASTROENTEROLOGIST should be consulted for treatment. Adults should be treated by a GASTROENTEROLOGIST.

The disease causes severe constipation, and sometimes the child who has Hirschsprung's disease (HD) is unable to have bowel movements; blockage and backup result. This condition may lead to abdominal distention and even perforation of the colon, which may be fatal to the child. The problem is caused by the damaged or destroyed nerve cells in the rectum/colon. The affected part does not relax to accommodate the passage of stool, causing functional obstruction. Only a small segment of the rectum and the sigmoid colon is involved in about 75 percent of cases; however, in about 10 percent of cases of Hirschsprung's disease, the entire colon is affected.

Hirschsprung's disease occurs in about one in every 5,000 births. About 20 percent of infants born with HD die in infancy.

### Risk Factors

Familial forms of Hirschsprung's disease stem from a genetic mutation that leads to lack of function in part of the colon; usually all children in a family do not have the disease. Several different genetic mutations have been identified in patients with HD. The disease may also occur sporadically, with no known familial relationship. Researchers say that it is not caused by anything that a pregnant woman does or does not do during her pregnancy.

Females are about four times more likely to be diagnosed with this medical problem than males. Hirschsprung's disease is associated with some cases of Down syndrome, and it occurs in about 6 percent of individuals diagnosed with Down syndrome.

### Symptoms

The majority of cases of Hirschsprung's disease present within the first few weeks of birth. Among newborns, infants with Hirschsprung's disease may vomit green bile after eating and may also have a swollen abdomen. There may be a delay in the passage of the first stool. These infants may have problems with DEHYDRATION and FAILURE TO THRIVE. These babies are usually very fussy because they are extremely uncomfortable as a result of both gas and constipation.

Small children and school-age children who have Hirschsprung's disease also have major problems with constipation, although some may have diarrhea at some times. In addition, children with this disease usually have slower growth and development rates than other children their own age.

Infants and children who have Hirschsprung's disease may contract a severe, life-threatening infection called enterocolitis. If a child who has the disease shows any of the following indicators, the physician should be called immediately:

- Bleeding from the rectum
- Swollen abdomen
- Vomiting
- Diarrhea
- Fever

Adults and adolescents who have Hirschsprung's disease may be severely constipated. Adults also may have a dilated colon and rectum caused by the disease.

### Diagnosis and Treatment

Doctors may suspect Hirschsprung's disease because of a patient's symptoms and/or a family medical history of HD, although other medical problems, such as IRRITABLE BOWEL SYNDROME (IBS), in adults may be diagnosed instead unless tests are ordered.

The barium X ray is one test used to diagnose Hirschsprung's disease; in this test, barium is inserted into the anus and the colon so that the physician can take X rays in which the barium highlights the colon. The barium enema reveals the narrow affected area of the colon/rectum and the proximal dilated colon. If a patient has a chronic problem with severe constipation, particularly a newborn baby who is suffering from chronic severe constipation, the physician may use diatrizoate meglumine (Gastrografin) rather than barium. Gastrografin is a water-soluble contrast dye that has the effect of a stool softener as well as a highlighter of the intestine on X rays.

Anorectal manometry to test for pressure–relaxation responses in the anorectal region is a test that is done on adults. A biopsy is considered to be the best diagnostic tool for HD. The biopsy result shows whether nerve cells are missing from the colon/rectum and definitively proves the presence of HD when it is present.

Surgery is usually the treatment of choice for HD. There are different methods of performing the procedure; all involve removing the damaged part of the intestine and then connecting the healthy intestine as close as possible to the anus to preserve the anal sphincter.

An estimated 70 to 90 percent of children are able to have five or fewer stools daily after the operation. Some children have diarrhea for a while, and others may subsequently have problems with constipation. These problems can usually be treated by a physician who orders stool softeners or other medications for the patient. There is a minimal operative mortality rate, and long-term problems, such as fecal soiling, occur in about 10 percent of patients.

For further information, contact the following organizations:

International Foundation for Functional
    Gastrointestinal Disorders, Inc. (IFFGD)
P.O. Box 170864
Milwaukee, WI 53217
(888) 964-2001 (toll-free)
http://www.iffgd.org

Pull-thru Network
2312 Savoy Street
Hoover, AL 35226
(205) 978-2930
http://www.pullthrough.org

See also DIARRHEA; FAILURE TO THRIVE.

Eng, Charis, M.D., "The *RET* Proto-Oncogene in Multiple Endocrine Neoplasia Type 2 and Hirschsprung's Disease." *New England Journal of Medicine* 335, no. 13 (September 20, 1996): 943–51.

Wynbrandt, James, and Mark D. Ludman, *The Encyclopedia of Genetic Disorders and Birth Defects.* 2d ed. New York: Facts On File, 2000.

**histamine-2 blockers**    Medications that block the acid secretion caused by body chemicals known as histamines. Histamine-2 blockers (H-2 blockers) are used to treat such patients as those who have chronic acid reflux problems, gastroesophageal reflux disease (GERD), or peptic ulcer. Treatment may be short term or long term, depending on the clinical situation. Patients who do not respond well to H-2 blockers are treated with more potent acid blockers called proton pump inhibitors.

The commonly known H-2 blockers include cimetidine (Tagamet), ranitidine (Zantac), famotidine (Pepcid), and nizatidine (Axid). H-2 blockers cut back on the production of acid in the stomach, allowing the ulcerated stomach to heal and helping the patient with GERD to feel better.

H-2 blockers are also available over-the-counter although the doses are lower than prescribed drugs. Studies have shown that prescribed H-2 blockers are effective in about half of cases of GERD. Sometimes over-the-counter H-2 blockers, including Tagamet HB, Zantac 75, and Pepcid AC, may be used for occasional indigestion.

See also ACID BLOCKING AGENTS; ACID REFLUX; GASTROESOPHAGEAL REFLUX DISEASE; PROTON PUMP INHIBITORS; ULCERS.

**hoarseness**    Difficulty with normal speaking. Hoarseness occurs as a result of disease of the voice box or larynx. Laryngitis may be caused by a viral infection or by a digestive disorder, such as GASTROESOPHAGEAL REFLUX DISEASE.

See also DYSPHAGIA.

**hormones**    Chemical messengers that are produced by the body or manufactured synthetically and that travel through the bloodstream to their site of action. For example, thyroid hormone is naturally produced by most people; however, in some people the body produces insufficient amounts of thyroid hormone and they need supplemental thyroid to survive. In contrast, others may produce too much thyroid hormone, and then the thyroid gland needs to be suppressed. Both President George H. W. Bush and his wife, Barbara Bush, had overactive thyroid gland, for which they were treated.

Adrenaline is a hormone that is naturally produced by the body, but in some cases, such as a severe allergic reaction, an injection of adrenaline or a similar substance is needed to supplement the sudden increase in demand for the body's adrenaline production to combat acute illness.

Insulin is a hormone that is produced by the pancreas and is required for glucose metabolism. A deficiency of insulin production leads to diabetes mellitus.

The key digestive hormones are cholecystokinin (CCK), gastrin, and secretin.

See also CHOLESCYSTOKININ; DIABETES MELLITUS; GASTRIN; HORMONE THERAPY; SECRETIN.

**hormone therapy**    Usually refers to the female hormones (estrogen or estrogen/progesterone combinations) that are given to women to resolve troubling symptoms of menopause; however, hormones may also be given as supplements for other conditions. Female hormones are also administered for the prevention of osteoporosis (the loss of bone density) to women who cannot tolerate the other drugs. Combination hormone replacement therapy increases the risk for the development of breast cancer, stroke and venous thrombosis.

Some people are deficient in thyroid hormone and need supplemental thyroid hormone to reach a normal level. Patients with type 1 diabetes are deficient in insulin and are treated with insulin injections, which they are trained to do themselves. Some men may become deficient in testosterone, which can be supplemented with testosterone hormone therapy. It is also true that women have a low level of testosterone present in their body, just as men have a low level of estrogen.

When female hormones are given, they are usually administered by a primary care physician or gynecologist. Other hormones, such as thyroid hormones or growth hormones, are likely to be monitored by an endocrinologist.

See also MENOPAUSE.

**human immunodeficiency virus**    The virus (HIV) that leads to acquired immunodeficiency syndrome (AIDS). HIV is transmitted through sexual contact as well as through sharing of contaminated needles or through blood, such as in a blood transfusion from contaminated blood. Individuals who have HIV are at risk for development of CACHEXIA, a state in which weight loss and body wasting occur.

Once AIDS develops, the patient's immune system is compromised and the person has a high risk for the development of infections that may become fatal. Until recently, all HIV was uniformly fatal. However, today once HIV is diagnosed, patients are started on treatment against HIV to suppress it, and they may live for a long time. The famous basketball star Earvin "Magic" Johnson was diagnosed with HIV in the late 1980s and as of 2004 appeared to be doing extremely well with treatment.

See also ACQUIRED IMMUNODEFICIENCY SYNDROME; KAPOSI'S SARCOMA.

**Hymenolepis nana (H. nana)**    A dwarf tapeworm that infects individuals worldwide and is spread by bad or insufficient sanitation and poor personal hygiene. It is most common in Asia and Latin America, although it is also found among some low-income children in the United States. It is more commonly found among children than adults.

Infected individuals have abdominal pain, diarrhea, pruritus ani (itching at the anus), and poor appetite. Some patients experience sleep disorders, dizziness, and seizures. The diagnosis is made by finding *H. nana* eggs in the stool.

Those who have *Hymenolepis nana* are treated with praziquantel given in a single dose and repeated in 10 days, which is effective in 95 percent of the cases of patients infected with this tapeworm.

See also PARASITIC INFECTIONS.

**hyperalgesia** A greatly increased sensitivity to pain; for example, a patient who has IRRITABLE BOWEL SYNDROME (IBS) may experience pain if the bowels are stimulated by the mild inflation of a balloon, whereas this same stimulus would not be perceived as painful by someone who does not have IBS. A similar condition is seen in many patients who have noncardiac chest pain or functional dyspepsia. FIBROMYALGIA patients may also experience hyperalgesia.

See also PAIN.

**hyperemesis gravidarum** A condition of severe vomiting that usually occurs in the first trimester of pregnancy and is far more severe than the expected "morning sickness" that many pregnant women experience. The cause of hyperemesis gravidarum is unknown, although the condition is considered a pregnancy-associated liver disease. In extreme cases of the disease, hyperemesis gravidarum may cause patients to experience DEHYDRATION, MALNUTRITION, and even death. Most women with hyperemesis gravidarum recover in the second trimester of pregnancy.

An estimated 1 percent of all pregnant women experience hyperemesis gravidarum.

### Risk Factors

Pregnant women who are below the age of 25 years have a greater risk of development of hyperemesis gravidarum than older pregnant women. In addition, women who have had multiple pregnancies also have a greater risk. The cause of hyperemesis gravidarum is unknown, but psychogenic as well as hormonal factors and nutritional deficiencies have been implicated.

### Symptoms and Signs

In addition to the nausea and the severe vomiting that are characteristic of hyperemesis gravidarum, abdominal pain and mild jaundice may be present. Many women with this condition also have GASTROESOPHAGEAL REFLUX DISEASE (GERD). Other symptoms and signs are as follows:

- Dehydration
- Deficiencies of vitamins and minerals
- Loss of more than 5 percent of body weight
- Abnormal liver enzyme values (in up to half of women who have hyperemesis gravidarum)
- Hyperbilirubinemia (high level of bilirubin in the blood, which is found in about half of women who are hospitalized for hyperemesis gravidarum)

### Diagnosis and Treatment

Physicians diagnose hyperemesis gravidarum on the basis of medical history, symptoms, and findings of a physical examination that is supplemented by laboratory tests, such as liver function tests. Blood levels may be abnormal among pregnant women with this condition, such as elevated levels of bilirubin, alkaline phosphatase, and aminotransferases.

Many women with hyperemesis gravidarum need to be hospitalized so that symptoms such as dehydration and electrolyte imbalance can be reversed with intravenous infusions of needed fluids. Pyridoxine (vitamin $B_6$), ginger and antihistamines are commonly prescribed as a treatment. Antiemetic medications are also administered to stop vomiting, and GERD patients may need to take PROTON PUMP INHIBITOR medications, prokinetic drugs, or histamine-2 receptor blocker drugs.

Some patients may need total PARENTERAL NUTRITION (feeding through the veins). Because most but not all women recover from hyperemesis gravidarum by the second trimester, the goal of most physicians is to stabilize their condition until that time.

See also LIVER ENZYMES/FUNCTION TESTS; NAUSEA AND VOMITING; PREGNANCY.

Knox, Tamsin A., M.D., and Lori B. Olans, M.D. "Liver Disease in Pregnancy." *New England Journal of Medicine* 335, no. 8 (August 22, 1996): 569–576.

**hypergastrinemia** Excessively high blood level of gastrin, a gastrointestinal hormone that stimulates the secretion of gastric acid. Blood tests such as the serum gastrin level can determine whether patients are within the normal range; among patients who have fasted, serum gastrin levels are usually less than 100 pg/ml (picograms per milliliter).

If patients have a higher level of serum gastrin, they may have ZOLLINGER–ELLISON SYNDROME. They may also have renal insufficiency, PERNICIOUS ANEMIA, or a gastric outlet obstruction. Hypergastrinemia patients may also have MULTIPLE ENDOCRINE NEOPLASIA. If patients are taking high doses of proton pump inhibitor medications, the test result indicates hypergastrinemia that is medication induced, which is not considered a problem.

See also GASTRIN; PROTON PUMP INHIBITORS.

**hypoalbuminemia** Below-normal level of albumin in the blood that is caused by liver disease, malnutrition, or severe kidney disease. Hypoalbuminemia may result in fluid buildup in the body including in the abdomen (ASCITES). Individuals who have a low serum albumin level have a high risk for complications of any surgery.

See also ALBUMIN.

**ileoanal pouch**   A pouch that comprises part of the small intestine and is connected to the anal canal. The procedure to create this pouch is usually done for ulcerative colitis patients. The ileoanal pouch is also known as the ileoanal reservoir. It is created in a process that is performed to remove the colon, the upper rectum, and most of the lower rectum. The surgeon then creates the ileoanal pouch from the small intestines so that it can hold the patient's stools, allowing continent function. Depending on how the pouch is constructed, it is sometimes called the J pouch, W pouch, or S pouch. The pouch may become inflamed in some cases, a condition called POUCHITIS.

See also ULCERATIVE COLITIS.

**imaging studies**   Radiologic diagnostic tests such as X rays, computed tomography (CT) scans, and magnetic resonance imaging (MRI) scans. Such tests are used to identify defects or diseases in the digestive system (as well as other systems). They are sometimes also used as part of therapy, for example, to assist a physician in performing a procedure such as a liver biopsy, PARACENTESIS, and drainage of an abscess. Radiologic imaging may be combined with endoscopic procedures, as in ERCP and endoscopic ultrasound.

**imperforate anus**   A defect that is present at birth in which the anal canal has not developed and the opening of the anus is closed. Surgery is required to create a normal anus.

**infants**   Babies may experience a broad range of digestive diseases and disorders, but of greatest concern are those illnesses that are severe or even life-threatening to the infant. Examples of such diseases and disorders include CELIAC SPRUE, food allergies, neonatal HEMOCHROMATOSIS (an iron overload in the blood of newborns), HIRSCHSPRUNG'S DISEASE, NECROTIZING ENTEROCOLITIS, and VITAMIN DEFICIENCIES. In addition, in some poor countries, untreated DIARRHEA and other infections may be sufficient to dehydrate and even kill some newborns.

See also ALLERGIES, FOOD; DEHYDRATION; INTUSSUSCEPTION.

**inflammatory bowel disease (IBD)**   A common disorder of the colon or the small intestine. It is often characterized by DIARRHEA, abdominal pain, bleeding, and other symptoms. The two primary types of illnesses that constitute chronic idiopathic inflammatory bowel disease are CROHN'S DISEASE and ULCERATIVE COLITIS.

Ulcerative colitis involves only parts of the colon and rectum, whereas Crohn's disease can involve any part of the gastrointestinal system from the mouth to the anus. As a result, the surgical removal of the colon and the rectum is curative for ulcerative colitis, whereas there is no known cure for Crohn's disease.

Inflammatory bowel disease patients can have involvement of the organs outside the gut, such as eye problems (uveitis, episcleritis), arthritis, kidney stones, a skin rash such as ERYTHEMA NODOSUM, autoimmune hepatitis, and PRIMARY SCLEROSING CHOLANGITIS. Individuals with inflammatory bowel disease also have an increased risk of development of colorectal cancer. In addition, researchers reporting their findings in 2000 in the *Annals of Internal Medicine* revealed that their patients with IBD (more than 6,000 subjects) had a significantly increased risk of having osteopenia (low bone density) and a 40 percent greater risk of experiencing hip fractures than those without IBD. They also had a higher rate of other bone fractures.

Although often confused with it, inflammatory bowel disease is not the same as irritable bowel syndrome (IBS), which is usually a condition of disturbed bowel habit (chronic constipation or diarrhea or constipation that fluctuates with diarrhea) associated with abdominal pain. IBS does not cause any grossly evident damage to the colon; nor does it cause an increased risk of development of colorectal cancer. In contrast, IBD is manifested with visible damage to the involved portions of the small and/or the large intestine and may also affect other organs such as the skin, the eyes, the liver, the gallbladder, and the joints.

See also CANCER, COLORECTAL; CELIAC SPRUE; ILEOANAL POUCH.

Bernstein, Charles N., M.D., et al. "The Incidence of Fracture among Patients with Inflammatory Bowel Disease: A Population-Based Cohort Study." *Annals of Internal Medicine* 133, no. 10 (November 21, 2000): 795–799.

Podolsky, Daniel K., M.D. "Inflammatory Bowel Disease." *New England Journal of Medicine* 347, no. 6 (August 8, 2002): 417–429.

**interferon**   A substance that is naturally produced by the body and is useful in maintaining the body's immune defenses. It can also be given in the form of a drug to combat some kinds of infections and cancers. Some patients who have forms of hepatitis, primarily hepatitis B, C, and D, are treated with interferon. The pegylated form of interferon is a long-acting interferon that is required only once a week, in contrast to conventional interferon given to treat hepatitis C, which is administered three times a week.

Patients who have some other diseases, including melanoma, advanced renal (kidney) cancer, certain kinds of leukemia, and multiple sclerosis, are also treated with interferon.

See also ACQUIRED IMMUNODEFICIENCY SYNDROME; HEPATITIS.

**intussusception**   A very severe medical problem in which part of the intestines becomes wrapped up by another part, causing an intestinal obstruction and sometimes bleeding. Some cases are fatal, if not treated quickly. When it occurs, intussusception is primarily a problem among infants ages three to five months old. Eighty percent of pediatric intussusceptions involve the ileum (the last part of the small intestine) and the colon. Infants who have this problem appear to be in abdominal distress. They vomit bilious material and have stools that resemble currant jelly.

In some cases, the baby has an intestinal defect, such as Meckel's diverticulum; in most cases, the cause of the intussusception is unknown.

Intussusception can also occur in adults; when it does, there is usually involvement of a distinct diseased part of the gut, and cancer occurs in up to one-half of these adults.

Some experts believe that respiratory adenovirus and rotavirus gastroenteritis can trigger intussusception. In one circumstance reported in 1999 in *Morbidity and Mortality Weekly Report*, a rotavirus vaccine that was given to infants apparently caused intussusception in some at a rate that was higher than was normally seen. The vaccine was withdrawn from the market.

Depending on the severity of the intussusception, some children can be treated with just an enema, whereas others will require hospitalization and may need surgery.

See also INFANTS.

Centers for Disease Control and Prevention. "Intussusception among Recipients of Rotavirus Vaccine—United States, 1998–1999." *Morbidity and Mortality Report* 48 (1999): 577–581.

Parashar, Umesh D., et al. "Trends in Intussusception-Associated Hospitalizations and Deaths among US Infants." *Pediatrics* 106, no. 6 (December 2000): 1,413–1,421.

**ipecac, syrup of**   Drug that is derived from the ipecacuanha plant grown in Brazil. Syrup of ipecac is used to induce vomiting and is sold as an over-the-counter drug in most pharmacies and supermarkets. It may also cause nausea and diarrhea, in addition to the expected copious vomiting.

Ipecac is an over-the-counter drug that is primarily used to treat children or others who have ingested certain poisons and overdoses, in order to eliminate the poison quickly. Pediatricians may recommend that parents have ipecac syrup on hand in the event their toddlers or small children ingest poison; however, the use of ipecac has declined in recent years.

Ipecac should only be given to children older than six months old who are alert and who may have taken a toxic level of poison. Ipecac should not be administered unless a physician or the Poison Control Center specifically recommends it, because inducing vomiting is not the best course of action in all cases of poison ingestion. In fact, ipecac may be harmful if used with certain poisons, such as when a person has ingested caustic items such as bleach. Ipecac must *not* be used for an unconscious person; the person should be active and moving about before ipecac should be considered.

Ipecac is sometimes used by patients who have EATING DISORDERS, in order to induce vomiting, especially among those who have BULIMIA NERVOSA. This is a dangerous use of a drug that should be used only rarely, if ever.

**iron**   A mineral that is necessary for health and in which some people may become deficient, as in iron deficiency anemia. The main role of iron is its involvement with the transport of oxygen throughout the body; iron is also an important part of many cell components as well as enzymes.

Heme iron and nonheme iron are the types of dietary iron. Foods that are rich in heme iron include cooked chicken liver, oysters, beef, turkey (dark turkey has a greater percentage of heme iron), and chicken. Foods that are rich in nonheme iron include soybeans, lentils, kidney beans, pinto beans, lima beans, spinach, grains, and fruit.

### Risk Factors for Iron Deficiency

People who are at risk for development of iron deficiency include individuals in the following categories:

- People who have kidney failure on kidney dialysis, especially those who are receiving erythropoietin
- Women who are *not* menopausal
- Older infants and toddlers
- People who have cancer
- Patients who have chronic gastrointestinal bleeding that may be difficult to cure, such as that caused by abnormal blood vessels in the bowel wall and radiation proctitis

Signs of an iron deficiency include the following:

- Chronic weakness and fatigue
- Slower or worse performance at work or at school
- Low body temperature
- Increased numbers of infections, indicating a decreased immune function

### Treatment of Iron Deficiency

Iron deficiency is usually treated with supplemental iron. Iron can be given orally or intravenously. Oral iron supplements may in some cases cause gastrointestinal problems, such as nausea and vomiting, and may cause either diarrhea or constipation. In patients for whom oral iron may cause problems, such as those who have inflammatory bowel disease, iron can be administered intravenously.

### Excessive Levels of Iron

Most people do not have toxic levels of iron in their body unless they are taking high and unnecessary supplemental doses of iron and/or are otherwise susceptible to an iron overload state. Over-the-counter iron supplements should not be taken unless recommended by a physician. Women who are postmenopausal rarely need to take iron supplements if they eat a well-balanced diet.

An iron overdose can be very dangerous in children. Even as little as one to three grams of iron can be fatal to a child weighing less than 22 pounds. For this reason, it is very important for people who take iron supplements and who have small children to keep the supplements securely capped and well out of reach of toddlers.

Some people suffer from a rare disease that causes an iron overload in the body called HEMACHROMATOSIS. They also have an increased risk of development of liver cancer.

People who need frequent blood transfusions are also at risk for development of an iron overload problem.

### Pregnant Women and Iron

Most women who are pregnant take vitamin pills with iron supplements to prevent anemia. Women who are anemic during pregnancy have an increased risk of having a baby who has low birth weight and/or is born prematurely. The mothers themselves are more likely to have complications from the delivery.

See also ANEMIA; VITAMIN DEFICIENCIES/EXCESSES.

**iron deficiency anemia**   See ANEMIA; IRON.

**irritable bowel syndrome (IBS)**   A common chronic medical problem that is usually characterized by abdominal pain plus disturbance of bowel function, either constipation or diarrhea, and sometimes by alternating conditions of both disorders. The colon of patients with IBS exhibits an abnormal pattern of colonic motility and contractions, although these findings are not consistent.

Also known as a spastic colon, IBS affects as many as 15 percent of adults at some point in their life; women have a greater risk of development of IBS than men. In Eastern cultures such as that in India, the prevalence of IBS is greater among men. Women who have been sexually or emotionally abused in the past appear to have an increased risk for development of irritable bowel syndrome. IBS is the most frequently diagnosed disease among patients seen by gastroenterologists in the United States.

IBS should not be confused with inflammatory bowel disease (IBD), which is an intestinal inflammation that stems from either Crohn's disease or ulcerative colitis. IBS is *not* associated with visible inflammation or cancer, and its presence does not increase the patient's risk of development of cancer. Some who are diagnosed with IBS may actually have other illnesses, such as CELIAC SPRUE or an intestinal bacterial overgrowth, which should be treated if identified.

Irritable bowel syndrome can be very aggravating for the patients who have it, and some patients must change jobs because they must use the toilet frequently. However, despite the aggravation IBS causes those who have it, the condition does not cause permanent grossly visible damage to either the colon or the digestive tract; nor does it appear to cause other diseases, although IBS patients have a lower quality of life and an increased risk for diagnosis with other medical problems, such as fibromyalgia, a chronic muscle pain disorder; noncardiac chest pain; psychiatric disorders; and/or interstitial cystitis, a chronic spasming and irritation of the bladder.

It is unknown what causes IBS, although those with IBS appear to have a very sensitive colon that may react spasmodically to some triggers, such as some foods or medications. Chocolate is an apparent trigger for some patients with IBS; milk and fatty foods or tomatoes may induce spasms in others. Large meals may trigger IBS for some patients. Some doctors believe that women's reproductive hormones may play a role, because IBS symptoms often worsen during menstrual periods. In most instances, however, no single trigger for IBS is identified.

The presence of increased stress makes IBS symptoms more likely to occur, although stress does not cause IBS. (Stress often exacerbates many chronic conditions, such as headaches, arthritis, and back pain.) Recent studies suggest that the IBS may be preceded or precipitated by an intestinal infection, which normally would be self-limited, but the symptoms tend to persist in patients who are predisposed to development of IBS. A composite biopsychosocial model for causation of the disease has been proposed. This model includes the involvement of the brain and spinal cord, the gut, and environmental influences.

### Symptoms of IBS

Physicians report that IBS patients usually have abdominal pain plus disturbed bowel function in the form of diarrhea, constipation, or alternating diarrhea and constipation, a condition that has been present for at least three months in the past year. The pain of IBS lessens with defecation.

The presence of the following symptoms further supports the diagnosis:

- Mucus that is present with the stool
- Straining during bowel movements
- Feelings of incompleteness after a bowel movement
- Hard stools or loose and watery stools
- Abdominal bloating

### Diagnosis and Treatment

Irritable bowel syndrome is diagnosed on the basis of symptoms that patients report, as well as the absence of any other disorder that may explain the symptoms. Frequently, patients have a SIGMOIDOSCOPY or a COLONOSCOPY. The physician may take a biopsy specimen of the bowel during the procedure to exclude other causes of the symptoms. Physicians also rule out other possible diseases with laboratory tests, such as a complete blood count and other common blood tests, such as a complete metabolic profile and thyroid function tests. The physician may also request a stool sample to analyze it for a possible PARASITIC INFECTION.

Patients who are diagnosed with IBS are often advised to keep a food diary as well as a stool diary, to help them note any apparent correlation between the day's events or the foods that they eat and subsequent symptoms. Some patients may benefit from avoiding caffeine and chocolate, as well as limiting their intake of fatty foods. If constipation is the primary problem, increasing fluid and fiber intake may help patients.

IBS is also treated with a variety of medications to help relax the bowel. Two drugs that are used to treat spasms are dicyclomine (Bentyl) and hyoscyamine sulfate (Levsin), both of which are anticholinergic agents. If patients are primarily troubled with diarrhea, other drugs, such as loperamide (Imodium), alosetron (Lotronex), diphenoxylate plus atropine sulfate (Lomotil), or cholestyramine resin, may be used. Alosetron, a drug formerly prescribed for IBS, was withdrawn

from the market in 2000 after reports of severe constipation and several deaths. It was approved again in 2002 on a restricted basis by the Food and Drug Administration (FDA) for women with IBS who have severe diarrhea-predominant IBS that is not responsive to other treatments.

Patients whose main problem is constipation may be given osmotic laxatives, such as magnesium hydroxide and lactulose. Polyethylene glycol solution may be used to flush out the stools. In 2002 the Food and Drug Administration approved tegaserod maleate (Zelnorm) for the short-term treatment of IBS among women whose primary problem is constipation. Some experts use the medication for longer periods for patients who are responding well to treatment.

Other types of drugs may be prescribed, such as low dosages of antidepressant medications. These drugs may help to calm patients, as well as help with sleep problems and relieve colonic cramping and spasms. Many patients actually have depression and anxiety, although the dosages of these drugs are much lower than those normally used to treat depression or anxiety.

Some physicians have found that patients may improve with Chinese herbal medicine. In a study reported in a 1998 edition of the *Journal of the American Medical Association,* the researchers compared the results of patients in three groups. In one group, the patients were treated with individualized Chinese herbal formulations; in a second group, the patients were treated with a standard Chinese herbal formulation. Patients in the third group received a placebo (no drugs). The patients who received either form of the Chinese herbal formulations improved significantly compared to the patients receiving placebo; however, in a follow-up that occurred 14 weeks after the end of the study, only the patients receiving the individualized Chinese herbal formulations maintained their improvement in their symptoms.

Hypnotherapy has also been shown in controlled trials to be helpful for some patients with IBS.

See also CONSTIPATION; CROHN'S DISEASE; DIARRHEA; HYPERALGESIA; INFLAMMATORY BOWEL DISEASE; ULCERATIVE COLITIS.

Bensoussan, Alan, M.Sc., et al. "Treatment of Irritable Bowel Syndrome with Chinese Herbal Medicine: A Randomized Controlled Trial." *Journal of the American Medical Association* 280, no. 18 (November 11, 1998): 1,585–1,589.

Horwitz, Brenda J., M.D., and Robert S. Fisher, M.D. "The Irritable Bowel Syndrome." *New England Journal of Medicine* 344, no. 24 (June 14, 2001): 1,846–1,850.

Jailwala, Jeegr, M.D., Thomas F. Imperiale, M.D., and Kurt Kroenke, M.D. "Pharmacologic Treatment of the Irritable Bowel Syndrome: A Systematic Review of Randomized, Controlled Trials." *Annals of Internal Medicine* 133, no. 2 (2000): 136–147.

Minocha, Anil, M.D., and David Carroll. *Natural Stomach Care.* New York: Penguin Putnam, 2003.

**ischemia**  A lack of blood supply that occurs because the blood supply is altogether blocked or because the blood supply is limited because the artery is severely narrowed, a condition that can lead to tissue damage or death. In the digestive system, intestinal ischemia can be caused by a hernia that becomes entangled or by adhesions from prior surgeries that entrap the intestines with scar tissue.

In mesenteric artery ischemia, the arteries that supply the blood to the intestines are narrowed or may undergo spasms. Mesenteric artery ischemia may be seen in patients with atherosclerosis and is more commonly found among smokers and individuals who have high cholesterol levels. According to Shaji Kumar and colleagues, in their 2001 article for the *New England Journal of Medicine*, mesenteric venous THROMBOSIS causes 5 to 15 percent of all mesenteric ischemia. Ischemic colitis occurs when a segment of the colon loses its blood supply.

Hepatic ischemia results from an inadequate blood supply to the liver, which causes damage or death to the liver cells. This condition, known as ischemic hepatitis or shock liver, can result from low blood pressure that results from abnormal heart rhythms, dehydration, severe bleeding, shock or other causes. Most patients with shock liver recover unless the underlying condition persists.

### Symptoms and Signs of Ischemia

Indicators of intestinal or mesenteric ischemia are abdominal pain, nausea, vomiting, and diarrhea. Abdominal pain is usually disproportionate to the physical findings elicited by the physician on examination. Overt or occult (microscopic) blood is found in the stools. Since these are common symptoms of many other digestive problems, the physician must determine the diagnosis and treatment.

In hepatic ischemia, liver enzyme levels are elevated. These abnormal liver test findings and the liver itself usually return to normal rapidly if the underlying condition causing it is resolved. However, liver failure may occur with hepatic ischemia, although it is very rare.

### Diagnosis and Treatment of Intestinal Ischemia

Laboratory tests may show an elevated white blood cell count when ischemia is the problem. An angiogram that uses dye injected into the arteries that supply the intestine will reveal whether there is an arterial blockage. If a narrowing is seen, it can be dilated. If a clot is identified, it can be dissolved with clot-busting drugs. If there is spasm, a vasodilator drug is injected directly into the narrowed vessel to dilate it. However, sometimes test results are inconclusive and physicians must perform exploratory surgery to identify the cause of the problem. CT scan is the test of choice to diagnose mesenteric venous thrombosis as the cause of mesenteric ischemia.

When surgery is performed, surgeons remove the dead part of the intestine and then reconnect the bowel to healthy tissue; however, in some cases, an osteomy is needed; in the procedure an opening is made and an external changeable pouch captures fecal material. The pouch is periodically changed by the patient.

In chronic mesenteric ischemia, physicians remove any blockage in the arteries that connect to the intestines.

If the patient has acute mesenteric ischemia, it is a medical emergency.

The treatment of ischemic colitis is supportive, and most patients recover.

Treatment for hepatic ischemia is supportive: the patient maintains good hydration by intravenous fluids or blood transfusion and oxygenation, as well as correcting any severe anemia. Correction of the underlying problem whenever possible, such as improving low blood pressure or another medical problem, is also important. Most patients recover completely from hepatic ischemia.

Brandt, L. J., and S. J. Boley. "A6A Technical Review on Intestinal Ischemia." *Gastroenterology* 118 (2000): 954–968.

Kumar, Shaji, M.D., Michael G. Sarr, M.D., and Patrick S. Kamath, M.D. "Mesenteric Venous Thrombosis." *New England Journal of Medicine* 345, no. 23 (December 6, 2001): 1,683–1,688.

**jaundice** Yellowing of the skin and eyes caused by an excessive level of bilirubin, a product of heme broken down by the liver. The condition is also known as hyperbilirubinemia. Jaundice may be a temporary problem faced by some newborn infants, who need pediatric treatment. It may also be a symptom of a serious liver disease, such as HEPATITIS or even CIRRHOSIS or PANCREATIC CANCER. The excessive hemolysis of red blood cells in hemolytic anemia is a non-liver-related cause of jaundice.

Any person whose skin appears more yellow than usual should consult a physician immediately for a medical evaluation. If the skin is bright yellow (for example, similar to a banana color), medical attention should be sought urgently. Note that yellow discoloration may also be seen in carotenemia (a high intake of vitamin A) and is best seen on the face, palms, and soles of the feet.

### Newborn Infants with Jaundice

Sometimes newborn babies have jaundice that needs to be treated. Jaundice may not be apparent on the first one or two days after birth for two weeks. It is important for an infant to be seen by a pediatrician within 24–48 hours after discharge if he or she is discharged from the hospital at any time before 48 hours after birth.

In one study of nearly 30,000 newborn infants in Michigan, reported in a 1998 issue of *Pediatrics,* 127 babies had to be readmitted to the hospital in the first two weeks of their life to be treated for jaundice. In addition, researchers found several factors that caused infants to be more likely to need readmission, including discharge from the hospital within 72 hours of birth.

See also CANCER, PANCREATIC; HEPATITIS.

Maisels, Jeffrey M., and Elizabeth Kring. "Length of Stay, Jaundice, and Hospital Readmission." *Pediatrics* 101, no. 6 (June 1998): 995–998.

**jejunitis** Inflammation of the jejunum, a part of the small intestine that lies between the duodenum and the ileum. It may be caused by CROHN'S DISEASE, ulcerative jejunitis, or severe infections, or other digestive diseases and disorders.

**jejunostomy** A procedure to create a hole in the abdominal wall and connecting to the jejunum (the middle section of the small intestine, between the duodenum and the ileum), so that enteral nutrition can be directly inserted. A jejunostomy can be performed with surgery as well as through an ENDOSCOPY.

**Kaposi's sarcoma**   Severe skin lesions of a vascular tumor that can occur in various parts of the body, including the digestive system. In the most extreme cases, Kaposi's sarcoma can result in gastrointestinal bleeding, which can rarely be fatal. It can also involve the respiratory system and the lymph nodes. Kaposi's sarcoma is caused by human herpesvirus 8 (HHV-8).

This condition was first described by the Hungarian dermatologist Moritz Kaposi in 1872. Variations of the condition that was described by Kaposi were subsequently identified; for example, a form of Kaposi's sarcoma was identified among homosexual men in New York in 1981.

### Risk Factors

Men have a greater risk for development of Kaposi's sarcoma than women by a ratio as high as 15 to one. Elderly Eastern European and Mediterranean men are at risk for Kaposi's sarcoma. Currently, Kaposi's sarcoma has been found in patients living in parts of Africa such as Uganda and Zambia. Gay men in the United States and other countries are at high risk for development of Kaposi's sarcoma.

Some people are at high risk for Kaposi's sarcoma, such as those who have acquired immunodeficiency syndrome (AIDS). In addition, organ transplantation recipients face an increased risk for Kaposi's sarcoma because of their impaired immune system.

### Diagnosis and Treatment

Trained physicians can usually identify the lesions of Kaposi's sarcoma by just looking at them. Physicians can also test the blood of patients with skin lesions for the presence of antibodies against HHV-8 or Kaposi's sarcoma–associated herpesvirus (KSHV), which would be indirect evidence of an infection. A biopsy specimen of the skin lesions will confirm the presence of Kaposi's sarcoma.

The presence of Kaposi's sarcoma is declining; the reasons for this decline are not well known. In the early stages, physicians concentrate on treating the symptoms and signs of Kaposi's sarcoma by shrinking the tumor to decrease swelling and to lessen psychological stress, as well as to prevent disease progression; for example, lesions can be removed with cryotherapy, freezing them off the skin. Other local treatments that can control tumor growth include injections of chemotherapeutic drugs such as vinblastine into the lesion. In addition, radiation therapy, laser therapy, and topical applications of various drugs such as Panretin gel may be used.

More aggressive treatment is used in the following cases:

- The number of lesions increases to more than 25 lesions on the skin.
- Kaposi's sarcoma is extensive and is not responding to local therapy.
- There is severe swelling.
- Internal organs are involved, causing symptoms such as bleeding from the digestive system.

Patients may be treated with radiation therapy, chemotherapy, or a combination of radiation therapy and chemotherapy. Current chemotherapy regimens employ liposomal doxorubicin (Doxil), liposomal daunorubicin (Dauno Xome), paclitaxel and vinorelbine. Drugs used in the past included bleomycin, vinblastine, vincristine, and etoposide. Some patients have been treated with interferon alfa. However, such treatments should not be undertaken in a patient who is already severely immunocompromised.

See also ACQUIRED IMMUNODEFICIENCY SYNDROME; HUMAN IMMUNODEFICIENCY VIRUS; INTERFERON.

Antman, Karen, M.D., and Yuan Chang, M.D. "Kaposi's Sarcoma." *New England Journal of Medicine* 342, no. 14 (April 6, 2000): 1,027–1,038.

**Lactobacillus**  Often considered to be one of the "friendly bacteria," *Lactobacillus* is a bacterium and the *Lactobacillus bulgaricus* is found in some products such as yogurt. Sometimes patients who are taking antibiotics experience an imbalance because friendly bacteria are killed along with harmful bacteria. Such an imbalance of insufficient friendly bacteria can cause diarrhea and even severe colitis. The administration of some types of *Lactobacillus* has been shown to be helpful in certain forms of diarrhea.

Eating yogurt with live cultures or taking over-the-counter tablets containing such probiotic bacteria can help restore the normal ecological balance in the gut; however, patients should consult their physician to obtain treatment of their disorder and to determine whether they should take such probiotics as *Lactobacillus*. They should not self-medicate.

See also ALTERNATIVE MEDICINE; THRUSH; YEAST.

**lactose intolerance**  A form of food intolerance; difficulty or inability related to digestion of the milk sugar (lactose) that is found in dairy products and in some other foods, which leads to the excessive production of fluid, gas, cramps, and diarrhea. The problem may be mild, moderate, or severe, depending on the patient.

Lactose intolerance is the result of an enzyme deficiency of lactase in the patient. The deficiency or lack of the enzyme lactase is called alactasia, hypolactasia, and lactase deficiency. Some patients may exhibit symptoms of lactose intolerance without evidence of a lactase deficiency.

Often confused with a food allergy, lactose intolerance is actually an inability to digest lactose, and there is no involvement with the immune system at all, as there is in the case of a food allergy. Worldwide, as much as 75 percent of the global population may be lactose-intolerant. The prevalence of lactose intolerance also varies considerably within countries; for example, about 70 percent of the people in the southern part of India are lactose-intolerant, in contrast to about 25 percent of the population in the northern portion of India, who are lactose-intolerant.

Very few infants are born lactose-intolerant. Most children up to the age of five years have the ability to tolerate lactose, but the level of their natural lactase enzyme starts to diminish in early childhood. For most people lactose intolerance does not become a problem until they reach adolescence or adulthood.

### Secondary Lactose Intolerance

Some children and adults acquire lactose intolerance as a result of a secondary medical problem, such as a severe gastrointestinal infection or other disease that damages the mucosa of the small intestines. In addition, chemotherapy or radiation therapy for cancer may also cause lactose intolerance. Some of the diseases or conditions that can cause secondary hypolactasia are

- Celiac sprue
- Whipple's disease
- Giardiasis
- Crohn's disease
- Human immunodeficiency virus (HIV) enteritis
- Zollinger-Ellison syndrome

Patients who have secondary lactose intolerance may recover with treatment of the underlying cause; for example, if patients have giardiasis, which can cause a secondary lactose intolerance, treatment with metronidazole (Flagyl) may resolve the problem. Patients who have lactose intolerance that is caused by excessive bacteria in the small bowel may improve after a course of antibiotics.

### Risk Factors

Males and females are about equally likely to be lactose-intolerant.

There are racial differences among those who are lactose-intolerant. Asians (depending on ethnicity) have one of the greatest risk of lactose intolerance and a 30 to 95 percent intolerance rate. In the United States, Native Americans follow Asians in the percentages of those who are lactose-intolerant: an estimated 79 percent of Native Americans have this condition. Many African Americans (about 75 percent) are also lactose-intolerant. They are followed by Hispanics (about 50 to 75 percent are intolerant) and then by whites in the United States (a range of from 6 to 30 percent).

### Symptoms

The common symptoms of lactose intolerance are as follows:

- Stomach cramps
- Bloating of the stomach
- Extreme gas
- Frothy and watery stool after consumption of products that contain lactose (however, most who have lactase deficiency can tolerate about one glass of milk per day without problems)

### Diagnosis and Treatment

If the physician or the patient suspects lactose intolerance to be a problem, the patient can have a hydrogen breath test and/or a blood test of the serum glucose level (both are administered after the patient consumes lactose), to confirm or refute the possible diagnosis. Some physicians also order biopsy examination of the small intestines to diagnose the level of lactase in the intestinal cells, although that test is only performed in research laboratories. Physicians who perform an intestinal biopsy may also be seeking to screen out other medical problems that may be causing malabsorption, such as celiac sprue.

Mild lactose intolerance can be managed with supplemental lactase enzyme oral supplements, which are over-the-counter drugs such as LactAid and Lactrase. These supplements may enable the patient who is moderately or severely lactose-intolerant to consume a glass of milk or several scoops of ice cream without incident.

In general, physicians do not advise lactose-intolerant patients to give up all dairy products because of concern that a calcium deficiency may develop. However, most lactose intolerance patients should carefully monitor their consumption of dairy products. They may also need to take supplemental calcium to ensure a healthy intake. Some patients drink lactose-reduced milk.

Patients with lactose intolerance are also advised to eat other foods when they consume products with lactose, to diminish the overall effect of the lactose. Some foods that include lactose may be well tolerated, such as yogurt with active cultures in it. The reason for this is that the bacterial lactase breaks down the lactose, and thus there is no remaining lactose to cause a reaction.

Milk and dairy products are not the only food items that include lactose, and patients who are extremely lactose-intolerant need to be aware of this fact. According to Dr. Swagerty and his colleagues in their 2002 article on lactose intolerance in *American Family Physician,* some products that include lactose are as follows:

- Bread
- Margarine
- Breakfast cereals
- Mixes for pancakes or cookies
- Breakfast drinks
- Salad dressings
- Some candies
- Packaged luncheon meats that are nonkosher
- Some medications (patients should advise their pharmacists that they are lactose-intolerant)

See also ALLERGIES, FOOD; CELIAC DISEASE/CELIAC SPRUE.

Srinivasan, R., and A. Minocha. "When to Suspect Lactose Intolerance." *Postgraduate Medicine* 105, no. 3 (1998): 109–123.

Swagerty, Daniel L., Jr., M.D., Anne D. Walling, M.D., and Robert M. Klein. "Lactose Intolerance." *American Family Physician* 65, no. 9 (May 1, 2002): 1,845–1,850.

**laparoscopy**   Procedure in which several small incisions are made in the abdomen so that an exploratory device called a laparoscope can be inserted and the patient can be examined or treated from the inside. Doctors use the laparoscope for diagnostic purposes as well as for minor and even some major surgeries. Examples of laparoscopic surgery include laparoscopic cholecystectomy and Nissen's fundoplication. The colectomy is an example of major surgery that may be performed laparoscopically at some centers.

See also CHOLECYSTECTOMY; FUNDOPLICATION; SURGERY.

**laxative abuse**   Extreme use of laxatives for the purpose of weight loss, as is seen in some people who have ANOREXIA NERVOSA. Laxative abuse can also be found among some people who are chronically constipated or obsessed with the idea that they are "constipated," and have become dependent on laxatives in order to have regular bowel movements. Some patients with laxative abuse complain of "diarrhea." A search of the patient's room and a laxative screen test may be in order in some cases to look for laxative abuse.

See also CONSTIPATION; DIARRHEA; LAXATIVES; NARCOTIC BOWEL SYNDROME.

**laxatives**   Over-the-counter or prescribed medications taken by people who are constipated. In most cases, the individual has not had a bowel movement for two to three days or longer. The excessive use of laxatives may lead to diarrhea. Some patients may constantly use laxatives; this practice is called LAXATIVE ABUSE. Such laxative abuse may be present with factitious diarrhea. The long-standing use of certain laxatives may lead to melanosis coli.

There are various types of laxatives. Bulk laxatives (psyllium, methyl cellulose) increase the bulk of the stool and promote bowel movement. They should be taken with plenty of water and avoided by patients who have GASTROPARESIS and MEGACOLON. The bulk laxative is initially tried for constipation. Other types of laxatives include stool softeners (docusate), stimulant cathartics (castor oil, bisacodyl, and senna), osmotic cathartics (Milk of Magnesia, lactulose, and sorbitol), and polyethylene glycol solutions (MiraLax).

Laxatives with a high concentration of MAGNESIUM or phosphorus should be avoided by those who have kidney failure.

See also CONSTIPATION; DIARRHEA.

**lipids**   Fats that are made in the body and that are also found naturally in some types of foods, such as fish, meat, poultry, eggs, and dairy products. Cholesterol circulates in the body as lipoproteins, in the form of low-density lipoproteins (LDLs) or high-density lipoproteins (HDLs). Lipid emulsions are administered as part of PARENTERAL NUTRITION to patients who are unable to have enteral feeding.

See also CHOLESTEROL.

**lipoma**   A slow-growing and benign fatty tumor that is painless and is generally located in the upper body, particularly the head, neck, shoulder, or back. When they occur, they are usually found among people ages 40 to 60 years old. Physicians need to differentiate lipoma from other medical problems such as neurofibroma and vascular nodules.

Lipomas can be removed by physicians. Sometimes they are removed without surgery, with steroid injections that cause a shrinking of the lipoma. A lipoma may also be seen inside the gut, for example, during a COLONOSCOPY; that finding usually has no clinical significance.

Salam, Gohar A. "Lipoma Excision." *American Family Physician* 65 (March 1, 2002): 901–904, 905.

***Listeria monocytogenes***   Common bacteria that cause food-borne illnesses. An infection with *Listeria* organisms is called listeriosis. According to the Centers for Disease Control and Prevention (CDC), about 1,700 severe cases of listeriosis are reported each year in the United States, and in these cases, as many as 450 patients die. In addition, listeriosis accounts for about 100 stillbirths each year.

When present, *Listeria* organisms may be found in cole slaw, luncheon meats, cold cuts, undercooked poultry, and dairy products. They are usually killed by cooking, or, in the case of dairy products, by pasteurization. The infection is treated with antibiotics. Epidemics may occur.

Most healthy people are unaffected by *Listeria* organisms; however, some groups of people are vulnerable to infection, particularly those in the following groups:

- Pregnant women (who can transmit the illness to the fetus, potentially causing severe health problems)
- Newborn babies
- Elderly individuals
- People who have a weakened immune system, such as those who have acquired immunodeficiency syndrome (AIDS) or have had organ transplantation
- Cancer patients

### Symptoms of Infection

People infected with *Listeria* organisms may experience fevers and chills and may believe that they have flu. Some individuals experience stomach upset. If the infection spreads farther to the brain (meningoencephalitis), patients may have headaches, stiff neck, and even loss of balance and convulsions.

### Diagnosis

Since many of the symptoms of listeriosis are nonspecific, a precise diagnosis is made by testing the blood or the cerebrospinal fluid of the patient. Cerebrospinal fluid is the fluid that bathes the brain and spinal cord.

### Treatment of Listeriosis

The infection is susceptible to many commonly used antibiotics. In most cases, a combination of antibiotics, such as ampicillin or penicillin G plus gentamicin, is used.

### Preventing Listeriosis

*Listeria* infections can often be prevented by the following simple actions:

- Washing hands before eating any ready-to-eat foods, such as cold cuts or deli-style meats
- Avoiding soft cheese such as feta cheese and brie
- Avoiding unpasteurized milk and unpasteurized cheese
- Reading and heeding expiration dates of all food products
- Reheating ready-to-eat foods such as hot dogs and cold cuts
- Refrigerating perishable foods within two hours

See also CONTAMINATED FOOD OR WATER; FOODBORNE ILLNESSES.

**lithotripsy**    A procedure that uses special shock waves to break up gallstones and kidney stones so that they may pass and not cause inflammation and harm to people. Not every patient who has gallstones or kidney stones is a good candidate for this procedure. In fact, lithotripsy for gallstones is used only for patients who are otherwise poor surgical candidates.

See also GALLSTONES.

**liver**    A digestive and metabolic organ that is necessary to sustain life. The liver is essential for numerous important functions in the body, including the digestion, absorption, and assimilation of nutrients, the synthesis of the building blocks of the body such as proteins, glucose metabolism, and drug detoxification. (Many medications are metabolized by the liver.)

Hepatitis is a disease that attacks the liver, as are hepatocellular carcinoma and other forms of liver cancer. Chronic alcoholism or alcohol abuse can cause CIRRHOSIS of the liver, a condition of severe scarring. Nonalcoholic steatohepatitis (also known as nonalcoholic fatty liver disease) may also cause damage to the liver. SARCOIDOSIS, HEMATOCHROMATOSIS, and WILSON'S DISEASE can also be very harmful to the liver.

Some rare diseases that can cause damage to the liver are AMYLOIDOSIS, BUDD-CHIARI SYNDROME, CYSTIC FIBROSIS, alpha$_1$-antitrypsin deficiency, PRIMARY SCLEROSING CHOLANGITIS, and glycogen storage disease. The acute fatty liver of pregnancy is a dangerous condition that some pregnant women experience.

If the liver fails because of severe disease or damage, the only way to continue to sustain a person's life in cases of advanced liver failure is through LIVER TRANSPLANTATION.

In the United States, about 1.8 million people have liver disease, according to information compiled by the National Center for Health Statistics for 1997. Of these, there are more males than females (975,000 males and 819,000 females). Most who have liver disease are younger than age 64, possibly because liver disease kills many people and thus they do not live to beyond age 64. In considering race and ethnicity, most people diagnosed with liver disease are white: there are 1,353,000 whites diagnosed with liver disease in the United States. Only 173,000 people with liver disease are black and 200,000 are Hispanic.

In looking at the geographic locations of people with liver disease in the United States, the predominance of the disease occurs in the South, with 661,000 people. The lowest number of patients with liver disease are in the Northeast, at 329,000. The reasons for these disparities are unknown. (See Appendix VII.)

See also ASCITES; CANCER, LIVER; CIRRHOSIS; HEPATITIS; HEPATOCELLULAR CANCER; JAUNDICE; LIVER FAILURE.

**liver abscess**   Severe bacterial, fungal, or parasitic infection of the liver. Generally, CHOLANGITIS (inflammation of the bile duct) that is caused by a blockage of the bile duct by gallstones or tumors is the most frequent cause of liver abscess. A spreading of an abscess from APPENDICITIS or DIVERTICULITIS may also result in a liver abscess.

### Signs and Symptoms

Patients who have a liver abscess experience abdominal pain, fever, sweating, nausea and vomiting, loss of appetite, and unintended weight loss. The physician's examination of the liver may find it swollen and tender.

### Diagnosis and Treatment

Laboratory tests of patients with liver abscesses are nonspecific and reveal an elevated white blood cell count. Patients may have an elevated erythrocyte sedimentation rate of the blood and may also have elevated alkaline phosphatase levels. The ultrasound and computed tomography (CT) scan are usually required for diagnosis. In addition, a gallium scan and magnetic resonance imaging (MRI) scan may be helpful. An endoscopic retrograde cholangiopancreatography (ERCP) can help to delineate the cause of the liver abscess in some cases and can allow insertion of a biliary stent to hold the bile duct open if it is blocked.

Drainage of the abscess is frequently undertaken, and patients need to take antibiotics, such as penicillin or metronidazole. Treatment is usually long: it may take weeks to months, depending upon the patient's response, which is monitored clinically by the physician as well as with CT scans.

In some cases, a liver abscess is caused by *Entamoeba histolytica,* an amebic parasite that is found more commonly in developing countries as well as in areas with poor sanitation and overcrowding. Results of stool tests in such cases are rarely positive for the amoeba. The abscess can spread to the lungs and the heart and can cause even worse problems that are related to these organs. The diagnosis of *E. histolytica* abscess is helped by imaging tests such as the CT scan. Serology testing for antibodies against the ameba yields positive findings in most cases. Liver abscesses that are caused by *E. histolytica* can usually be resolved with metronidazole treatment, although occasionally drainage may also be necessary. The individual treatment of each patient must be decided by his or her doctor.

See also CAROLI'S DISEASE; LIVER.

Krige, J. E. J. "Liver Abscesses and Hydatid Diseases." *British Medical Journal* 322 (March 3, 2001): 537–540.

**liver cancer**   See CANCER, LIVER.

**liver enzymes/function tests**    Laboratory blood tests that are specifically helpful in identifying possible liver diseases because they provide markers of liver damage and, thus, they can lead the physician to further investigations of potential problems.

Elevated levels of serum aminotransferases (alanine aminotransferase [ALT]) and aspartine aminotransferase (AST), alkaline phosphatase, and gamma-glutamyltransferase may indicate possible liver disease. For example, above-normal levels of aminotransferase may indicate the presence of HEPATITIS B or C, HEMOCHROMATOSIS (iron overload), ALCOHOLIC HEPATITIS, OR nonalcoholic steatohepatitis. Aminotransferases are also produced by the kidney and the muscles, and elevated levels may also indicate a non-liver-related medical problem, such as kidney disorders, or muscle problems such as myoscitis, or even a prior period of excessive exercise. Above-normal levels of aminotransferase may also be caused by numerous medications or even by heart attack.

Elevated levels of alkaline phosphatase, another marker for liver disease, may indicate a bone disorder or a variety of cholestatic diseases, such as bile duct obstruction, choledocholithiasis, or PRIMARY BILIARY CIRRHOSIS; in some cases it may be medication induced (such as by chlorpromazine). It may also indicate the presence of SARCOIDOSIS or another granulomatous disease, such as TUBERCULOSIS. On occasion, high alkaline phosphatase level indicate the presence of advanced liver cancer.

As with conventional medications, herbal remedies, including chaparral, Chinese herbs, gentia, senna, and shark cartilage, may elevate liver enzyme level. Some illegal drugs, such as cocaine and anabolic steroids, can also raise an individual's liver enzyme level.

Beckingham, I. J., and S. D. Ryder. "Investigation of Liver and Biliary Disease." *British Journal of Medicine* 322 (January 6, 2001): 33–36.

Pratt, Daniel S., M. D., and Marshall M. Kaplan, M. D. "Evaluation of Abnormal Liver-Enzyme Results in Asymptomatic Patients." *New England Journal of Medicine* 342, no. 17 (April 27, 2000): 1,266–1,271.

**liver failure**    Condition in which liver function is not present or is reduced significantly enough to cause severe problems. This is a life-threatening condition, and only liver transplantation can sustain life if the entire liver fails. The liver may fail because of medications, CIRRHOSIS, HEPATITIS or other liver diseases, or liver cancer.

In a study of 308 patients with liver failure reported in 2002 in *Annals of Internal Medicine,* overdose of acetaminophen was the most common cause of acute liver failure (representing 39 percent of all cases), followed by overdoses of or reactions to other drugs (13 percent) and infection with hepatitis A and B (12 percent). The survival rate for patients with acetaminophen-induced liver failure was 68 percent compared to only 25 percent survival rate of patients whose liver failed as a result of ingestion of other drugs. In addition, when the cause of the liver failure was unknown, only 17 percent of the patients survived. According to the researchers, "Acetaminophen overdose and idiosyncratic drug reactions have replaced viral hepatitis as the most frequent cause of acute liver failure."

### Risk Factors

Clearly, it is important to prevent overdosage of acetaminophen, since it is a common cause of liver failure. Other risk factors are hepatitis and/or alcoholism.

### Symptoms

When the liver is failing, it can no longer function correctly or cannot function at all. Signs and symptoms of liver failure include the following indicators:

- Jaundice (yellowed skin and eyes)
- Extreme fatigue
- Itching of the skin
- Easy bruising and bleeding
- Slow blood clotting
- Mental confusion or, at worst, coma
- Bleeding

### Diagnosis and Treatment

The diagnosis of liver failure is based on the patient's signs and symptoms as well as liver function laboratory test results. In severe cases, the presence of JAUNDICE makes it clear that the patient has a liver disease, although jaundice in itself does not signify an irreversible liver failure. In addition, the physician must rule out the presence of HEPATITIS, pancreatic cancer, and other diseases that cause jaundice.

Transplantation of a new liver is the only cure for advanced liver failure, and patients who have fulminant liver failure receive the highest priority. Some very specialized intensive care facilities offer interim artificial support systems before liver transplantation; this practice is comparable to dialysis for kidneys that fail before a kidney transplantation can be accomplished.

An article in 2003 in the *Journal of the American Medical Association* described a review of 12 clinical trials of such interim bioartificial support systems. According to the authors, the meta-analysis of these trials revealed that such artificial support systems were successful in reducing the rate of death of liver failure by 33 percent.

Said the authors, "The objective of artificial and bioartificial support systems is to 'bridge' patients with liver failure to transplantation or recovery. Liver support must include removal of toxins, synthesis of products, and treatment of inflammation."

See also ALCOHOL ABUSE AND DEPENDENCE/ALCOHOLISM; LIVER; LIVER TRANSPLANTATION.

Kjaegard, Lise L., M.D., et al. "Artificial and Bioartificial Support Systems for Acute and Acute-on-Chronic Liver Failure." *Journal of the American Medical Association* 289, no. 2 (January 8, 2003): 217–222.

Ostapowicz, G., et al. "Results of a Prospective Study of Acute Liver Failure at 17 Tertiary Care Centers in the United States." *Annals of Internal Medicine* 137 (December 2002): 947–954.

**liver transplantation**   Replacement of a damaged liver with a donor liver from a recently deceased person or, in a very few cases, with the donated partial liver of a live person. Usually the patient has liver failure, usually because of severe hepatitis or cirrhosis, and is anticipated to die without transplantation. Hepatitis C is the leading indication of liver transplantation in the United States.

According to the U.S. Scientific Registry of Transplant Recipients, 5,261 people in the United States had liver transplantations in the year ending June 30, 2002. Of these, only 476 livers were transplanted from living donors. (The first adult-to-adult liver transplantation from a live donor was performed in the United States in 1997.) There were also 17,379 people on a waiting list for a liver transplantation in the United States. The registry reported a one-year survival rate for liver transplantation of 86 percent in 2002.

### Key Reasons for Liver Transplantation

In most cases of a need for a liver transplantation, the patient has extremely severe liver disease and the liver is failing as a result of HEPATITIS C, alcoholic liver disease, liver cancer, or PRIMARY BILIARY CIRRHOSIS. Patients who have primary liver cancer (HCC) are usually not considered as candidates for liver transplantation if their tumor is larger than five centimeters in the case of a single lesion or there are more than 3 smaller tumor lesions because the cancer is likely to recur.

The signs suggesting the need for liver transplantation include recurrent episodes of bleeding esophageal or gastric varices (enlarged veins that usually occur in the esophagus or stomach), spontaneous bacterial peritonitis, and encephalopathy. The Model for Endstage of Liver Disease (MELD) is used to triage patients who have the greatest need for immediate transplantation.

### Study of Patient Characteristics

In 1999 physicians reported on a demographic and clinical analysis of 711 patients who had had liver transplantation between 1991 and 1994 in California, Minnesota, and Nebraska in the *Journal of the American Medical Association*. In this study, 55 percent of the patients were male and most (81 percent) were white. The average hospital stay for patients was 21.2 days.

The researchers found a correlation between the age of the deceased donor and cost; for example, they found that patients who had liver transplantation from older donors (age 60 and older) were hospitalized several days longer and hospital costs were significantly higher. The researchers also found that alcoholic liver disease patients required more time (5.5 days more) in the hospital than other liver transplantation patients. Patients who were severely ill at the time of transplantation also required more time in the hospital and incurred more costs than other liver recipients.

### Using Living Adult Donors

Some patients receive partial liver donations; this procedure is only performed at a few medical centers. The reason for the donation may be that the patient is on a waiting list for a liver transplantation and the family and friends fear that the patient will die before a donor is found; consequently, one of them donates part of his or her liver. Children who need liver donations receive a partial liver, but the practice of partial liver donation in an adult is considered controversial. Researchers reported on information they obtained on patients (donor and recipients) involved in adult-to-adult partial liver donations in 2003 in the *New England Journal of Medicine.*

According to this study, most of the donors (74.4 percent) were related to the recipient. In 13.4 percent of the cases, friends donated part of their liver, and in 10.9 cases, the donors were spouses. In the remaining cases (1.3 percent) the donors were "good Samaritans" who were not relatives, friends, or spouses. In nearly all cases, the donors were screened by a hepatologist (medical liver expert), social worker, and a psychiatrist or psychologist before the procedure was approved and performed.

Among the donors, 14.5 percent had one or more complications of surgery, and 8.5 percent had to be rehospitalized because of complications from the procedure. A bile leak was the most common complication reported. Some patients needed blood transfusions or additional surgery. One donor died. The patients who *received* partial liver donations from live donors also had some complications: 22 percent had biliary complications and 9.8 percent had vascular complications.

### Immune System Rejection Problems

One key problem of liver transplantation (or any transplantation) is that the immune system rejects an organ from another person. To combat this rejection, patients must receive medications such as cyclosporine and tacrolimus to suppress their immune system; however, when the immune system is suppressed, the patient is more susceptible to infection as well as development of cancer and other complications. In addition, even with immune system–suppressing drugs, sometimes the immune system overcomes the effect and the transplanted organ is rejected.

For further information on liver transplantation, contact the following organizations:

American Liver Foundation
75 Maiden Lane
Suite 603
New York, NY 10038
(800) 465-4837 (Toll-free)
http://www.liverfoundation.org

Hepatitis Foundation International
504 Blick Drive
Silver Spring, MD 20904
(800) 891-0707 (Toll-free)
http://www.hepfi.org

United Network for Organ Sharing
1100 Boulders Parkway
Suite 500
P.O. Box 13770
Richmond, VA 23225
(888) 894-6361 (Toll-free)
http://www.unos.org

See also CANCER, LIVER; HEPATITIS; HEPATOCELLULAR CARCINOMA; LIVER; LIVER FAILURE.

Brown, Robert S., Jr., M.D., et al. "A Survey of Liver Transplantation from Living Adult Donors in the United States." *New England Journal of Medicine* 348, no. 9 (February 27, 2003): 818–825.

Prasad, K. R., and J. P. A. Lodge. "Transplantation of the Liver and Pancreas." *British Medical Journal* 322 (April 7, 2001): 845–847.

Showstack, Jonathan, et al. "Resource Utilization in Liver Transplantation: Effects of Patient Characteristics and Clinical Practice." *Journal of the American Medical Association* 281, no. 15 (April 21, 1999): 1,381–1,386.

**lower gastrointestinal series**   X rays taken of the lower part of the colon and the rectum; it is also called a barium enema. In the lower gastrointestinal series barium is introduced into the rectum in sufficient quantity to fill the entire colon so that the barium highlights the inside of the colon/rectum. Air may also be injected into the rectum to improve the visualization. In contrast to this test, an upper gastrointestinal series is the X ray of the esophagus, stomach, and upper part of the small intestine. In that test, the patient drinks the barium and then X rays are taken of the upper gastrointestinal tract. Similarly, the small bowel series examines the small intestines.

See also BARIUM STUDIES; UPPER GASTROINTESTINAL X RAY.

**lymphoma**   A form of cancer that starts in the lymphatic system. The two key forms of lymphoma are Hodgkin's disease (HD) and non-Hodgkin's lymphoma (NHL). Non-Hodgkin's lymphoma may develop in the liver or other organs. About 7,400 people in the United States are diagnosed with Hodgkin's disease each year and about 57,000 with non-Hodgkin's lymphoma.

NHL may be considered indolent: that is, it is not curable with treatment, but at the same time, patients have a long survival period even if they are untreated for years. In contrast, the aggressive and the highly aggressive forms of lymphoma are curable, but patients with those forms of lymphoma can die quickly if they are untreated or do not respond to treatment.

Burkitt's lymphoma is a form of non-Hodgkin's lymphoma, first identified by David Burkitt in 1958, which is found in children as well as among acquired immunodeficiency syndrome (AIDS) patients. When diagnosed, it is often found in the digestive system.

The digestive system is frequently involved in non-Hodgkin's lymphoma, but it is rarely affected in Hodgkin's disease. For example, NHL may be seen in the stomach, the small or large intestine, or the liver. A computed tomography (CT) scan, barium studies, and/or an endoscopy with biopsy may be needed for diagnosis. Sometimes, lymphoma occurring outside the gut in the surrounding lymph nodes may cause an obstruction of the gut by extrinsic compression; for example, dysphagia

(difficulty swallowing) may occur if the lymphoma surrounds the esophagus. In addition, the bowel may become obstructed if the lymphoma surrounds any loop of the bowel.

Mucosa associated lymphoid tissue (MALT) lymphoma is a specific form of lymphoma that frequently occurs in the gut. When it is found in the stomach, MALT lymphoma is frequently associated with a HELICOBACTER PYLORI infection. The eradication of the *H. pylori* can induce remission in the majority of these cases.

*Risk Factors for NHL*

According to Baris and Hoar Zahm in their 2000 article on the epidemiological characteristics of lymphomas in *Current Opinion in Oncology,* the key risk factor for NHL is immunosuppression, either primary or acquired. Lymphomas develop in as many as 25 percent of individuals with congenital immunosuppressive problems. The risk for development of lymphoma is greatest among individuals who have a first-degree relative (parent, child, or sibling) who has also been diagnosed with NHL. In addition, if a first-degree relative is diagnosed with leukemia or Hodgkin's disease, this diagnosis indicates an increased risk for NHL among other family members.

Individuals who have an acquired immune illness, such as AIDS, also face an increased risk of development of lymphoma.

Other individuals at risk for NHL development are those who are taking medications to suppress the immune system because they have received kidney, heart, or bone marrow transplantation. In one study of more than 18,000 patients worldwide who had had bone marrow transplantation, lymphomas developed in 78 patients compared to 1.5 cases in the general population.

Some infections increase the individual's risk of development of lymphoma; for example, infection with the Epstein-Barr virus increases the risk for Burkitt's lymphoma.

People who have some disorders have a greater risk for development of lymphoma, including individuals who have CELIAC SPRUE, DIABETES MELLITUS, rheumatoid arthritis, and Sjögen's syndrome. Some studies have also found a linkage between having malaria or tuberculosis and later diagnosis of NHL.

Individuals in some occupations appear to experience a greater risk of development of NHL, including farmers, pesticide workers, and some manufacturing workers. The exposure to pesticides appears to be the common denominator among these individuals.

Other workers are also at greater risk for NHL than most individuals, including employees in the rubber, petroleum refining, chemical, dry cleaning, and aircraft maintenance fields. Chronic exposure to organic solvents appears to be the factor that unites these workers. Laboratory technicians also face an increased risk of development of lymphoma.

See also ACQUIRED IMMUNODEFICIENCY SYNDROME; MULTIPLE LYMPHOMATOUS POLYPOSIS.

Baris, Dalsu, M.D., and Sheilia Hoar Zahm. "Epidemiology of Lymphomas." *Current Opinion in Oncology* 12 (2000): 383–394.

Zebrack, Brad J., et al. "Psychological Outcomes in Long-Term Survivors of Childhood Leukemia, Hodgkin's Disease, and Non-Hodgkin's Lymphoma: A Report from the Childhood Cancer Survivor Study." *Pediatrics* 110, no. 1 (July 2002): 42–52.

**macroglossia** The presence of an abnormally large and protruding tongue, which is usually associated with diseases or hereditary syndromes, such as AMYLOIDOSIS, acromegaly, and Down syndrome. It is also associated with hypothyroidism. Macroglossia may make feeding infants and children who have this problem difficult. As children grow, they may have speech and dental problems. In some cases, the tongue may be reduced by surgery; in other cases, the condition may resolve itself as the baby grows older.

See also THYROID DISEASE.

**magnesium** An essential mineral needed by humans for many different biochemical reactions. Some researchers believe that a slightly low level of magnesium may result in migraine headaches and in many other symptoms, and supplemental magnesium has been used to treat acute migraine headaches.

Foods that are high in magnesium include wheat germ, almonds, pumpkin seeds, dry roasted cashews, nuts, cooked spinach, baked potato with the skin, peanut butter, chocolate bars, and bananas.

Magnesium is the key ingredient in many LAXATIVES that are given to treat constipation. Magnesium-containing antacids and laxatives should be avoided by patients who have renal failure.

### Magnesium Deficiencies

A magnesium deficiency is more likely to occur in elderly individuals, although younger people may also become deficient. People who are taking diuretic drugs (water pills) are at risk for magnesium deficiency. Other groups of people who are at risk for magnesium deficiency include the following:

- People with poorly controlled diabetes
- People who are alcoholics or heavy drinkers
- People who take some anticancer drugs, such as Cisplatin
- People with gastrointestinal malabsorption disorders
- Individuals with chronic vomiting and diarrhea

Indications of a severe magnesium deficiency include the following:

- Seizures
- Mental confusion
- Appetite loss
- Depression
- Involuntary muscle contractions
- Numbness and tingling
- Abnormal heart rhythms

Low levels of magnesium can be present in the body despite normal serum levels. If individuals are deficient in magnesium, they should increase their dietary intake of foods that are rich in magnesium. They may also need to take magnesium supplements. If the magnesium level is dangerously low, the individual should be hospitalized to receive magnesium intravenously. A severe magnesium deficiency can be fatal.

### Hypermagnesemia

Few people have toxically high levels of magnesium, but such toxicity can occur; for example, people who are taking large doses of laxatives are at risk for development of magnesium toxicity, as are those who have kidney failure.

High levels of magnesium may cause indicators ranging from sleepiness to coma as well as dizziness, muscle paralysis, slow heart, and heart blocks. People with toxic levels of magnesium may also have extremely low blood pressure (hypotension) and may also have breathing problems.

See also IRON; VITAMIN DEFICIENCIES/EXCESSES.

**magnetic resonance cholangiopancreatography (MRCP)**   A noninvasive test that uses magnetic resonance imaging (MRI) technology to examine the pancreatic and bile ducts. The MRCP is noninvasive; however, it is a diagnostic procedure only, and consequently, physicians must perform endoscopic retrograde cholangiopancreatography (ERCP) if they wish to have subsequent access to the area to treat any abnormalities or blockages.

An MRCP may be used if a stone or a tumor in the bile duct or CHOLEDOCHAL CYSTS are suspected but not confirmed. It may also be a test that is used if the physician suspects CAROLI'S DISEASE or a patient has already undergone a failed ERCP.

In one study of patients with suspected CHOLEDOCHOLITHIASIS, reported in the *Mayo Clinic Proceedings* in 2002, the researchers found that the MRCP was a useful tool in detecting risk for choledocholithiasis. Said the researchers, "Magnetic resonance cholangiopancreatography seems to be effective in diagnosing choledocholithiasis. It plays a fundamental role in patients with a low or intermediate risk of choledocholithiasis, contributing to the avoidance of purely diagnostic ERCP."

Calvo, M. M., et al. "Role of Magnetic Resonance Cholangiopancreatography with Suspected Choledocholithiasis." *Mayo Clinic Proceedings* 77, no. 5 (May 2002): 422–428.

**malabsorption syndrome**   A condition in which an individual's intestines are unable to absorb sufficient nutrients from food that leads to nutrient, vitamin, and mineral deficiencies.

Among causes of malabsorption are the following diseases or conditions:

- CROHN'S DISEASE
- CELIAC disease
- PANCREATITIS
- Extensive small bowel resection
- Overgrowth of bacteria in the small intestine
- WHIPPLE'S DISEASE

See also VITAMIN DEFICIENCIES/EXCESSES.

**Mallory-Weiss syndrome**   A medical problem that some people with ALCOHOLISM experience, although not everyone who has Mallory-Weiss tear is an alcoholic. The primary symptom of Mallory-Weiss tear is internal bleeding (mild to heavy) in the area where the esophagus joins the stomach. It may be caused by vomiting and retching, which are common among people who are alcoholics. This vomiting or retching causes tears at the gastroesophageal junction and in turn causes bleeding. (However, about half of Mallory-Weiss syndrome patients do not have a history of prior vomiting or retching.)

Most Mallory-Weiss syndrome patients heal on their own; for others, cauterization or an injection of epinephrine into the damaged area through endoscopy is necessary to stop the hemorrhaging.

Mallory-Weiss syndrome is suspected clinically on the basis of a patient's history and is diagnosed with endoscopy.

See also NAUSEA AND VOMITING.

**malnutrition/starvation**   A serious condition in which nutritional intake is so low that if it is not corrected, an individual becomes sick and predisposed to many illnesses such as infection. The individual may also die. The condition may be caused by a famine, in which there is insufficient food for many people. It may also be caused by other problems, such as poverty or even by an elderly person's inability to feed him- or herself. In some cases, people who have eating disorders, such as anorexia nervosa, become malnourished and may actually starve to death. In other cases, malnutrition may be a result of a sickness, such as uncontrolled CROHN'S DISEASE and MALABSORPTION SYNDROME. Patients who are unable to be fed through the gut may need to receive PARENTERAL NUTRITION.

Although malnutrition is frequently seen in hospitalized patients, malnutrition due to a lack of sufficient food is not a common problem in the United States, Canada, and other developed countries.

See also BERIBERI; VITAMIN DEFICIENCIES/EXCESSES.

**manometry** A diagnostic procedure that tests for resting pressure as well as for contractions and relaxations of the muscles of different parts of the digestive tube; for example, in esophageal manometry, the pressures in the esophagus and the upper and lower esophageal sphincters in both fasting and response to swallowing are each measured with a specific type of catheter. The findings of this test may aid surgeons in planning anti-reflux surgery on what kind of operation to perform.

See also ACHALASIA; HIRSCHSPRUNG'S DISEASE; ZENKER'S DIVERTICULUM.

**Meckel's diverticulum** A congenital small pouch in the small intestine (similar to the appendix in the cecum) that is found in about 2 percent of all individuals. It is usually asymptomatic, but Meckel's diverticulum can cause or lead to an obstruction and to bleeding. This condition, which is frequently difficult to diagnose, is correctable with surgery.

See also ZENKER'S DIVERTICULUM.

**medications** Over-the-counter or prescribed drugs that are used to treat acute or chronic ailments. Most illnesses of the stomach or colon, as well as disorders in other digestive organs, require medication. Some people also use alternative medicines to treat common digestive diseases, such as IRRITABLE BOWEL SYNDROME, heartburn, ULCERATIVE COLITIS, CROHN'S DISEASE, viral hepatitis, and CIRRHOSIS.

Sometimes medications taken for non-digestion-related illnesses have digestive side effects, such as diarrhea, constipation, or dyspepsia. These side effects may subside or may be very difficult to tolerate. In such cases, patients should advise their doctor, who can frequently change the medication or the dosage. Some medications can lead to digestive diseases; for example, nonsteroidal anti-inflammatory drugs (NSAIDs), which are often prescribed for arthritis, may cause ulcers in susceptible individuals.

See also ACID BLOCKING AGENTS; ANTACIDS; ANTIBIOTICS; ANTIDIARRHEALS; ANTIEMETICS; ANTISPASMODICS; BETA BLOCKERS; CYCLOOXYGENASE-2 INHIBITORS; HISTAMINE-2 BLOCKERS; LAXATIVES; NONSTEROIDAL ANTI-INFLAMMATORY DRUGS; PROTON PUMP INHIBITORS.

**megacolon** Very enlarged large intestine (colon), which may cause abdominal distension and constipation. Megacolon may be caused by impaired PERISTALSIS, the wavelike process that moves digesting food and waste through the digestive system. Megacolon may also be caused by an inflammation or blockage stemming from a tumor or volvulus (a type of obstruction that occurs when the gut twists, producing obstruction as well as interruption of the blood supply to the region). A diatrizoate meglumine (Gastrografin) enema or colonoscopy may be ordered to exclude a blockage. In the case of an acute megacolon, decompression of the colon can be carried out, for example, by colonoscopy, in order to reduce the risk of perforation.

**men and digestive diseases** Digestive ailments that occur in males. In many cases, men and women have about an equal risk of development of digestive diseases and disorders; however, some higher risks are based on gender. For example, men have a much greater risk of cancer of the esophagus than women. Similarly, they are more likely to have KAPOSI'S SARCOMA (15 men to one woman). Men also have a higher risk of CIRRHOSIS of the liver, liver cancer, stomach cancer, alcoholic pancreatitis, and HEMOCHROMATOSIS than women. In contrast, women have a higher risk for development of GALLSTONES, gallbladder cancer, HIRSCHSPRUNG'S DISEASE, IRRITABLE BOWEL SYNDROME (IBS), and WATERMELON STOMACH.

See also CANCER, ESOPHAGEAL; CANCER, GALL-
BLADDER; CANCER, LIVER; CANCER, STOMACH.

**Ménétrier's disease**    A rare disease that is characterized by large reddened folds of gastric tissue
inside the stomach. This disease also causes a
depletion of the stomach glands and the acid-pro-
ducing cells, as well as a loss of proteins from the
stomach wall. Ménétrier's disease also increases the
risk of stomach cancer. It is not known what causes this disease. It may involve transforming growth
factor-alpha (TGf-alpha) which increases gastric
mucous production and inhibits acid secretion.

### Symptoms
Ménétrier's disease patients experience the following symptoms:

- Appetite loss
- Pain in the upper middle of the abdomen
- Nausea and vomiting, including vomiting of
  blood
- Ulcerlike pain that occurs after eating
- Fluid build up in the body, resulting in swelling

### Diagnosis and Treatment
The diagnosis of Ménétrier's disease is based on the
patient's symptoms and signs as well as the results
of X rays, endoscopy, and biopsy of tissue from the
stomach.

A variety of medications have been used to treat
Ménétrier's disease, including anti-ulcer medications, but the results have been inconsistent.
Patients are also placed on a high-protein diet.
Patients who have *Helicobacter pylori* infection
require antibiotics to eradicate the infection.
Octreotide may help to reduce protein loss. In some
severe cases of Ménétrier's disease, surgery to
remove part or all of the stomach is required.

See also CANCER, STOMACH; *HELICOBACTER PYLORI*;
ULCERS, PEPTIC.

**menopause**    The time of life in a middle-aged or
older woman (usually in her 40s or older) when
hormonal balance changes. She ceases to menstru-

ate and other body and hormonal changes occur.
These changes can also affect the digestive system;
for example, calcium absorption may be reduced
during menopause, thus increasing the risk for
osteoporosis (bone density loss). Diseases such as
HEMOCHROMATOSIS (iron overload) may become
unmasked when the blood loss due to menstruation ceases. Older women are also more likely to
have problems with OBESITY.

Some women who experience difficult problems
with menopause, such as hot flashes, insomnia,
and mood swings, take hormone replacement therapy to resolve these problems. They may take combination therapy (estrogen and progesterone) or
may take estrogen only. Studies released in 2002
reported on potential health problems associated
with combination therapy, such as an increased
risk of heart disease and breast cancer. Women
should consult their own physician to obtain individualized advice on dealing with menopausal
medical problems that they experience.

See also HORMONE THERAPY.

**mesenteric circulation**    Blood supply to and
drainage from the large intestines and the stomach.
In mesenteric artery ISCHEMIA, arteries that supply
the blood to the intestines may be narrowed. In
extreme cases, the blood flow is completely blocked,
because of a thrombosis or an embolism. If the
blockage is not cleared, it can be fatal to the patient.

Patients who have problems with mesenteric
circulation experience abdominal pain that is usually disproportionate to the physical findings.
Bleeding may be present. Patients with colonic
ischemia (ischemic colitis) primarily have bleeding
or bloody diarrhea. Patients with atherosclerosis
are at risk for mesenteric artery ischemia. Elderly
individuals also have an increased risk for vascular
problems of the bowel and the digestive system.

The treatment depends upon the type of disorder involved and may include observation, medications, angioplasty, or surgery.

See also ISCHEMIA; VASCULITIS.

**microlithiasis**    Gallstones that are so small that
they may not be detectable in imaging studies. The

stones are usually less than five millimeters in diameter. Most patients who have such small stones do not have any symptoms; however, some do experience pain. In some cases, microlithiasis can lead to pancreatitis.

On an ultrasound, microlithiasis may appear as "biliary sludge," or a suspension of fluid that contains tiny crystals or granules of stone. The presence of biliary sludge is more commonly found among patients who are receiving total parenteral nutrition. If patients have repeated attacks and biliary sludge is identified, physicians may determine that cholecystectomy (the surgical removal of the gallbladder) is the best treatment.

See also CHOLECYSTECTOMY; CHOLECYSTITIS; CHOLESTATIS; GALLSTONES; PANCREATITIS; PARENTERAL NUTRITION.

**migrating motor complex (MMC)**    A complex sequence of myoelectrical gastrointestinal events in the fasting state involved in the propelling of the contents of the gut downward. Myoelectric patterns of the gut are divided into two distinct parts: fasting and feeding. Migrating motor complex occurs during the fasting phase of digestion.

In the fasting phase, the electro muscular activity of the gastrointestinal system is relatively quiet. The only exception to this quiet is the occurrence of periodic waves of electrical and muscular activity that causes propagation of the luminal contents of the gut. This is called the migrating myoelectric complex (MMC), which often begins in the esophagus or stomach and may transmit regular contractions for variable distances through the stomach and the small intestine and even into the colon.

MMC starts about four to six hours after a meal is consumed, and it occurs throughout the day in the fasting state, including during sleep. This cycle usually occurs about every 90 to 120 minutes.

### Phases of Migrating Motor Complex

There are four phases of migrating motor complex. In the first phase, there is little motor activity; it is often called the quiescent (quiet) phase. In phase II, a series of seemingly random and erratic contractions occur. Then in phase III, continuous contractions occur. Phase IV is a transition between phase III and phase I. The entire cycle of phases I through IV takes one to two hours, affecting the entire digestive system. The MMCs perform a "housekeeping" function by clearing the intestines of cellular and useless bacterial debris. When eating occurs, the MMC is interrupted by a burst of chaotic contractions, and the fed phase of myoelectric activity then starts.

### After Eating Occurs

During and after a meal, when a person is in the "fed" state, the kinetics of the system change drastically. It is then primarily a mixing flow, as opposed to a migrating motor, that propels the luminal contents downward.

The stomach in the fed state provides regular contractions, usually at a maximum of three contractions per minute. These contractions perform the functions of both mixing and propagation, for example, emptying of small particles from the stomach and into the small intestine. The fed phase of myoelectric activity usually lasts two to three hours postprandially (after a meal); then the fasting phase resumes.

See also DIGESTION AND ABSORPTION.

**milk–alkali syndrome**    A condition of very high calcium blood level that is caused by a combination of an excessive amount of both milk and calcium-containing antacids plus alkaline antacids. Milk–alkali syndrome was once very common, when antacids alone were used to treat ulcers. Then this treatment declined, as did milk–alkali syndrome. However, the incidence of milk–alkali syndrome is again rising, because of an increased emphasis on calcium intake for the prevention of osteoporosis as well as the increased availability of calcium-containing antacids. Milk–alkali syndrome occurs predominantly among women.

In past years, before it was known that nearly all ulcers are caused by either *HELICOBACTER PYLORI* bacteria or chronic consumption of NONSTEROIDAL ANTI-INFLAMMATORY DRUGS (NSAIDs), many patients used very high doses of antacids and some physicians also believed that milk had a soothing influence on the medical problem. As a result, some patients experienced milk–alkali syndrome. However, patients today who do not see a doctor for chronic digestive disorders, such as ulcer or heartburn, and who attempt to treat themselves by using high doses of over-the-counter antacids and drinking large quantities of milk are still at risk for development of milk–alkali syndrome.

Milk–alkali syndrome can cause calcium deposits in the kidneys, which are seen in computed tomography (CT) scans, magnetic resonance imaging (MRI) scans, X rays, or ultrasound of the kidneys.

In severe cases (which are rare), the kidney is damaged and the patient may experience kidney failure and require dialysis or kidney transplantation.

### Symptoms and Signs

Most milk–alkali syndrome patients have acute symptoms, although some may remain asymptomatic. The acute form of the syndrome occurs after about one week of self-treatment with milk and antacids; patients report nausea, vomiting, weakness, and mental changes. Kidney failure may also occur. Stopping the milk and antacids resolves the problem.

In its subacute or intermediate form, milk–alkali syndrome is called Cope's syndrome. It occurs after months to years of intermittent treatment. Kidney function may not always return to normal, even after stopping both milk and antacids.

The chronic form of milk–alkali syndrome is called Burnett's syndrome. Burnett's syndrome patients have a long-standing history of treatment; they report increased thirst and urination, muscle aches, and itchy skin. They may have calcium deposits in the eyes and kidneys. Their kidney function does not return to normal after stopping of the treatment that caused the milk–alkali syndrome.

See also ULCERS, PEPTIC.

**multiple endocrine neoplasia (MEN)**  A genetic condition that causes hyperactivity of the endocrine organs and results in endocrine cancers, such as thyroid cancer and tumors of the adrenal gland, pituitary, and parathyroid glands.

If one family member is diagnosed with multiple endocrine endoplasia (MEN), all first-degree relatives (parents, siblings, and children) should be tested for this condition.

MEN is categorized into MEN I and II. In MEN I, patients are at risk for multiple tumors, starting with the parathyroids, then the pancreas and pituitary, whereas in MEN II, the thyroid, parathyroid, and adrenals may be involved. MEN II is further classified into MEN IIa and IIb, depending on the clinical presentation of the condition.

ZOLLINGER-ELLISON SYNDROME, also known as gastrinoma, is a pancreatic tumor that leads to a severe peptic ulcer disease that is caused by the body's overproduction of gastrin from a tumor in the pancreatic islet cells. It may occur sporadically or can result from MEN I.

Treatment of MEN is usually a combination of medical and surgical therapies, depending upon the site involved and the symptoms of the disease.

See also ULCERS, PEPTIC.

Brandi, Maria Luisa, et al. "Guidelines for Diagnosis and Therapy of MEN Type 1 and Type 2." *Journal of Clinical Endocrinology & Metabolism* 86, no. 12 (2001): 5,658–5,671.

Wynbrandt, James, and Mark D. Ludman. *The Encyclopedia of Genetic Disorders and Birth Defects.* 2d ed. New York: Facts On File, 2000.

**multiple lymphomatous polyposis (MLP)**  A rare form of gastrointestinal non-Hodgkin's lymphoma that occurs primarily among middle-aged to elderly individuals. It occurs more commonly among men than among women.

Patients with multiple lymphomatous polyposis (MLP) have ABDOMINAL PAIN as well as DIARRHEA, which may be bloody. The colon and the rectum are involved in about 90 percent of cases of MLP and show numerous polyps of varying sizes.

MLP is a very aggressive tumor, and the prognosis for MLP is generally poor for most patients, with a mean survival time of less than three years.

However, a 60 percent five-year survival rate is found with some treatment regimens. In one study of 31 patients with multiple lymphomatous polyposis, reported in a 1997 issue of *Gastroenterology*, the prognosis for patients was improved with high-dose radiochemotherapy and stem cell autotransplantation.

Ruskone-Fourmestrauz, A., et al. "Multiple Lymphomatous Polyposis of the Gastrointestinal Tract: Prospective Clinicopthologic Study of 31 Cases." *Gastroenterology* 112, no. 1 (January 1997): 7–16.

**myotomy** A surgical procedure in which the muscle layer of the digestive tube is cut, for example, when a patient suffers from ACHALASIA. Then a Heller's myotomy is performed to allow the lower esophageal sphincter to stay open so that food can pass from the esophagus into the stomach. Similarly, a myotomy may be carried out for infantile pyloric hypertrophic stenosis, to relieve gastric outlet obstruction. This is called Ramstedt pyloromyotomy.

See also ESOPHAGITIS; GASTROESOPHAGEAL REFLUX DISEASE.

**narcotic bowel syndrome** A medical problem that is caused by the chronic and long-term use of opiate painkillers that physicians have prescribed for patients who have a variety of painful medical problems. Narcotic bowel syndrome is characterized by the following symptoms and signs:

- Severe constipation
- Nausea and vomiting
- Excessive gas, which leads to abdominal bloating
- Abdominal pain
- Weight loss

Patients may also appear to have intestinal obstructions, although no obstruction is present (intestinal pseudo-obstruction).

### *Diagnosis and Treatment*

Physicians may suspect the presence of narcotic bowel syndrome if a patient has been taking large doses of narcotics for pain relief for two weeks or more, although not all patients who use narcotics experience this medical problem. X rays of the abdomen show dilated loops of the small and large bowels, with a lot of stool but no evidence of any obstruction.

In most cases, narcotic bowel syndrome patients need to stop taking narcotics, although they should consult the physician about slow tapering off the drug to prevent a severe withdrawal reaction. Naltrexone is frequently used as part of a narcotic detoxification program. During the initial withdrawal from the narcotic, patients may also experience vomiting, diarrhea, and cramps, which can be reduced by taking clonidine. For patients who have an absolute requirement for the continued use of narcotics (such as those who have severe cancer pain), metoclopramide and laxatives may be tried.

Narcotic bowel syndrome can be treated successfully in most cases.

See also CONSTIPATION; LAXATIVES; MEDICATIONS; PAIN.

**nausea and vomiting** Nausea is a subjective complaint that may be described as the feeling or sensation that immediately precedes vomiting. Patients may say that they are about to vomit or may describe themselves as "sick to the stomach" or feeling "queasy." Vomiting is a physical event, involving the rapid, forceful expulsion of the gastric contents from the stomach and up and out of the mouth. Nausea may also precede vomiting that is followed by retching, which creates abdominal pressure to cause further vomiting.

Just as with nausea, retching may occur alone, without actual vomiting of the stomach contents. Similarly, vomiting need not be preceded by nausea.

Vomiting is different from regurgitation, which is a passive phenomenon of the backward flow of the esophageal or gastric contents out of the mouth, such as regurgitation of the acid in GAS-TROESOPHAGEAL REFLUX DISEASE (GERD).

Rumination, on the other hand, is the effortless regurgitation of recently ingested food, which is then followed by rechewing and reswallowing. No nausea or retching occurs in rumination. Although rumination is usually seen in developmentally disabled patients or in those who have psychiatric problems, it may also occur among some patients without such problems.

Nausea and vomiting may accompany relatively minor viruses and illnesses. They are often also symptoms present in the first trimester of pregnancy.

Persistent nausea and vomiting may indicate a serious illness, such as a form of ulcer or cancer or one of many different digestive diseases; however, often nausea and vomiting are signs that are present in common gastrointestinal infections that resolve themselves within a day or two.

If nausea and vomiting become severe, patients are in danger of dehydration and electrolyte imbalances and may require hospitalization. The treatment of nausea and vomiting is directed at identifying the cause and relieving the symptoms. Drugs used to treat nausea and vomiting include metoclopramide (Reglan), promethazine (Phenergan), granisetron (Kytril), and ondansetron (Zofran).

See also CANCER; RUMINATION SYNDROME.

**necrotizing enterocolitis**    A severe form of colon inflammation in which all or part of the colon is damaged by severe inflammation and infection. This rare condition, which occurs primarily in underweight newborn infants, is due to a combination of factors, including prematurity, milk feeding, poor blood circulation, infection, and impaired immune defenses. Necrotizing enterocolitis may also occur in adults who are immune suppressed, especially after chemotherapy for cancer treatment.

Treatment for necrotizing enterocolitis includes antibiotics, bowel rest, PARENTERAL NUTRITION, and sometimes surgery.

**neoplasm**    A tumor or abnormal growth that may be benign or malignant (cancerous). Although many neoplasms are suspected on clinical grounds, in many cases, only a biopsy can determine for certain whether a neoplasm is cancerous.

**nerve block**    A procedure involving the injection of a medication, usually a local anesthetic, to produce short-term pain relief or of a chemical, such as phenol or alcohol, to disrupt the nerve over a longer term. A nerve block is usually injected at the site of a nerve to stop the nerve from functioning, and it is used to stop severe chronic pain. For example, nerve blocks are used for the pain of Herpes zoster, chronic PANCREATITIS, and CANCER.

**neurotransmitters**    Chemicals that act as chemical messengers inside the nervous system, including the brain, spinal cord, and nerves. The part of the nervous system that involves the gut is known as the enteric nervous system. Serotonin and norephinephrine are two of the numerous neurotransmitters in the body, and their actions depend upon the organ, nerves, and nerve cells that are involved. In the gut, the neurotransmitters participate in the regulation of peristalsis (the wavelike movements that push food through the gastrointestinal system), gut immune function, and intestinal secretions.

See also PERISTALSIS.

**nocturnal acid breakthrough**    A digestive problem that is faced by some people who also have GASTROESOPHAGEAL REFLUX DISEASE (GERD), in which there is a surge of stomach acid production leading to ACID REFLUX in the middle of the night, usually when the person is asleep. This may occur despite patients' taking the standard doses of acid blocker medications to block acid production overnight. In considering the problem, doctors ask patients questions about the timing of their acid-related symptoms, and physicians may also prescribe additional doses of the acid blockers in the evening or recommend additional medications at bedtime. Doctors may also recommend over-the-counter drugs to supplement the acid blocker medications that patients already use.

As in any case of GERD, patients are also usually urged to avoid foods such as orange juice, chocolate, and cola drinks, especially before going to bed at night. GERD patients should not go to bed for at least two to four hours after eating their evening meal. They should also sleep on the left side, and with the head of the bed elevated.

**nonalcoholic steatohepatitis/nonalcoholic fatty liver disease (NASH/NAFLD)**    An illness that is characterized by an enlarged liver that is caused by the accumulation of fat in the liver and may be associated with inflammation and scarring (fibrosis) and, in some cases, even with cirrhosis. The disease has also previously been called "fatty liver hepatitis," "alcohol-like liver disease," and, among patients who have diabetes, "diabetes hepatitis."

Although NAFLD does not lead to significant medical symptoms or problems in most patients, it may in the long run in some cases lead to liver cirrhosis and even to liver failure. Predicting in which patients the condition will progress to cirrhosis and in which it will not is difficult.

It is unknown how many people in the United States and other countries have NASH or NAFLD. The condition may be seen in about 7 to 9 percent of patients who have liver biopsy in the United States, and it also occurs more commonly among women. In the majority of cases, patients are between 40 and 60 years old.

Although the biopsy findings are similar for NAFLD and alcoholic hepatitis, the prognosis is different in the two conditions. In about 40 to 50 percent of alcoholic hepatitis patients, cirrhosis develops over a period of 7 years; in 8 to 26 percent of NAFLD patients, cirrhosis develops over the same period.

### Causes of Nonalcoholic Fatty Liver Disease

This disease may stem from many different causes. About 70 percent of NAFLD patients are overweight by about 10 to 40 percent above their ideal body weight. As many as 75 percent of NAFLD patients may have DIABETES MELLITUS. Medications may also induce the disease, including such drugs as aspirin, estrogens, calcium channel blockers, glucocorticoids, synthetic estrogens, methotrexate, tetracycline, tamoxifen, amiodarone, and some antiviral agents as well as some pesticides.

The disease is also associated with extremely rapid weight loss, as well as with bariatric surgery to treat obesity, and with gallbladder and pancreatic surgery, human immunodeficiency virus (HIV), small intestinal DIVERTICULOSIS, and total PARENTERAL NUTRITION. It is also associated with overexposure to some environmental toxins, such as phosphorus, toxic mushrooms, organic cleaning solvents, and oil-based chemicals.

### Risk Factors

Conditions that are commonly associated with nonalcoholic steatohepatitis are obesity, type 2 diabetes, and hyperlipidemia. Some children diagnosed with this medical problem have type 1 (insulin-dependent) diabetes. The excessive weight of the patient is generally centered around the abdomen, among obese people who also have nonalcoholic steatohepatitis, and thus, they are "apple"-shaped rather than "pear"-shaped. Diabetes, obesity, and hyperlipidemia patients are frequently labeled as having *insulin resistance syndrome.*

There are no racial or ethnic differences among people with this condition, who may be either male or female. There appears to be a genetic risk for the disease, although little is known about the genetic transmission, and it has simply been observed that the condition seems to "run in families."

### Symptoms and Signs

There are usually few or no symptoms or signs of nonalcoholic fatty liver disease. Some patients may feel some pain in the right side at the location of the liver, and others complain of tiredness.

### Diagnosis and Treatment

Physicians perform a physical examination, noting the enlarged liver that is seen in nonalcoholic fatty liver disease. Blood tests show mild to moderate elevations of liver enzymes (aspartate aminotransferase [AST] and alanine aminotransferase [ALT]) levels. Other blood tests may be done to exclude other causes of abnormal liver enzyme level, such as viral hepatitis.

An ultrasound reveals the excessive fat of the liver. However, the ultrasound may not provide information on inflammation and scarring and does not distinguish NAFLD from other diseases that may be similar. Magnetic resonance imaging (MRI) can also help to determine the presence of nonalcoholic fatty liver disease. However, imaging studies cannot show the extent of damage to the liver, which can only be determined by liver biopsy.

It is controversial whether a liver biopsy should be performed in all cases. The liver biopsy can definitively confirm the presence of nonalcoholic fatty liver disease, assuming that alcohol has been excluded as a factor by the taking of a medical history. Liver biopsy may be deferred by the doctor, pending a therapeutic trial of weight loss.

Treatment is usually directed to the associated problems; for example, if the patient is obese, the liver test findings may improve with weight loss.

Diabetes patients should be treated with medications to achieve optimal glucose level control.

It is best to prevent very rapid weight loss with this disease because sudden major weight loss can also cause NAFLD. Instead, it is generally recommended that patients gradually lose about 10 to 15 pounds. Adults should lose no more than 1,600 grams (3.5 pounds) per week, and ideally no more than one to two pounds per week, and children with NAFLD should lose about 500 grams per week.

Some improvement may also occur if patients with diabetes improve their blood sugar level, maintaining the level at as close to normal as possible.

There are no medications definitively proved to treat nonalcoholic fatty liver disease, as of this writing. Physicians frequently recommend medications such as ursodeoxycholic acid, vitamin E supplements, and trimethylglycine (Betaine). Metformin may be recommended for patients who also have diabetes.

See also BARIATRIC SURGERY; CIRRHOSIS; HEPATITIS; LIVER ENZYMES/FUNCTION TESTS; LIVER FAILURE; STEATORRHEA.

Angulo, Paul, M.D. "Nonalcoholic Fatty Liver Disease." *New England Journal of Medicine* 346, no. 16 (April 18, 2002): 1,221–1,231.

**nonerosive reflux disease (NERD)** Gastroesophageal reflux disease (GERD) with an absence of esophagitis (inflammation of the esophagus). About half of GERD patients have no esophagitis. Patients with nonerosive reflux disease (NERD) have normal endoscopy results but still have GERD which can be confirmed by esophageal biopsy. They must be diagnosed on their symptoms with or without esophageal biopsy and treated with the same medications and lifestyle recommendations as GERD patients.

See also GASTROESOPHAGEAL REFLUX DISEASE.

**nonsteroidal anti-inflammatory drugs (NSAIDs)** Over-the-counter and prescribed medications that are taken to decrease the pain and inflammation that are caused by illnesses such as arthritis or muscle pain. Stomach distress, gastritis, and even ulcers are often side effects of use of these medications. In a small number of patients, these side effects can lead to life-threatening gastrointestinal bleeding.

The side effects of NSAIDs can be particularly risky for individuals who are 65 years and older, who may have many medical problems and may also may be taking a wide variety of medications. Patients who are elderly or have a history of severe heart disease, prior ulcers, or prior gastrointestinal bleeding and who have chronic pain that would normally be relieved by an NSAID should take, in addition to the NSAID, a medication protective against its ulcerogenic effects, such as misoprostol (Cytotec) or a proton pump inhibitor medication. Alternately, cyclooxygenase-2 (COX-2) inhibitors such as rofecoxib (Vioxx) and valdecoxib (Bextra) may be used instead of traditional NSAIDs, since they have lower gastrointestinal toxicity. Some high risk patients may be prescribed prophylactic medication (misoprostol or a proton pump inhibitor) even when taking COX-2 inhibitors.

See also PAIN; PROSTAGLANDINS; PROTON PUMP INHIBITORS; ULCERS, PEPTIC.

**nonviral liver disease** A liver ailment that is not caused by a virus, such as HEPATITIS, or by CIRRHOSIS, that results from alcoholism. Examples of nonviral liver diseases are HEMOCHROMATOSIS (iron overload), WILSON'S DISEASE (copper overload), PRIMARY BILIARY CIRRHOSIS, NONALCOHOLIC STEATOHEPATITIS (NASH), autoimmune hepatitis, and liver cancer.

See also ALCOHOL ABUSE AND DEPENDENCE/ALCOHOLISM; CANCER, LIVER.

**obesity**   Excessive weight for one's height, which is an increasing health problem in the United States, Canada, and many other developed nations and even among people in many developing countries because it increases risk for diabetes, gallstones, cancer, heart disease, and other illnesses.

According to the World Health Organization, there are about 300 million obese adults in the world, and at least 115 million live in developing nations. This may be in large part due to the increased caloric intake of many people. For example, according to the World Health Organization in their 2003 report, in the period 1974 to 1976, the worldwide per capita food consumption in calories per day was 2,435. By 1997 to 1999 that number had increased to 2,803 calories, and it is projected to increase to 2,940 calories per day by 2015. In industrialized countries, calorie intake has also increased; for example, in the period 1974 to 1976, per capita daily calorie consumption was 3,065. That calorie intake increased to 3,380 by the 1997 to 1999 period, and the World Health Organization projects a further increase to 3,440 calories per day by 2015.

Obesity leads to death in some people. According to the United States surgeon general, about 300,000 deaths per year in the United States may be attributable to obesity. In addition, people who are obese have at least a 50 percent greater risk of premature death of all causes than that of nonobese individuals.

In the United States as well as in many other countries, obesity is defined in terms of the individual's BODY MASS INDEX (BMI): people are obese when they have a body mass index that is equal to or greater than 30 kilograms per square meter (meters of height squared, or the number multiplied times itself). BMI is usually expressed without units, for example, a BMI of 30.

The BMI is based on a mathematical formula; to compute BMI in inches, an individual can take his or her own weight in pounds, multiply that number by 704.5, and then divide the result by his or her height in inches. That number is then divided *again* by the height in inches to determine the BMI. However, most people simply look at a chart of height and weight to look up their individual BMI. (See APPENDIX IX for BMI information on adults and APPENDIX X for the BMI charts on boys and girls of all ages.)

### *Considering Weight Ranges and Obesity*

Individuals who have a BMI between 25 and 29 are considered to be overweight but are not regarded as obese. As mentioned earlier, a BMI of 30 or more indicates obesity. (This information is summarized in the chart that follows.) In addition, individuals who have a BMI of 40 or greater are considered morbidly obese; they are at an especially high risk for development of many severe health problems, such as diabetes, hypertension, and heart disease.

| BMI | Weight Status |
|---|---|
| Less than 18.5 | Underweight |
| 18.5 to 24.9 | Normal weight |
| 25.0 to 29.9 | Overweight |
| 30.0 to 39.9 | Obese |
| 40.0 and greater | Morbidly obese |

### *A Prominent Problem Nationwide and Worldwide*

Many Americans are overweight or obese: according to the Centers for Disease Control and Prevention (CDC), about 45 million Americans, or 25 percent of the entire adult U.S. population, are obese. Since 1990 alone, the number of obese people has risen by about 60 percent. About two-thirds of obese adults have a BMI more than 25, 30 percent have a BMI greater than 30, whereas as many as 5 percent have a BMI exceeding 40. The prevalence of obesity amongst American children has more than doubled over the last twenty years. Despite these facts some studies have shown that most people in the United States are not told by their doctor that they should lose weight. A study reported in 2000 in *Archives of Internal Medicine* revealed that most patients who are told to lose weight are middle-aged individuals who have other medical problems. Yet many younger and elderly individuals have severe weight problems and also need such weight counseling.

### Abdominal Obesity

Many people who are obese carry much of their weight in their abdomen and they are considered "apple"-shaped rather than pear-shaped (in which most of the extra fat is carried in the hips rather than the abdomen). Yet studies have shown that abdominal obesity (the apple shape) greatly increases the risk of development of diabetes, hypertension, and other medical problems.

In a related issue, some researchers believe that the waist–hip ratio is a better predictor than the body mass index of poor health or even mortality among obese people when abdominal obesity is the problem. In one study, reported in 2000 in *Archives of Internal Medicine,* the researchers compared the waist-to-hip ratio of deceased subjects with their body mass index to determine which measure was ultimately a better predictor of death among obese individuals. They found that the waist–hip ratio was a significantly better predictive measure.

### Obesity and Disease

Obesity causes or contributes to the development of many serious and chronic digestion-related illnesses, such as DIABETES MELLITUS, CANCER, GALLSTONES, and NONALCOHOLIC STEATOHEPATITIS, as well as other nondigestive illnesses, such as hypertension, heart disease, kidney disease, arthritis, sleep disorders, and stroke. Obesity also increases the risk for heart failure. Several of these health issues are discussed in this section.

***Diabetes and obesity***  The risk in obese people of development of diabetes is very well document-ed by many researchers. An article in a 1999 issue of *Diabetes Care* reported on a study in which researchers followed nearly 7,000 men with no diabetes history over 12 years. During that time, in 237 of the men developed type 2 diabetes. The researchers found that a weight gain greater than 10 percent was significantly associated with the development of diabetes.

Said the researchers: "This study confirms the critical importance of overweight and obesity, particularly of long duration, in the development of type 2 diabetes. The data support current public health recommendations to reduce the risk of type 2 diabetes by preventing weight gain in middle-aged men who are not overweight and by encouraging weight loss in overweight and obese men." (Of course, obese and overweight women should also lose weight, because they too are at risk for type 2 diabetes. The study emphasized weight loss among obese men because the subjects were males.)

***Cancer and obesity***  Obesity apparently also increases the risk of development of many different types of cancer. A study that was reported by researchers in the *New England Journal of Medicine* in 2003 attributed 14 percent of the cancer deaths in men and 20 percent in women in part to either overweight or obesity. Many of the cancers that subjects died of were digestion-related cancers, and the risk of death of these cancers increased proportionately with the patient's body mass index.

In this study, more than 900,000 adults were enrolled in 1982. Over the next 16 years, 57,145 of the subjects died of cancer. In considering the various forms of cancer and the deceased person's BMI, the findings were as follows: For esophageal cancer, the risk was 13.97 per 100,000 people for subjects with a BMI of 18.5 to 24.9 (normal weight for height). For overweight individuals (BMI of 25.0 to 29.9), the death rate increased even more, to 15.74 per 100,000 people. The risk of death increased further, to 18.07 per 100,000 subjects, for those who had a BMI between 30.1 and 34.9, and to 24.18 for those with a BMI of 35.0 to 39.9.

The risk of cancer development among those who are overweight or obese was even more marked for colorectal cancer. Normal-weight subjects had a colorectal cancer death rate of 53.51 per 100,000 subjects. That rate climbed to 64.43 for overweight subjects (with a BMI of 25.0 to 29.9) and still further to 79.50 per 100,000 for subjects with a BMI of 30.0 to 34.9. For even more obese subjects, the risk was 101.25, nearly double the risk for those who had normal body weight.

Another area of an even more marked risk of death from cancer was seen for liver cancer, although liver cancer is relatively rare. In the study, the liver cancer death rate was 9.24 per 100,000 individuals for people of normal body weight. It more than doubled to 19.22 for those with a BMI of 30.0 to 34.9 and dramatically rose to 47.80 for those subjects who had a BMI of 35.0 to 39.9, or more than five times the rate among those individuals with normal BMI.

The researchers concluded:

The large size of our cohort [study group] allowed us to investigate the effect of overweight and obesity on the occurrence of 57,000 deaths from cancer among 900,000 men and women who were free of cancer at base line. Overweight and obesity are associated with the risk of death from all cancers and with death from cancers at many specific sites. From our results, we estimate that 90,000 deaths due to cancer could be prevented each year in the United States if men and women could maintain normal weight.

### Causes of Obesity

In most cases, the basic and obvious cause of obesity is overeating combined with insufficient physical activity; however, rarely, there are other prevailing causes, such as hypothyroidism (low thyroid level), Cushing's syndrome, and other medical problems. Some endocrinological researchers believe that there may be a link between problems with the secretion of cortisol, a hormone that is secreted by the adrenal glands, and obesity, and research is ongoing.

**Emotional issues**  Some doctors and therapists believe that obesity is both maladaptive behavior and a response to stress. It may also be learned behavior, based on childhood experiences; for example, perhaps cake or cookies were used as a reward by parents as well as a comfort food for distressing events. This learned behavior may become incorporated into the patient's basic habits, and overeating may continue to be a pattern when the person is struggling with problems or celebrating successes. Patients may need to resolve their underlying emotional conflicts and fully explore these issues before they can successfully lose a significant amount of weight.

**Ghrelin may affect obesity**  In 1999 ghrelin, a hormone that is released by the stomach and that appears to affect appetite directly, was discovered. Some preliminary studies indicate that one key problem that many dieters face is that their blood level of ghrelin rises in response to dieting: that is, dieters are much more hungry, even ravenous, than nondieters, and thus they find losing weight very difficult. Some experts hope that an "antighrelin" medication can be developed as a diet medication.

A study by Cummings and colleagues of patients who had gastric bypass surgery for weight reduction (also known as BARIATRIC SURGERY) showed that the level of ghrelin of those who had surgery was significantly lower than the ghrelin level of the dieters in the study who did not have surgery. In fact, the postoperative ghrelin levels of the patients were even lower than those of control subjects of normal weight. These findings were reported in 2002 in the *New England Journal of Medicine*. Apparently the result of the gastric bypass surgery was to impede somehow the secretion of ghrelin; further studies are needed to determine how this occurs, whether the effect continues, and other key issues.

**Genetics and obesity**  Obesity may be caused by a genetic problem; research on an association is ongoing. Genes contributing to the more common forms of obesity in humans have not been identified. To date, only a tiny proportion of obesity has been directly attributed to genetic factors, such as mutations in single genes that affect fat storage. Continuing research may uncover further human genetic links to obesity. Some researchers have found a genetic link to both type 2 diabetes and obesity on chromosome 18p11; it was described in a 2001 issue of *Diabetes*.

## HEALTHY WEIGHT, OVERWEIGHT, AND OBESITY AMONG PERSONS 20 YEARS OF AGE AND OLDER, ACCORDING TO SEX, AGE, RACE, AND HISPANIC ORIGIN: UNITED STATES, 1960–62, 1971–74, 1976–80, AND 1988–94

[Data are based on measured height and weight of a sample of the civilian noninstitutionalized population]

| Sex, Age, Race, and Hispanic Origin[1] | Overweight[2] | | | | Obesity[3] | | | |
|---|---|---|---|---|---|---|---|---|
| | 1960–62 | 1971–74 | 1976–80[4] | 1988–94 | 1960–62 | 1971–74 | 1976–80[4] | 1988–94 |
| 20–74 years, age adjusted[5] | Percent of population | | | | | | | |
| Both sexes[6,7] | 44.8 | 47.7 | 47.4 | 56.0 | 13.3 | 14.6 | 15.1 | 23.3 |
| Male | 49.5 | 54.7 | 52.9 | 61.0 | 10.7 | 12.2 | 12.8 | 20.6 |
| Female[6] | 40.2 | 41.1 | 42.0 | 51.2 | 15.7 | 16.8 | 17.1 | 26.0 |
| White male | 50.2 | 55.4 | 53.8 | 62.3 | 10.5 | 11.8 | 12.5 | 21.0 |
| White female[6] | 37.5 | 38.8 | 39.4 | 49.4 | 14.2 | 15.4 | 15.5 | 24.3 |
| Black male | 43.9 | 50.4 | 51.4 | 58.0 | 14.0 | 16.8 | 16.7 | 21.1 |
| Black female[6] | 59.2 | 60.5 | 63.2 | 68.5 | 26.8 | 29.7 | 31.3 | 39.0 |
| White, non-Hispanic male | — | — | 53.4 | 61.6 | — | — | 12.4 | 20.7 |
| White, non-Hispanic female[6] | — | — | 38.7 | 47.2 | — | — | 15.4 | 23.3 |
| Black, non-Hispanic male | — | — | 51.3 | 58.2 | — | — | 16.5 | 21.3 |
| Black, non-Hispanic female[6] | — | — | 62.6 | 68.5 | — | — | 31.0 | 39.1 |
| Mexican male | — | — | 61.6 | 69.4 | — | — | 15.7 | 24.4 |
| Mexican female[6] | — | — | 61.7 | 69.6 | — | — | 26.6 | 36.1 |
| 20–74 years, crude | | | | | | | | |
| Both sexes[6,7] | 45.2 | 47.0 | 46.4 | 55.0 | 13.5 | 14.4 | 14.7 | 22.7 |
| Male | 49.4 | 53.5 | 51.5 | 59.6 | 10.7 | 12.0 | 12.3 | 19.9 |
| Female[6] | 41.2 | 41.0 | 41.6 | 50.5 | 16.1 | 16.7 | 16.8 | 25.5 |
| White male | 50.2 | 54.3 | 52.5 | 61.1 | 10.4 | 11.7 | 12.1 | 20.4 |
| White female[6] | 38.9 | 39.1 | 39.4 | 49.0 | 14.7 | 15.4 | 15.3 | 24.0 |
| Black male | 43.9 | 49.3 | 48.5 | 56.7 | 14.1 | 16.0 | 15.0 | 20.9 |
| Black female[6] | 58.8 | 58.2 | 60.0 | 65.9 | 26.6 | 28.7 | 29.8 | 37.0 |
| White, non-Hispanic male | — | — | 52.2 | 60.8 | — | — | 12.0 | 20.3 |
| White, non-Hispanic female[6] | — | — | 38.9 | 47.1 | — | — | 15.2 | 23.1 |
| Black, non-Hispanic male | — | — | 48.4 | 57.0 | — | — | 14.9 | 21.1 |
| Black, non-Hispanic female[6] | — | — | 59.4 | 66.2 | — | — | 29.5 | 37.2 |
| Mexican male | — | — | 57.0 | 64.0 | — | — | 14.6 | 20.7 |
| Mexican female[6] | — | — | 57.4 | 66.2 | — | — | 23.8 | 33.6 |
| Male | | | | | | | | |
| 20–34 years | 42.7 | 42.8 | 41.2 | 47.5 | 9.2 | 9.7 | 8.9 | 14.1 |
| 35–44 years | 53.5 | 63.2 | 57.2 | 65.5 | 12.1 | 13.5 | 13.5 | 21.5 |
| 45–54 years | 53.9 | 59.7 | 60.2 | 66.1 | 12.5 | 13.7 | 16.7 | 23.2 |
| 55–64 years | 52.2 | 58.5 | 60.2 | 70.5 | 9.2 | 14.1 | 14.1 | 27.2 |
| 65–74 years | 47.8 | 54.6 | 54.2 | 68.5 | 10.4 | 10.9 | 13.2 | 24.1 |
| 75 years and over | — | — | — | 56.5 | — | — | — | 13.2 |
| Female[6] | | | | | | | | |
| 20–34 years | 21.2 | 25.8 | 27.9 | 37.0 | 7.2 | 9.7 | 11.0 | 18.5 |
| 35–44 years | 37.2 | 40.5 | 40.7 | 49.6 | 14.7 | 17.7 | 17.8 | 25.5 |
| 45–54 years | 49.3 | 49.0 | 48.7 | 60.3 | 20.3 | 18.9 | 19.6 | 32.4 |
| 55–64 years | 59.9 | 54.5 | 53.7 | 66.3 | 24.4 | 24.1 | 22.9 | 33.7 |
| 65–74 years | 60.9 | 55.9 | 59.5 | 60.3 | 23.2 | 22.0 | 21.5 | 26.9 |
| 75 years and over | — | — | — | 52.3 | — | — | — | 19.2 |

—Data not available

[1]The race groups, white and black, include persons of Hispanic and non-Hispanic origin.
[2]Body mass index (BMI) greater than or equal to 25.
[3]BMI greater than or equal to 30.
[4]Data for Mexicans are for 1982–84.

[5]Age adjusted to 2000 population using 5 age groups.
[6]Excludes pregnant women.
[7]Includes persons of all races and Hispanic origins, not just those shown separately.
[8]BMI of 18.5 to less than 25 kilograms/m².

| Sex, Age, Race, and Hispanic Origin[1] | Healthy Weight[8] | | | |
|---|---|---|---|---|
| | 1960–62 | 1971–74 | 1976–80[4] | 1988–94 |
| **20–74 years, age adjusted[5]** | Percent of population | | | |
| Both sexes[6,7] | 51.2 | 48.8 | 49.6 | 41.7 |
| Male | 48.3 | 43.0 | 45.4 | 37.9 |
| Female[6] | 54.1 | 54.3 | 53.7 | 45.3 |
| White male | 47.6 | 42.4 | 44.8 | 36.7 |
| White female[6] | 56.5 | 56.6 | 56.1 | 47.2 |
| Black male | 53.2 | 47.3 | 46.4 | 40.3 |
| Black female[6] | 36.0 | 34.9 | 34.4 | 28.6 |
| White, non-Hispanic male | — | — | 45.3 | 37.4 |
| White, non-Hispanic female[6] | — | — | 56.7 | 49.2 |
| Black, non-Hispanic male | — | — | 46.6 | 40.0 |
| Black, non-Hispanic female[6] | — | — | 35.0 | 28.9 |
| Mexican male | — | — | 37.1 | 29.8 |
| Mexican female[6] | — | — | 36.4 | 29.1 |
| **20–74 years, crude** | | | | |
| Both sexes[6,7] | 50.8 | 49.3 | 50.5 | 42.6 |
| Male | 48.3 | 44.1 | 46.8 | 39.3 |
| Female[6] | 53.2 | 54.1 | 53.9 | 45.9 |
| White male | 47.6 | 43.4 | 46.1 | 37.8 |
| White female[6] | 55.4 | 56.1 | 55.9 | 47.5 |
| Black male | 53.5 | 48.5 | 49.5 | 41.7 |
| Black female[6] | 36.4 | 36.5 | 37.2 | 30.9 |
| White, non-Hispanic male | — | — | 46.4 | 38.1 |
| White, non-Hispanic female[6] | — | — | 56.4 | 49.2 |
| Black, non-Hispanic male | — | — | 49.6 | 41.4 |
| Black, non-Hispanic female[6] | — | — | 37.7 | 31.1 |
| Mexican male | — | — | 41.6 | 35.2 |
| Mexican female[6] | — | — | 40.1 | 32.2 |
| **Male** | | | | |
| 20–34 years | 55.3 | 54.7 | 57.1 | 51.1 |
| 35–44 years | 45.2 | 35.2 | 41.3 | 33.4 |
| 45–54 years | 44.8 | 38.5 | 38.7 | 33.6 |
| 55–64 years | 44.9 | 38.3 | 38.7 | 28.6 |
| 65–74 years | 46.2 | 42.1 | 42.3 | 30.1 |
| 75 years and over | — | — | — | 40.9 |
| **Female[6]** | | | | |
| 20–34 years | 67.6 | 65.8 | 65.0 | 57.9 |
| 35–44 years | 58.4 | 56.7 | 55.6 | 47.1 |
| 45–54 years | 47.6 | 49.3 | 48.7 | 37.2 |
| 55–64 years | 38.1 | 41.1 | 43.5 | 31.5 |
| 65–74 years | 36.4 | 40.6 | 37.8 | 37.0 |
| 75 years and over | — | — | — | 43.0 |

Notes: Percentages do not sum to 100 because the percentage of persons with BMI less than 18.5 is not shown and the percentage of persons with obesity is a subset of the percentage with overweight. Height was measured without shoes; two pounds was deducted from data for 1960–62 to allow for weight of clothing. Initial results from the 1999 NHANES indicate that 61 percent of U.S. adults were overweight and 27 percent were obese in 1999. The 1999 data are preliminary estimates from the 1999 NHANES. The 1999 data are limited in sample size and geographic coverage and, therefore, are subject to more sampling error than multiyear NHANES data. As a result, annual prevalence estimates may fluctuate more than those from multiyear NHANES data. See www.cdc.gov/nchs/products/pubs/ pubd/hestats/obese/obes99.htm.
Source: Centers for Disease Control and Prevention, National Center for Health Statistics, National Health Examination Surveys, and National Health and Nutrition Examination Surveys (NHANES).

Obesity related genes that have been identified to date, according to the Centers for Disease Control and Prevention (CDC), include the following gene products and genes:

- *LEP* (164160) (leptin)
- *LEPR* (601007) (leptin receptor)
- *POMC1* (176830) (proopiomelanocortin)
- SIM1 (human homolog of *Drosophilia* single-minded 1) (603128)
- *PC1* (prohormone convertase 1) (162150)
- *MC4R* (melanocortin-4 receptor) (155541)

### Risk Factors for Obesity

Men and women are equally likely to be obese in the United States; however, there are some interesting gender differences to consider when looking at some aspects of obese people, such as their marital status, education, and age, some of which are summarized here.

*Marital status and obesity* Studies by the Centers for Disease Control and Prevention (CDC) have shown that married men are *more* likely to be obese (20.4 percent were obese in 1997) than separated or divorced men (16.8 percent were obese). In contrast, the situation is reversed among females: married women are *less* likely to be obese (18.4 percent) than are separated or divorced women (23.2 percent). The underlying causes of these differences are unknown and are certainly worthy of further exploration.

*Race and ethnicity* There are some other significant demographic differences among obese people in the United States; for example, non-Hispanic blacks and Hispanic whites are more likely to be obese than are whites or people of other races or ethnicities. (See table on pages 188–189.)

In addition, some groups, such as the Pima in Arizona, have high rates of obesity, as well as diabetes, hypertension, and kidney disease. Other populations in the world, such as people living in the Pacific Islands, have an extremely high rate of obesity. According to the World Health Organization in their 2003 report "Diet, Food Supply and Obesity in the Pacific," as much as 75 percent of the population is overweight or obese in Samoa, American Samoa, French Polynesia, and other areas.

*Age and obesity* Age is another factor in obesity statistics. Adults who are ages 18 to 24 years are less likely to be obese (12.9 percent were obese) than are older individuals. (See tables.)

*Education and obesity* Education is another significant factor that apparently affects who is obese. Obesity rates decrease with education; for example, CDC statistics have shown that 24.7 percent of men with less than a high school diploma were obese compared to 11.3 percent of men with a master's degree or other advanced degree beyond a bachelor's degree. Thus, poorly educated men have more than twice the risk of obesity of very well-educated men.

The impact of education is even greater among women. Among women, 27.4 percent who had not graduated from high school were obese, compared to 10.5 percent who had completed a graduate degree. Thus, poorly educated women are more than two and a half times more likely to be obese than are very well-educated women.

The lower rate of obesity among more educated people may stem from a more nutritious diet consumed by educated people and more opportunities (in terms of time and money) for exercise and physical activity. However, the reasons are not really known, and, thus, these are only speculations.

*Income and obesity* Family income is another factor related to obesity. According to data provided by the CDC, 26 percent of individuals living below the poverty level were obese in 1997, compared to 15.8 percent whose income was four times the poverty level. Low-income people may be more likely to eat a diet that is high in carbohydrates, especially sweets, as well as in fats; further investigation is needed to explore the reasons for higher levels of obesity among low-income individuals.

*Geographic area* The geographic region in the United States where a person lives also apparently plays some role in the levels of obesity among Americans. According to the CDC data, people in the West had the lowest level of obesity (17 percent of adults), followed by those in the Northeast (18.9

percent). The Midwest and the South were nearly tied, at 20.8 percent for those in the Midwest who were obese and 20.4 percent for the people living in the South. The reasons for these geographic disparities are unknown.

**Disabilities and obesity**  Some studies have shown that individuals who are disabled are more likely to be obese. In a study reported in a 2002 issue of the *Journal of the American Medical Association,* the researchers analyzed subjects who had a variety of disabilities, including blindness or severe difficulties with sight, deafness or impaired hearing, and inability to walk without difficulty. The researchers found that nearly 25 percent of the disabled individuals were obese, compared to 15.1 percent of individuals without disabilities who were obese.

Some patients who are ill or disabled may find it very difficult to have sufficient exercise. Their physician may also feel sorry for them or not wish to take the time to help them create a plan of exercise that is within the scope of their abilities. Such a plan is important because patients can become even less active and more obese, worsening a disability, in a vicious cycle.

### Children and Obesity

Many children and adolescents in the United States and other countries have problems with obesity, and some are morbidly obese. Often they have parents and other family members who are obese, although not always. It is important that parents and others help children overcome problems with obesity to prevent a lifelong problem of obesity; however, at the same time, it is also important to prevent stigmatizing of children who are overweight.

According to the 2003 report by the World Health Organization, "Diet, Nutrition and the Prevention of Chronic Diseases," birth weights among babies in industrialized countries have risen only slightly and cannot account for a much greater incidence of obesity among children. Said the authors:

The "obesogenic" environment appears to be largely directed at the adolescent market, making healthy choices that much more difficult. At the same time, exercise patterns have changed and considerable parts of the day are spent sitting at school, in a factory, or in front of a television or computer. Raised blood pressure, impaired glucose tolerance and dyslipidaemia are associated in children and adolescents with unhealthy lifestyles, such as diets containing excessive intakes of fats (especially saturated), cholesterol and salt, an inadequate intake of fibre and potassium, a lack of exercise, and increased television viewing.

The percentages of overweight and obese children in the United States have increased dramatically over time; for example, in the period 1963 to 1970, only about 4.2 percent of all children and adolescents ages six to 19 were overweight, and the percentage dropped slightly to 4.0 percent during the 1971 to 1974 period. Since then, the percentage of obese children has risen dramatically. In the period 1999 to 2000, an estimated 15.3 percent of children and adolescents were overweight: nearly a fourfold increase over 1963 through 1974.

The reasons for obesity among children may and probably do mirror the reasons for obesity among adults, as indicated by studies that have been performed to date, such as spending too much time watching television, eating large quantities of carbohydrates, and exercising only infrequently; however, the solution may be even trickier because children are still growing (hence, medications such as diet drugs may be inadvisable) and are more emotionally vulnerable than adults.

A study of Pima children in Arizona reported in 2002 in *Pediatrics* indicated that they have a greater obesity problem than other children. (The Pima are noted for their severe problems with obesity and with the highest rate of type 2 diabetes worldwide.) The researchers found that prominent factors for obesity were a low rate of participating in sports and a higher rate of watching television than those of peers.

Researchers have analyzed many aspects of childhood obesity, seeking solutions. In one study, researchers studied obesity in parents and their children and found that having an obese parent doubles the risk of growing up to be obese. These findings were reported in a 1997 issue of the *New*

## PERCENTAGE OF OVERWEIGHT CHILDREN AND ADOLESCENTS 6–19 YEARS OF AGE, ACCORDING TO SEX, AGE, RACE, AND HISPANIC ORIGIN: UNITED STATES, SELECTED YEARS 1963–65 THROUGH 1988–94

[Data are based on measured height and weight of a sample of the civilian noninstitutionalized population]

| Age, Sex, Race, and Hispanic Origin[1] | 1963–65 1966–70[2] | 1971–74 | 1976–80[3] | 1988–94 |
|---|---|---|---|---|
| **6–11 years of age:** | | | | |
| Both sexes | 4.2 | 4.0 | 6.5 | 11.4 |
| Boys | 4.0 | 4.3 | 6.6 | 11.8 |
| White | 4.4 | 4.1 | 6.7 | 11.6 |
| Black | 1.6 | 5.3 | 6.7 | 12.3 |
| White, non-Hispanic | — | — | 6.1 | 10.9 |
| Black, non-Hispanic | — | — | 6.8 | 12.3 |
| Mexican | — | — | 13.3 | 17.7 |
| Girls | 4.5 | 3.6 | 6.4 | 11.0 |
| White | 4.5 | 3.7 | 5.7 | 9.8 |
| Black | 4.5 | 3.3 | 11.1 | 16.9 |
| White, non-Hispanic | — | — | 5.2 | 9.8 |
| Black, non-Hispanic | — | — | 11.2 | 17.1 |
| Mexican | — | — | 9.8 | 15.3 |
| **12–19 years of age:** | | | | |
| Both sexes | 4.6 | 6.1 | 5.0 | 10.5 |
| Boys | 4.5 | 6.1 | 4.8 | 11.3 |
| White | 4.7 | 5.5 | 4.6 | 12.1 |
| Black | 3.1 | 5.0 | 4.8 | 10.4 |
| White, non-Hispanic | — | — | 3.6 | 11.6 |
| Black, non-Hispanic | — | — | 4.9 | 10.7 |
| Mexican | — | — | 7.7 | 14.1 |
| Girls[4] | 4.7 | 6.2 | 5.3 | 9.7 |
| White | 4.5 | 6.1 | 4.7 | 9.0 |
| Black | 6.4 | 10.1 | 10.0 | 16.3 |
| White, non-Hispanic | — | — | 5.0 | 8.9 |
| Black, non-Hispanic | — | — | 10.3 | 16.3 |
| Mexican | — | — | 9.1 | 13.5 |

—Data not available.

[1]The race groups, white and black, include persons of Hispanic and non-Hispanic origin. Conversely, persons of Hispanic origin may be of any race.

[2]Data for 1963–65 are for children 6–11 years of age; data for 1966–70 are for adolescents 12–17 years of age, not 12–19 years.

[3]Data for Mexicans are for 1982–84.

[4]Excludes pregnant women starting with 1971–74. Pregnancy status not available for 1963–65 and 1966–70.

Notes: Overweight is defined as body mass index (BMI) at or above the sex- and age-specific 95th percentile BMI cutoff points from the 2000 CDC Growth Charts: United States. Advance data from vital and health statistics; no. 314. Hyattsville, Maryland: National Center for Health Statistics. 2000. Age is at time of examination at mobile examination center. Crude rates, not age-adjusted rates, are shown. Initial results from the 1999 NHANES indicate that 13 percent of children ages 6–11 years and 14 percent of children ages 12–19 years were overweight in 1999. The 1999 data are preliminary estimates from the 1999 NHANES. The 1999 data are limited in sample size and geographic coverage and, therefore, are subject to more sampling error than multiyear NHANES. As a result, annual prevalence estimates may fluctuate more than those from multiyear NHANES. See www.cdc.gov/nchs/ products/pubs/pubd/hestats/overwght99.htm.

Source: Centers for Disease Control and Prevention, National Center for Health Statistics, National Health Examination Surveys, and National Health and Nutrition Examination Surveys (NHANES).

Table will be updated with 1999–2000 data on the Web. Go to www. cdc.gov/nchs/hus.htm.

*England Journal of Medicine.* The possible effect on obese children of their obese parent's attaining normal weights is not known; however, logically, it would seem to be a positive step and children might model their behavior on their parent's actions.

### Diagnosing and Treating Obesity

Some doctors specialize in assisting patients with weight loss, but most patients who try to lose weight see an internist or a general practitioner. Most doctors can readily identify obesity on the basis of a patient's weight and body mass index. Treatment is more difficult. Many physicians believe that chronic obesity is a very complex problem. For a normal-weight or slightly over-weight person who gains five or 10 pounds, eating less and exercising more to lose the weight are relatively simple. However, for an obese person who needs to lose 50 pounds or more, that task is far more daunting for both the patient and the physician.

*Dieting attempts* Millions of dollars are spent each year by individuals seeking an easy and quick way to lose a lot of weight, including money spent on DIET DRUGS and other weight loss items, as well as purportedly easy-to-use exercise devices. Some patients use hypnotherapy to lose weight.

Medications for weight loss are recommended for patients with a BMI of greater than 30 or greater than 27 if they have obesity-related problems for which conservative management with diet and exercise have failed. Drugs should not be used by children or the elderly (older than age 65 years); nor should they be used by women who are pregnant or are breastfeeding. Individuals who have pulmonary hypertension, uncontrolled systemic hypertension, or unstable heart disease should also avoid diet drugs.

Orlistat (Xenical) prevents the digestion of fat in the gut and thus reduces its absorption in the body. Subutramine (Meridia) increases norepinephrine and serotonin at the nerve terminals, reduces food intake, and may increase body metabolism. Phentermine is another diet drug that is approved for short-term use.

*Weight reduction surgery* Some obese individuals choose to have weight reduction surgery, also known as BARIATRIC SURGERY, although this procedure is considered controversial by some physicians because of the health risks associated with this surgery as well as potential postsurgical risks. Surgery is an effective method for weight control. As many as 90 percent of patients lose greater than 20 percent of their body weight, and a majority of them maintain the weight loss over a period of five years. Many insurance companies do not pay for bariatric surgery. Bariatric surgery is indicated for patients who have a BMI of greater than 40 or patients whose BMI exceeds 35 and is associated with obesity-related conditions that are also present (such as diabetes or hypertension).

The weight reduction operations that are commonly used by bariatric surgeons include Roux-en-Y (gastric bypass or RYGB). Biliary-pancreatic diversion (duodenal switch) and laparoscopic adjustable lap band (Lap-Band) and these can be performed laparoscopically. In the case of gastroplasty, only about 40 percent of patients have lost significant excessive weight at the end of three years. The gastric bypass is superior in producing sustained weight loss among morbidly obese patients.

See also EXERCISE; GHRELIN; WALKING; YO-YO DIETING.

Barlow, Sarah E., M.D., et al. "Treatment of Child and Adolescent Obesity: Reports from Pediatricians, Pediatric Nurse Practitioners, and Registered Dietitians." *Pediatrics* 110, no. 1 (July 2002): 229–235.

Blanck, Heidi Michels, Laura Kettel Khan, and Mary K. Serdula, M.D. "Use of Nonprescription Weight Loss Products: Results from a Multistate Survey." *Journal of American Medical Association* 286, no. 8 (August 22/29, 2001): 930–935.

Calle, Eugenia E., et al. "Overweight, Obesity, and Mortality from Cancer in a Prospectively Studied Cohort of U.S. Adults." *New England Journal of Medicine* 348, no. 17 (April 24, 2003): 1,625–1,638.

Cummings, David E., M.D., et al. "Plasma Ghrelin Levels after Diet-Induced Weight Loss or Gastric Bypass Surgery." *New England Journal of Medicine* 346, no. 21 (May 23, 2002): 1,623–1,630.

Field, Alison E., et al. "Impact of Overweight on the Risk of Developing Common Chronic Diseases during a 10-Year Period." *Archives of Internal Medicine* 161 (July 9, 2001): 1,581–1,586.

Flegal, Katherine M., et al. "Prevalence and Trends in Obesity among US Adults, 1999–2000." *Journal of the American Medical Association* 288, no. 14 (October 9, 2002): 1,723–1,727.

Folsom, Aaron R., M.D., et al. "Associations of General and Abdominal Obesity with Multiple Health Outcomes in Older Women." *Archives of Internal Medicine* 160 (July 24, 2000): 2,117–2,128.

Fontaine, Kevin R., et al. "Years of Life Lost Due to Obesity." *Journal of the American Medical Association* 289, no. 2 (January 8, 2003): 187–193.

Jacobsen, Bjarne K., et al. "Increase in Weight in All Birth Cohorts in a General Population: The Tromso Study, 1974–1994." *Archives of Internal Medicine* 161 (February 12, 2001): 466–472.

Kenchaiah, Satish, M.D., et al. "Obesity and the Risk of Heart Failure." *New England Journal of Medicine* 347, no. 5 (August 1, 2002): 305–313.

List, James F., M.D., and Joel F. Habener, M.D. "Defective Melanocortin 4 Receptors in Hyperphagia and Morbid Obesity." *New England Journal of Medicine* 348, no. 12 (March 20, 2003): 1,160–1,163.

McTigue, Kathleen M., M.D., et al. "The Natural History of the Development of Obesity in a Cohort of Young U.S. Adults between 1981 and 1998." *Annals of Internal Medicine* 136, no. 12 (June 2002): 857–864.

National Center for Chronic Disease Prevention and Health Promotion, "The Burden of Chronic Diseases and Their Risk Factors: National and State Perspectives." Centers for Disease Control and Prevention, 2002.

National Task Force on the Prevention and Treatment of Obesity. "Overweight, Obesity, and Health Risk." *Archives of Internal Medicine* 160 (April 10, 2000): 898–904.

Parker, Alex, et al. "A Gene Conferring Susceptibility to Type 2 Diabetes in Conjunction with Obesity is Located on Chromosome 18p11." *Diabetes* 50 (March 2001): 675–680.

Salbe, Arline D., et al. "Assessing Risk Factors for Obesity between Childhood and Adolescence. I. Birth Weight, Childhood Adiposity, Parental Obesity, Insulin, and Leptin." *Pediatrics* 110, no. 2 (August 2002): 299–306.

Salbe, Arline D., et al. "Assessing Risk Factors for Obesity between Childhood and Adolescence. II. Energy Metabolism and Physical Activity." *Pediatrics* 110, no. 2 (August 2002): 307–314.

Schoenborn, Charlotte A., Patricia F. Adams, and Patricia M. Barnes. "Body Weight Status of Adults: United States, 1997–1998." *Advance Data from Vital and Health Statistics* no. 330 (September 6, 2002).

Sciamanna, Christoper N., M.D. et al. "Who Reports Receiving Advice to Lose Weight? Results from a Multistate Survey." *Archives of Internal Medicine* 160 (August 14/28, 2000): 2,334–2,339.

Stewart, Paul M., et al. "Cortisol Metabolism in Human Obesity: Impaired Cortisone [arrow] Cortisol Conversion in Subjects with Central Adiposity."
*Journal of Clinical Endocrinology & Metabolism* 84, no. 3 (1999): 1,022–1,027.

Story, Mary T. "Management of Child and Adolescent Obesity: Attitudes, Barriers, Skills, and Training Needs among Health Care Professionals." *Pediatrics* 110, no. 1 (July 2002): 210–214.

Wannamethee, S. Goya, and A. Gerald Shaper. "Weight Change and Duration of Overweight and Obesity in the Incidence of Type 2 Diabetes." *Diabetes Care* 22, no. 8 (August 1999): 1,266–1,272.

Weil, Evette, et al. "Obesity among Adults with Disabling Conditions." *Journal of the American Medical Association* 288, no. 10 (September 11, 2002): 1,265–1,268.

Whitaker, Robert C., M.D., et al. "Predicting Obesity in Young Adulthood from Childhood and Parental Obesity." *New England Journal of Medicine* 337, no. 13 (September 25, 1997): 869–873.

Wing, Rena R., et al. "Behavioral Science Research in Diabetes: Lifestyle Changes Related to Obesity, Eating Behavior, and Physical Activity." *Diabetes Care* 24, no.1 (January 2001): 117–123.

World Health Organization. "Diet, Nutrition and the Prevention of Chronic Diseases." WHO Technical Report Series 916, Geneva, 2003.

World Health Organization. "Diet, Food Supply and Obesity in the Pacific." Geneva, 2003.

Yanovski, Susan Z., M.D., and Jack A. Yanovski, M.D. "Obesity." *New England Journal of Medicine* 346, no. 8 (February 21, 2002): 591–602.

**occult gastrointestinal bleeding**  Microscopic or "hidden" (not visible to the naked eye) gastrointestinal bleeding that may indicate the presence of medical problems or diseases, such as ulcers and COLORECTAL CANCER. This bleeding is not usually noticed by the patient but is sufficient to be detected in specific tests for occult blood. Fecal occult bleeding may be an indication of the presence of colorectal cancer, which should be ruled out.

Other diseases that may produce occult gastrointestinal bleeding include the following:

- Crohn's disease
- Watermelon stomach
- Tuberculosis enterocolitis
- Parasitic infections

- Celiac disease
- Ulcer
- Esophagitis
- Colitis
- Telengiectasia (abnormal blood vessels in the gut that may bleed slowly or heavily)

In addition, use of some medications can cause occult bleeding, such as chronic use of aspirin or nonsteroidal anti-inflammatory drugs (NSAIDs).

### Testing for Occult Bleeding

Most physicians recommend that individuals who are age 50 and older have an annual fecal occult blood test (FOBT) to check for microscopic blood in the stool. In this test, the person smears a small sample of feces on a card to be tested in a laboratory for blood by adding a chemical reagent to the card. A change of color to blue indicates the presence of blood. A negative FOBT result does not entirely rule out cancer, but screening by using this noninvasive test has been shown to decrease the rate of colorectal cancer mortality. Only a colonoscopy can rule out colorectal cancer. Note, however, that no test is perfect and, rarely, cancers can be missed even during colonoscopy.

Some patients are resistant to performing this test, finding it repugnant, and sometimes physicians have had considerable difficulty convincing patients to comply with this test requirement.

See also CANCER, COLORECTAL; FECAL OCCULT BLOOD TEST; GUAIAC; NONSTEROIDAL ANTI-INFLAMMATORY DRUGS.

Rockey, Don C., M.D. "Occult Gastrointestinal Bleeding." *New England Journal of Medicine* 341, no. 1 (July 1, 1999): 38–46.

**Ogilvie's syndrome**   An extreme dilation of the right side of the colon when no obstruction is present. Sometimes the whole colon may be involved. The syndrome is also known as acute colonic pseudoobstruction. This condition was first described by Dr. Ogilvie in 1948. Ogilvie's syndrome may occur among hospitalized patients who

have experienced recent surgery, trauma, or a severe infection.

Ogilvie's syndrome patients experience nausea, vomiting, and abdominal distention with constipation. The diagnosis is based on the patient's medical history and a physical examination, plus the results of X rays.

Treatment for this medical problem involves identification and correction of the cause, if possible, for example, treatment of an existing infection or correction of any fluid and electrolyte abnormalities. A nasogastric tube with or without a rectal tube may be placed for suctioning air from the gastrointestinal system.

In one study of patients with an acute form of Ogilvie's syndrome who were treated with the medication neostigmine, reported in a 1999 issue of the *New England Journal of Medicine,* the patients responded well and the colon rapidly downsized to normal. Erythromycin has also been used with beneficial results by Ogilvie's syndrome patients.

If conservative measures fail, Ogilvie's syndrome patients are treated with decompression done by colonoscopy, or, in some cases, by cecostomy by the surgeon. Major abdominal surgery may rarely be required.

See also FLUID AND ELECTROLYTE BALANCE.

Ponec, Robert J., M.D., Michael D. Saunders, M.D., and Michael B. Kimmey, M.D. "Neostigmine for the Treatment of Acute Colonic Pseudo-Obstruction." *New England Journal of Medicine* 341, no. 3 (July 15, 1999): 137–141.

**oral cancer**   See CANCER, ORAL.

**outlet obstruction**   A blockage that prevents the normal flow of digestive juices or the outflow of solids such as food or fecal matter; for example, in gastric outlet obstruction, food contents are prevented from passing in an antegrade fashion from the stomach to the intestine by a blockage of the pylorus. Gastric outlet obstruction may be due to a complication of an ulcer or CANCER.

See also ADHESIONS; GALLSTONES; POLYPS.

**pain**  Mild, moderate, or severe discomfort. Pain may be acute: generally short-term pain lasting several minutes, hours or as long as a day. For many patients, pain is chronic: the person experiences continuous or intermittent pain that may increase and decrease in severity.

Pain varies not only in intensity, but in its very nature. For example, pain may be stabbing or burning. It may also feel like dull or stronger pressure. For this reason, physicians usually ask patients to describe *how* the pain feels, as well as specifically which area hurts.

### Rating the Pain

In the United States, many physicians ask patients to rate their pain on a scale of one to 10: one is the mildest pain that they have experienced and 10 is the worst they can imagine ever feeling. This subjective rating helps doctors to know how severe the patient considers his or her own pain and aids the physician in determining the treatment: the type of drug to use, the dosage, and so forth. For patients who cannot use such ratings, such as children or those who have trouble with the scale, doctors may show a series of simple drawings of a person in pain and ask the patient to select which drawing illustrates his or her pain.

### Causes of Pain

There are many causes of pain, ranging from organ damage or injury due to infection, to inflammation and other causes. Sometimes pain is caused by a disease, such as an ulcer or appendicitis. Sometimes it is difficult for the doctor to determine the underlying cause of the pain, even with results of laboratory tests or findings of imaging studies such as magnetic resonance imaging (MRI) or computed tomography (CT) scans.

Determining the source of pain can be challenging in some cases. One reason for this is that sometimes pain is *referred:* stemming from one part of the body but actually experienced as pain elsewhere. Heart pain may be experienced as pain in the chest, arms, or other locations, such as the upper abdomen. Some people who think they are having a heart attack may be experiencing severe heartburn or ulcer. On the other hand, they may also be having a heart attack, and sometimes even a physician has difficulty in determining the difference without testing.

### Purpose of Pain

Pain is necessary to life, because it is the body's warning system of a problem. Without pain, severe injuries would be unnoticed and could ultimately lead to death.

It can be hard to understand the purpose of chronic pain; pain may stem from an untreated or insufficiently treated ailment, such as GASTROESOPHAGEAL REFLUX DISEASE, an ULCER or CROHN'S DISEASE. Sometimes physicians cannot determine the exact cause of pain and can only treat the pain and other related symptoms the patient experiences.

### Treatment of Pain

When individuals have severe acute pain, in addition to their need for the underlying problem to be diagnosed and treated, they may require strong painkilling drugs, such as meperidine (Demerol) or morphine. Over-the-counter medications such as acetaminophen (Tylenol) or ibuprofen (Advil) may be sufficient to manage the pain that is less severe.

If the pain is a chronic problem that has occurred for weeks, months, or even longer, the doctor may prescribe a variety of different analgesic medications. For example, if the physician believes that the pain is inflammatory in nature (as in rheumatoid arthritis), he or she may prescribe non-steroidal anti-inflammatory drugs (NSAIDs).

If chronic pain is severe, the doctor may prescribe narcotics, such as oxycodone (OxyContin, Oxy Fast) or a codeine-based drug. In the United States, narcotics are medications that are *scheduled,* or controlled by the Drug Enforcement Administration. The federal government requires that careful records be kept on such drugs by both physicians and pharmacies, and there are both federal and state laws governing the prescribing of narcotic painkillers.

A key reason for these laws is that some people abuse painkilling drugs, taking them to obtain an artificial high or using excessively high doses. Another reason is that these drugs can be physically and psychologically addicting, and physicians need to maintain a careful watch over their patients who take them. Sometimes patients become dependent on such narcotics and may develop severe constipation, abdominal distention, and other symptoms associated with narcotic bowel syndrome. Physicians who are pain specialists are best at managing chronic pain, especially when narcotics are needed.

See also HYPERALGESIA; NARCOTIC BOWEL SYNDROME; NONSTEROIDAL ANTI-INFLAMMATORY DRUGS; PROSTAGLANDINS.

**pancreas**  A large combined exocrine–endocrine gland that secretes digestive juices, including enzymes that help to digest foods. The endocrine function of the pancreas involves secretion of the hormone insulin in the bloodstream. Endocrine glands produce hormones. An exocrine gland secretes through ducts, such as the digestive juices secreted by the pancreas.

Major medical diseases of the pancreas include pancreatitis (inflammation of the pancreas) and pancreatic cancer. Diabetes mellitus occurs when the pancreas secretes too little insulin for the metabolism of glucose or the body is unable to respond to all the insulin that is produced, as in insulin resistance.

See also CANCER, PANCREATIC; DIABETES MELLITUS; PANCREATITIS.

**pancreatic cancer**  See CANCER, PANCREATIC.

**pancreatic cholera**  A condition of diarrhea, hypokalemia (a potassium deficiency), and a neuroendocrine tumor of the pancreas. The diarrhea causes a loss of fluids and electrolytes from the intestine and is severe and watery. It is caused by an excessive secretion of vasoactive intestinal peptide (VIP) from the tumor, which is usually located in the pancreas. Pancreatic cholera is also known as Verner-Morrison syndrome, named for Verner and Morrison, who described the condition in 1958.

The treatment of pancreatic cholera involves preventing fluid and electrolyte depletion, as well as controlling the diarrhea and the tumor. The treatment of choice for controlling the diarrhea is octreotide. Some patients need a combination of a corticosteroid drug and octreotide. The surgical excision of the tumor may be an option in selected cases. Patients may also be treated with interferon alfa.

In contrast to treatment of many cases of pancreatic cancer, aggressive treatment of pancreatic cholera can often be lifesaving. The five-year survival rate is 90 percent, and the 10-year survival rate is 25 percent. Survival rate is better in cases of small tumors and tumors that have not spread.

See also CANCER, PANCREATIC; PANCREAS; PANCREATITIS.

**pancreatic insufficiency**  A condition in which the pancreas does not make enough digestive enzymes for the normal digestive process. In the most severe cases, pancreatic insufficiency leads to malabsorption, in which the nutrients are not digested and, therefore, cannot be absorbed from the small intestine. Clinically significant pancreatic insufficiency usually does not occur until about 80 to 90 percent of the pancreas is destroyed or nonfunctional.

Pancreatic insufficiency is seen in patients who have chronic pancreatitis or cystic fibrosis. Sometimes DIABETES MELLITUS may also occur in association with pancreatic insufficiency.

### Symptoms and Signs
The symptoms and signs of pancreatic insufficiency include fatty, and loose stools; vitamin deficiencies; and unintended weight loss. Some patients have muscle cramps and abdominal pain.

### Diagnosis and Treatment

The diagnosis of pancreatic insufficiency is based on the patient's clinical signs, a physical examination, and laboratory tests. Patients who are diagnosed with pancreatic insufficiency are given pancreatic enzyme supplements, and they are also advised to consume a low-fat diet. Patients who drink are advised to avoid all alcohol, especially since alcohol exacerbates pancreatitis and may worsen the pancreatic insufficiency. Patients who develop diabetes would need to be treated appropriately.

See also ALCOHOL ABUSE AND DEPENDENCE/ALCOHOLISM; CANCER, STOMACH; CANCER, PANCREATIC; CELIAC SPRUE; CROHN'S DISEASE; CYSTIC FIBROSIS; DIABETES MELLITUS; MALABSORPTION; PANCREATITIS; ULCERS, PEPTIC.

**pancreatic juice**   Secretions that include water; electrolytes such as sodium, potassium, and bicarbonate; plus digestive enzymes such as lipase, amylase, and trypsin that are produced by the pancreas to aid digestion of food.

**pancreatitis**   Painful and acute or chronic inflammation of the pancreas, which may be caused by disease, stones that are blocking the bile duct, pancreatic tumors, or a chronic illness that has caused damage to the pancreas. Sometimes a physical trauma, such as a blunt trauma to the abdomen, causes pancreatitis. In about 10 percent of acute cases of pancreatitis, patients become severely ill and are at risk for death.

Chronic alcoholism may also cause pancreatitis. An estimated 80 percent of all cases of pancreatitis are due to either gallstones or alcoholism. In addition, an estimated 85 different medications, particularly sulfa drugs, metronidazole, and valproic acid, can induce pancreatitis. The presence of high triglyceride blood levels (hypertriglyceridemia) is another cause of pancreatitis among patients.

Rarely, hypercalcemia, which is a condition of excessively high blood levels of calcium that is frequently caused by hyperparathyroidism, causes pancreatitis. A penetrating peptic ulcer is another rare cause of pancreatitis.

### Risk Factors

Patients who are at highest risk for development of pancreatitis include the following groups:

- Patients who have abused alcohol for several years
- Patients who have gallstones
- Patients who have a family history of pancreatitis
- Patients who have acquired immunodeficiency syndrome (AIDS)
- Patients who have hypertriglyceridemia (high blood levels of triglycerides)

### Symptoms

Patients report severe pain, and nausea and vomiting. They may enter a hospital emergency room for treatment of the symptoms.

### Diagnosis and Treatment

Laboratory tests are performed in cases of suspected pancreatitis. If pancreatitis is present, blood levels of pancreatic enzymes (such as amylase and lipase) are usually elevated. Normal levels of pancreatic enzymes cannot exclude pancreatitis, but they make it less likely. An ultrasound of the gallbladder is also done, to check for gallstones. A computed tomography (CT) scan may be ordered to assess the severity of the pancreatitis and to look for complications.

Chronic pancreatitis can be diagnosed with a plain X ray of the abdomen if pancreatic calcifications are visible or with endoscopic retrograde cholangiopancreatography (ERCP) or an endoscopic ultrasound procedure that uses endoscopic ultrasonography. This procedure usually follows a CT scan of the pancreas. Normal findings on imaging studies do not exclude chronic pancreatitis but make it less likely.

The treatment of pancreatitis involves control of the symptoms, such as control of pain with analgesics (painkilling medications). It also includes treatment of the causes of the pancreatitis, such as infections or other medical problems. For example, if gallstones have caused the pancreatitis, they are removed, along with the gallbladder. If alcoholism appears to be the primary cause, the patient is urged to refrain from drinking all alcohol and is warned about the consequences of failure to comply with the recommendation, which are more attacks of pancreatitis and a shortened life span. If medications appear to be the cause of pancreatitis, they are discontinued. If high triglyceride levels are the cause, the patient is instructed on how to change his or her diet, and appropriate medications are prescribed.

Chronic pancreatitis patients may have reduced levels of the pancreatic enzymes that are needed for digestion and may require exogenous enzyme supplementation. Surgery is required in some cases of acute and chronic pancreatitis.

See also ALCOHOL ABUSE AND DEPENDENCE/ALCOHOLISM; HEPATITIS; HEREDITARY PANCREATITIS; ULCERS, PEPTIC.

Sandberg, Ake Andren, and Anders Borgstrom. "Early Prediction of Severity in Acute Pancreatitis. Is it Possible?" *Journal of the Pancreas* 3, no. 5 (September 2002): 116–125.
Steinberg, William, and Scott Tenner. "Acute Pancreatitis." *New England Journal of Medicine* 330, no. 17 (April 28, 1994): 1,198–1,210.

**papillotomy**  An endoscopic procedure used to widen the papilla by making a cut so as to facilitate the removal of stones from the bile duct. This procedure is performed during ENDOSCOPIC RETROGRADE CHOLANGIOPANCREATOGRAPHY (ERCP). The ERCP alone is considered a diagnostic test; the papillotomy is regarded as more invasive and is used for therapeutic purposes. Early ERCP and endoscopic papillotomy are beneficial in the case of acute biliary pancreatitis. However, patients who do not have biliary obstruction do not benefit from the procedure.

According to a study published in 1997 in the *New England Journal of Medicine,* patients who have acute biliary pancreatitis but do not have obstructive jaundice do not benefit from this procedure. In this study, of the 126 patients in the ERCP group, some had severe complications, including death in the case of 14 patients, during the course of three months. Among the 112 subjects who were in the conservative treatment group, seven died during the same period.

Although the overall complication rates for both groups of patients were similar, the group who had the invasive procedure experienced more severe complications. Concluded the researchers, "Our controlled, randomized trial of early ERCP and papillotomy in patients with acute biliary pancreatitis demonstrated that patients without biliary obstruction or biliary sepsis did not benefit from these interventions."

See also ENDOSCOPIC RETROGRADE CHOLANGIOPANCREATOGRAPHY; GALLSTONES; PANCREATITIS.

Folsch, Ulrich R., M.D., et al. "Early ERCP and Papillotomy Compared with Conservative Treatment for Acute Biliary Pancreatitis." *New England Journal of Medicine* 336, no. 4 (January 23, 1997): 237–242.

**paracentesis**  A procedure in which a needle is inserted into the abdomen to remove excess fluid that has been caused by ASCITES. The most common cause of ascites is liver cirrhosis. The extracted fluid is analyzed for abnormalities to determine the cause of the ascites as well as to see whether any infection is present. In some cases, there may be so much fluid in the abdomen that it causes the patient difficulty with breathing. In such cases, a therapeutic large-volume paracentesis is performed by removing several liters of fluid (as many as 10 to 20 liters) to ease the patient's breathing difficulties. Paracentesis is usually a relatively risk-free procedure, and complications are uncommon. However, death may occur rarely as a complication of the procedure.

See also ALCOHOL ABUSE AND DEPENDENCE/ALCOHOLISM; CIRRHOSIS.

Minocha, A. "A Fatal Case of Paracentesis." *American Journal of Gastroenterology* 94 (1999): 856.

**parasitic infection**  An illness that is caused by a nonbacterial and nonviral organism, such as by an Entameba histolytica (AMEBIASIS), an *Enterobius* (pinworm), or a hookworm, tapeworm, roundworm, or another parasite. The diagnosis may be made by a variety of laboratory tests, such as tests of the blood or stool, depending on the parasite.

Medications can usually cure or at least improve the condition in most instances.

See also CHAGA'S DISEASE; CHOLANGITIS; *CRYPTOSPORIDIUM PARVUM;* DIARRHEA; DIGESTIVE ABSORPTION; DIGESTIVE ENZYMES; ENZYME-LINKED IMMUNOSORBENT ASSAY; EOSINOPHILIC GASTROENTERITIS; FAILURE TO THRIVE; FOOD-BORNE ILLNESSES; IRRITABLE BOWEL SYNDROME; LIVER ABSCESS; OCCULT GASTROINTESTINAL BLEEDING; TRICHINOSIS.

**parenteral nutrition**   Provision of food through a tube that is connected to a catheter that is inserted into the veins. Thus, nutrition is introduced directly into the blood rather than taken by mouth or by a tube into the stomach or small intestine. Parenteral nutrition is used when the person is too ill to have oral nutrition or an abnormality of the gastrointestinal system makes it difficult or impossible for the person to eat normally or to handle nutrients fed into the gut, such as an intestinal obstruction. Long-term parenteral nutrition may lead to complications, such as catheter sepsis, venous thrombosis, and NONALCOHOLIC STEATOHEPATITIS/NONALCOHOLIC FATTY LIVER DISEASE.

See also ENTERAL NUTRITION; FEEDING TUBE.

**pasteurization**   A food processing procedure that removes microbes that can cause disease. Pasteurization improves the quality of food by making it safer and by prolonging its shelf life. The process was named after Louis Pasteur, a 19th-century researcher who discovered that beer and wine could be preserved by heating them to below the boiling point, then rapidly cooling them.

Pasteurization techniques were later used to eradicate the bacteria in milk, cheese, and other products, which are heated and then cooled rapidly. For example, the pasteurization of milk removes an estimated 97 to 99 percent of such bacteria as *Mycobacterium tuberculosis,* SALMONELLA, and *Streptococcus* species.

The temperature and duration used in pasteurization vary by product; for example, milk must be heated to 63°C for 30 minutes or to 72°C for 16 seconds, then rapidly cooled. Ice cream must be heated to 69°C for 30 minutes or 80°C for 25 seconds. The addition of other products, such as sugar or chocolate, changes both the temperature and duration requirements.

See also CONTAMINATED FOOD OR WATER.

**pediatric gastroenterologist**   Physician who is specially trained to diagnose and treat digestive diseases and disorders that occur in infants, children, and adolescents.

See also ADOLESCENTS AND DIGESTIVE DISEASES; CHILDREN AND DIGESTIVE DISEASES; GASTROENTEROLOGIST.

**perforation**   A hole in the wall of an organ or other body part. An ulcer is said to be perforated when there is a hole at the site of the ulcer, for example, in the stomach or duodenum. This perforation, which would cause the contents of the stomach to leak into the patient's abdominal cavity and cause a life-threatening emergency, usually requires surgery. Similarly, the intestines may perforate, especially when they are inflamed and/or totally obstructed, as in APPENDICITIS, DIVERTICULITIS, CROHN'S DISEASE, and toxic MEGACOLON.

See also ULCERS, PEPTIC.

**peristalsis**   A digestive process that moves food downward through the gastrointestinal tract in a continuous and sinuous, wavelike muscular motion. While the upper part of the gut squeezes to push the food downward, the immediately lower part relaxes to receive it. This wave contraction and relaxation are continued and coordinated throughout the digestive tract.

See also ACHALASIA; MEGACOLON; NEUROTRANSMITTERS.

**peritoneum**   A lining that protects the organs in the abdominal cavity. An infection of the peritoneum, called peritonitis, can be life-threatening. Such infections may be due to digestive problems such as a PERFORATION or to rupture in the case of acute APPENDICITIS. These infections are more likely to occur in elderly patients or individuals who have a compromised immune system.

See also PERITONITIS.

**peritonitis**  A dangerous and possibly life-threatening infection of the peritoneum, which is the lining that protects the internal abdominal organs. Individuals who have peritonitis require antibiotics and hospitalization, and, depending upon the cause of the peritonitis, may need surgery. Those who have a weakened immune system, such as liver CIRRHOSIS patients, are at risk for contracting peritonitis.

See also INFECTION; PERFORATION; PERITONEUM.

**pernicious anemia**  A major cause of vitamin $B_{12}$ deficiency. Pernicious anemia as a cause should be excluded in all cases of vitamin $B_{12}$ deficiency, since 75 percent of the cases of this deficiency are caused by pernicious anemia. Pernicious anemia is an autoimmune attack on gastric intrinsic factor, which is a chemical that is necessary for the absorption of vitamin $B_{12}$. The lack of functional intrinsic factor contributes to vitamin $B_{12}$ deficiency. Pernicious anemia also causes atrophic gastritis, which causes decreased production of intrinsic factor, thereby further exacerbating the condition. There is also an increased risk for gastric cancer associated with pernicious anemia.

There are numerous other causes of vitamin $B_{12}$ deficiency, such as *Helicobacter pylori* infection, human immunodeficiency virus (HIV) infection, or an inherited disorder. Some individuals who consume only vegetables, avoiding all meat and dairy products, may have a vitamin $B_{12}$ deficiency.

### Risk Factors

Pernicious anemia is a common problem, especially among elderly subjects. In fact, some older individuals are misdiagnosed with Alzheimer's disease or dementia when their true medical problem is actually a vitamin $B_{12}$ deficiency.

Pernicious anemia is more common in women than in men (4.1 percent of women versus 2.1 percent of men). It is rare among Hispanic and Asian Americans.

### Symptoms and Signs

The symptoms and signs of pernicious anemia vary; they may include numbness and tingling in the hands and feet, weakness, as well as mood swings and memory loss. If the illness is untreated for years, it may also produce irreversible nerve damage.

### Diagnosis and Treatment

If a deficiency is suspected, laboratory tests may be done to confirm it. A deficiency of vitamin $B_{12}$ is characterized by large red blood cells (macrocytosis). Anti-intrinsic factor antibodies are present in most patients. A Schilling test confirms the diagnosis. A pernicious anemia–related vitamin $B_{12}$ deficiency is treated with either injections of vitamin $B_{12}$ or, in some cases, high doses of oral tablets of vitamin $B_{12}$. It can also be given sublingually (under the tongue) or in the form of nasal sprays, but the extent of $B_{12}$ absorption for these forms is not reliable.

See also ANEMIA; VITAMIN DEFICIENCIES/EXCESSES.

Ban-Hock Toh, M. B., Ian R. van Direl, and Paul A. Gleeson. "Pernicious Anemia." *New England Journal of Medicine* 447, no. 20 (November 13, 1997): 1,441–1,448.

**Peutz-Jeghers syndrome**  A hereditary disorder that is characterized by the presence of intestinal polyps and skin lesions. This syndrome is mapped to chromosome 19p13.3. Patients are also at an increased risk for intestinal cancers, as well as pancreatic cancer, lung cancer, breast cancer, uterine cancer, ovarian cancer, and testicular cancer. For Peutz-Jeghers syndrome patients, the risk of dying of cancer approaches 45 to 50 percent by the age of 60 years. The syndrome was named after J. L. A. Peutz, a Dutch physician who first described it in 1921. Dr. Jeghers, an American doctor, provided further details in 1944 and the condition was subsequently named after both men.

The polyps that are characteristic of this syndrome usually begin to develop in childhood, although the newborn infant may also have the identifiable black freckle-like lesions on the body, especially on and around the lips and the mouth, that are characteristic of this disease.

## Symptoms and Signs

Peutz-Jeghers syndrome patients may have frequent attacks of mild to severe abdominal pains. As mentioned, they also have polyps of the gastrointestinal tract, which are benign, usually multiple, and of variable size. The polyps may be present in the stomach and the small and/or large intestine and can lead to intestinal blockage as well as to gastrointestinal bleeding. Only a minority of these polyps (1 to 13 percent) become cancerous. However, the syndrome is associated with an increased risk of gastrointestinal as well as non-gastrointestinal tumor malignancies and the risk of cancer is about 50 percent by the age of sixty.

## Diagnosis and Treatment

Diagnosis is made by observing the classic skin/buccal lesions and by finding polyps in the gut. The doctor orders a colonoscopy and upper endoscopy, as well as a small bowel endoscopy or X ray to look for these polyps. If polyps are found, they are excised, especially the large ones, while biopsies may be taken from the small polyps. Periodic surveillance by colonoscopy and upper endoscopy is recommended for those who have Peutz–Jeghers syndrome, as well as a surveillance for breast and testicular tumors.

See also COLONOSCOPY; ENDOSCOPY; POLYPS; SIGMOIDOSCOPY.

Wynbrandt, James, and Mark D. Ludman. *The Encyclopedia of Genetic Disorders and Birth Defects.* 2d ed. New York: Facts On File, 2000.

**photodynamic therapy**   Treatment that uses the administration of drugs to cause body tissues to become very sensitive to certain wavelengths of light and enables physicians to treat diseases such as Barrett's esophagus by using wavelengths to destroy precancerous cells. As of this writing, the efficacy of photodynamic therapy in preventing the progression from Barrett's esophagus to cancer has not been established.

See also BARRETT'S ESOPHAGUS.

**physical activity**   See EXERCISE; OBESITY.

**pica**   A strange desire or compulsion to eat non-food items, such as paper, clay, laundry detergent, baking soda, or dirt, a compulsion that lasts for at least a month. Pica may stem from iron deficiency ANEMIA. Sometimes pica for ice, or papophagia, may be seen even when patients are not anemic, and even in such cases, patients often respond promptly to treatment with IRON.

Although actual pica may develop during pregnancy, food cravings, such as the intense desire to eat pickles or other foods, are not a form of pica; eating of nonfood is true pica.

Pica may sometimes be associated with a psychotic disturbance, such as schizophrenia or another severe emotional disorder. Pica is also behavior that is sometimes exhibited by mentally retarded adults.

It is unknown how many children and adults have pica and why it occurs.

Some preschool children experience a form of pica in that they consume paper or paint chips. (This is not the same type of behavior as when infants put virtually everything into their mouth in an exploration phase.) Eating paint chips can cause lead poisoning and lead to irreversible brain damage to the child.

It is important that parents and other caregivers monitor the behavior of young children because it is impossible to predict which children will exhibit pica (unless they have already been known to have such symptoms in the past). The child exhibiting pica should be corrected and kept away from the desired nonfood as much as possible.

**pneumatosis intestinalis (PI)**   A condition of digestive gas that is found inside the wall of either the colon or the small intestine. It may be seen in infants or adults. Among infants with pneumatosis intestinalis (PI), most have NECROTIZING ENTEROCOLITIS, although some infants and children may have very severe gastroenteritis. Among adults, pneumatosis intestinalis more commonly appears from about age 50 to 80 years.

## Signs and Symptoms

Most patients have no symptoms or signs. Usually the signs and symptoms of pneumatosis intestinalis, if any are present, pertain to the underlying disorder involved. When the condition occurs in the small intestine and symptoms result, patients may have nausea and vomiting, unintended weight loss, diarrhea, and abdominal pain. When PI is present in the colon and symptoms occur, patients may have diarrhea, abdominal pain, enlarged abdomen, and constipation.

### Diagnosis and Treatment

Generally, pneumatosis intestinalis is identified in plain X rays of the abdomen; however, computed tomography (CT) scans are more effective at diagnosing PI. The condition may also be diagnosed during a routine sigmoidoscopy or colonoscopy. A magnetic resonance imaging (MRI) scan can also reveal gas inside the bowel wall.

If patients are not symptomatic and there is no apparent emergency, physicians may decide to continue to observe the condition over time and prescribe no medication or treatment. The condition may resolve. If patients do have symptoms, some physicians treat them with hyperbaric oxygen; others treat with antibiotics, particularly metronidazole, for as long as three months.

Some patients may need surgery; most do not. Surgery is indicated, however, if the patient experiences an obstruction or a perforation of the intestine or the colon. The puncture of these gas-filled lesions can be accomplished during an endoscopy for patients who are otherwise symptomatic but are poor candidates for surgery.

St. Peter, Shawn D., M.D., Maher A. Abbas, M.D., and Keith A. Kelly, M.D. "The Spectrum of Pneumatosis Intestinalis." *Archives of Surgery* 138, no. 1 (January 2000): 68–75.

**Poison Information Centers**  State offices in the United States or other countries that are prepared to provide emergency medical information over the telephone in the event of ingestion of poisons and drug overdoses, particularly when young children have consumed poisonous items. Centers offer such advice as whether a caller should try to make an individual vomit or take other emergency actions. The person who has ingested poison should see a physician as soon as possible, preferably at the nearest hospital emergency room, in most cases.

In 2000 Congress passed a law establishing a national poison control number: (800) 222-1222. Individuals in the United States who call this number are routed to the nearest center. (See APPENDIX V for a listing of poison control centers nationwide.)

See also POISONS/POISONING.

**poisons/poisoning**  Fatal or dangerous substances that may be ingested. Poisons may be artificial substances, such as pesticides, or may be naturally occurring, such as poisonous plants or the venom of some snakes or spiders. Individuals can also be poisoned by purposely or accidentally ingesting overdoses of medications, both prescription and over-the-counter drugs.

According to the Food and Drug Administration (FDA), many medications and household products can poison a person. In the case of children, the FDA reports that the primary cause of childhood death of poisoning is the ingestion of vitamin pills with iron. Death can result after a small child takes as few as five such pills. As a result, it is very important for parents to place all drugs, including vitamin pills, well out of the reach of small children, preferably in a locked cabinet.

In adults, one of the most common causes of poisoning is acetaminophen (Tylenol). Sleeping aids that are taken with or without alcohol are another common culprit. In short, people take whatever is handy or easily available and may accidentally or purposely overdose themselves.

### Risk Factors for Ingesting Poisons among Children

Children below age 12 have the highest rate (13 per 1,000 children) of incidents of poisoning. An estimated three of every four poisoning incidents involving children younger than age six are reported to a poison control center. However, adults also are at a risk for ingesting poison. (See table on page 205 for annual rates of poisoning by age and sex.)

### Symptoms of Poisoning

There are no symptoms early or during the preclinical phase. There are some indications that a patient may have ingested poison; the classic sign is

## ANNUAL RATE OF POISONING PER 1,000 POPULATION, UNITED STATES, 1997

| Sex and Age | Rate Per 1,000 Population | Standard Error |
|---|---|---|
| **Both sexes:** | | |
| All | 7.3 | 0.6 |
| All, age adjusted | 7.2 | 0.6 |
| Under 12 years | 13.0 | 1.8 |
| 12–21 years | 5.6 | 1.4 |
| 22–44 years | 6.7 | 1.0 |
| 45–64 years | 5.5 | 1.3 |
| 65 years and over | 5.4 | 1.6 |
| **Male:** | | |
| All | 6.9 | 0.9 |
| All, age adjusted | 6.7 | 0.9 |
| Under 12 years | 11.3 | 2.1 |
| 12–21 years | *4.8 | 1.7 |
| 22–44 years | 7.6 | 1.6 |
| 45–64 years | *5.2 | 1.7 |
| 65 years and over | *2.9 | 1.8 |
| **Female:** | | |
| All | 7.7 | 0.8 |
| All, age adjusted | 7.7 | 0.8 |
| Under 12 years | 14.7 | 2.9 |
| 12–21 years | *6.4 | 2.3 |
| 22–44 years | 5.9 | 1.2 |
| 45–64 years | 5.8 | 1.6 |
| 65 years and over | *7.2 | 2.4 |

*Figure does not meet standard of reliability or precision.

## NUMBER OF POISONING EPISODES, NUMBER AND PERCENTAGE OF POISONING EPISODES INVOLVING A CALL TO A POISON CONTROL CENTER, AND STANDARD ERROR BY SEX AND AGE: UNITED STATES, 1997

| | Poisonings | Poison Control Center Called | | |
|---|---|---|---|---|
| Sex and Age | Number of Episodes in Thousands | Number of Episodes in Thousands | Percentage | Standard Error |
| **Both sexes:** | | | | |
| All ages | 1,945 | 877 | 45.1 | 4.3 |
| Less than 6 years | 551 | 415 | 75.5 | 6.0 |
| 6 years and older | 1,394 | 461 | 33.1 | 4.9 |
| **Male:** | | | | |
| All ages | 898 | 346 | 38.6 | 6.7 |
| Less than 6 years | 212 | 155 | 72.9 | 9.9 |
| 6 years and older | 685 | *191 | *27.9 | 7.4 |
| **Female:** | | | | |
| All ages | 1,047 | 531 | 50.7 | 5.5 |
| Less than 6 years | 338 | 261 | 77.1 | 7.5 |
| 6 years and older | 709 | 270 | 38.1 | 6.4 |

*Figure does not meet standard of reliability or precision.

a spilled or opened pill bottle. Other signs and symptoms of poisoning in a child or adult are as follows:

- The person is very sleepy even though he or she would not normally be tired at this time.
- The person cannot follow another person with the eyes.
- The person's eyes are moving around in circles.
- The person has stains or burns around the mouth.
- The person's breath smells odd.

If a patient exhibits one or more of these symptoms, the person who notes these symptoms should contact the poison control center immediately. If the name of the poison is known, it should be reported, as well as the way in which the poison was ingested (swallowing, sniffing, splashing, or other method). The child's or adult's age, weight, and height should be reported, if known. If the person who has ingested poison has any other known medical problems, this information should also be provided.

### Diagnosis and Treatment of Poisoning

The parent, family member, or other person who is concerned about possible poisoning should always take the suspected poison to the emergency room or doctor's office. Sometimes after ingesting the poison, the patient may drive himself to the emergency room and provide a history. A physician who suspects poisoning may induce vomiting in the patient, if it is indicated. However, it is important to understand that causing vomiting is *not* always the best procedure. The physician may need to pump the patient's stomach.

Many patients are administered ACTIVATED CHARCOAL with a cathartic to bind to the poison and prevent its absorption into the body. In some cases, the physician may observe the patient for an hour or more and if the patient is behaving normally, release the patient to another person, such as a parent, for continued observation.

### *Date Rape Drugs and Other Illegal Drugs*

In rare cases, adolescents and adults consume drugs that were placed in their drink without their knowledge by a predatory person. The drug that is usually used is colorless and odorless and induces unconsciousness and amnesia. The drug is usually given to achieve the aim that gave it the name: date rape.

Later a woman may feel sore or notice torn clothes but feel confused. She may not report anything to authorities until days later or may never report it. Placing drugs in the drink of another person is a felony.

In other cases, adolescents or young adults consume illegal drugs such as "Ecstasy," which is 3,4-methylenedioxymethamphetamine (MDMA), which can induce severe dehydration, irregular heartbeat, and even death. Hospital emergency rooms have seen an increase in such symptoms, particularly among teenagers and adults who attend "rave" parties, which are all-night dance parties that are largely unsupervised and where illegal drugs are often freely available. People at such parties may take drugs without knowing what they are or mix drugs. These drugs are dangerous for everyone but are particularly dangerous for individuals who have medical conditions such as diabetes.

Combining illegal drugs with alcohol is another dangerous and very common practice among some younger individuals.

### *Suicide Attempts*

Sometimes very depressed individuals purposely ingest drugs, household cleaners, or other items in an attempt to commit suicide. As with other patients, the concerned family member or other person should provide poison control center staff and emergency room personnel with as much information as possible.

See also POISON CONTROL CENTERS.

Barnes, Warner, PM and L. A. Fingerhut. "Injury and Poisoning Episodes and Conditions: National Health Interview Study: 1997." *Vital Health Statistics* 10, no. 202, July 2000.

Spyker, D. A., and A. Minocha. "Toxicodynamic Approach to Management of Poisoned Patients." *Journal of Emergency Medicine* 6 (1988): 117–120.

**polyps** Nodule or mushroomlike growths that are usually benign but may sometimes become cancerous if they are not removed in a timely fashion. Polyps are most frequently found in the colon and can be detected and removed by a physician while a patient is having a COLONOSCOPY. If they are not removed, these polyps may become cancerous within the colon in about 10 years; however, not all polyps are precancerous; nor do all become cancerous.

Most polyps do not cause symptoms; however, large polyps may cause abdominal pain and gastrointestinal bleeding. Colon cancer screening is generally recommended for average-risk patients after the age of 50 years so that physicians can look for precancerous polyps and remove any they find.

See also CANCER, COLORECTAL.

**portal circulation** The transmission of blood from the portal vein, which accounts for 75 percent of the blood flow to the liver. The portal vein is formed by the union of the superior mesenteric vein from the intestines and the splenic vein from the spleen. In some cases, the resistance to the blood flow in the portal vein is increased, resulting in increased portal pressure; which is also known as portal hypertension, for example, in liver cirrhosis or a blockage in the portal or splenic vein by a clot that leads to elevated pressure in the portal vein.

See also CIRRHOSIS; LIVER.

**pouchitis** A complication of some surgeries involving the formation of an artificial reservoir for stool from the small intestine, particularly the ileal pouch created in ileoanal anastomosis, an operation used for patients who have ULCERATIVE COLITIS.

The symptoms of pouchitis are bloody stools, an increased frequency and urgency of defecation, and fever and lethargy. Pouchitis may be acute or chronic, and it can usually be treated with metronidazole. Antibiotics have been used to treat pouchitis, as well as corticosteroids and aminosalicylate enemas. If medications are not effective, patients may need additional surgery.

See also INFLAMMATORY BOWEL DISEASE; ULCERATIVE COLITIS.

**pregnancy** Period during which a human fetus grows inside a woman, approximately nine months. In the early part of pregnancy (the first trimester, or first three months), many women experience nausea and some also experience periodic vomiting as well. In an extreme and unusual case, the vomiting and dehydration become dangerous and life-threatening, as with HYPEREMESIS GRAVIDARUM.

As many as 75 percent of all pregnant women may also experience GASTROESOPHAGEAL REFLUX DISEASE. Women in their third trimester may experience digestive problems such as CONSTIPATION, because of hormonal influences as well as the pressure of the growing fetus on the internal organs. The liver can also be affected by diseases that are unique to pregnancy, such as the acute fatty liver of pregnancy and other syndromes that may be life-threatening.

See also NAUSEA AND VOMITING.

**primary biliary cirrhosis (PBC)** A progressive liver disease that mainly affects women and can lead to liver failure.

The illness is apparently caused by an immunological defect, and both genetic and environmental factors have been implicated. Primary biliary cirrhosis (PBC) is unique among autoimmune diseases because it never occurs in childhood and it is also rare in young adults. Many primary biliary cirrhosis patients also have another autoimmune disease, such as rheumatoid arthritis, SCLERODERMA, or thyroid disease (hypothyroidism), or other illnesses, such as CREST SYNDROME. Patients who have primary biliary cirrhosis have liver inflammation and scarring as well as damaged intrahepatic bile ducts, which ultimately lead to liver cirrhosis and liver failure. The rate of progression to liver failure is variable.

### Risk Factors

Nearly 95 percent of primary biliary cirrhosis patients are females, and most of them are between 30 and 65 years old. The disease is rare: it has an estimated incidence of 3.9 to 15 individuals per million. It is found among women of all races worldwide. There is an apparent genetic risk, and individuals in families in which parents or siblings have the disease have a significantly increased risk of development of primary biliary cirrhosis.

### Symptoms and Signs

Patients with primary biliary cirrhosis may have no symptoms or signs in the early stages of the illness, or they may have some vague indicators, such as fatigue and pruritus (itching of the skin). The pruritus may become severe, with no apparent cause, and sometimes patients who have not been diagnosed with primary biliary cirrhosis are sent to dermatologists for diagnosis and treatment. As the disease progresses further, the patient's liver becomes enlarged (hepatomegaly). Many patients have pain on the right upper quadrant of the body.

About a third of patients who have this illness also have an enlarged spleen, particularly as the disease progresses. Some patients have jaundice in the early stages, and many are jaundiced at the later stages of the illness. Patients with advanced primary biliary cirrhosis may also have edema (water retention) and ascites. Some patients experience unintended weight loss.

### Diagnosis and Treatment

According to Kaplan in his 1996 article in the *New England Journal of Medicine,* there are usually four stages of primary biliary cirrhosis, and cirrhosis is clearly apparent in the fourth stage. It is possible, however, to see several different stages at the same time in different parts of the patient's liver.

Routine liver enzyme and function tests may help the physician to suspect the problem. Patients who have primary biliary cirrhosis have elevated blood levels of alkaline phosphaste and gamma-glutamyltransferase. Another test, the antimitochondrial antibody test, has a positive result in nearly all (95 percent) of patients who have this condition. Blood cholesterol level is also usually mildly to significantly elevated in primary biliary cirrhosis patients.

Doctors should carefully question patients about the medications that they take, because a wide variety of medications can cause fatigue, pruritus, and other signs that are also characteristic of primary biliary cirrhosis.

Physicians usually order an ultrasound of the patient's liver to look for any other causes of liver disease. In some cases, however, a computed tomography (CT) scan may be needed; in others, an ENDOSCOPIC RETROGRADE CHOLANGIOPANCREATOGRAPHY (ERCP) is required to determine the cause of abnormal liver test findings. A liver biopsy specimen is usually taken to make the diagnosis.

There is no medical cure for primary biliary cirrhosis, but medications may help treat the symptoms. Ursodiol is the most commonly used medication. It helps relieve symptoms and slows the progression of the disease, and it has essentially no side effects. Physicians may also try such medications as colchicine and methotrexate. A combination of ursodiol plus colchicine may be superior to either drug alone. However, most patients eventually experience LIVER FAILURE, and the only known cure is a LIVER TRANSPLANTATION.

See also LIVER; LIVER ENZYMES/FUNCTION TESTS.

Kaplan, Marshall M., M.D. "Primary Biliary Cirrhosis." *New England Journal of Medicine* 335, no. 21 (November 21, 1996): 1,570–1,580.

**primary sclerosing cholangitis**  A severe and chronic liver disease that involves inflammation and scarring of the bile ducts of the liver. These ducts can become so narrow that they are blocked and cannot effectively transport bile out of the liver. With this increasing bile buildup, frequent infections occur, and the liver becomes damaged. The cause of primary sclerosing cholangitis (PSC) is unknown; it may be caused by an infection of the bile duct. Some experts believe that it may be an autoimmune disease.

### Risk Factors

Most primary sclerosing cholangitis patients are 30 to 60 years old, and the majority are male.

According to Kaplan's 1997 article in the *New England Journal of Medicine,* the majority of primary sclerosing cholangitis patients (75 percent) have INFLAMMATORY BOWEL DISEASE (IBD). CROHN'S DISEASE and ulcerative colitis are the two forms of an inflammatory bowel disease.

IBD and PSC may not have the same underlying cause, since the two diseases may occur at different times during life. PSC can occur long after colectomy for ULCERATIVE COLITIS. Similarly, the onset of ulcerative colitis may follow a liver transplantation for PSC. Also, it should also be pointed out that primary sclerosing cholangitis develops in only a minority (less than 5 percent) of inflammatory bowel disease patients.

### Symptoms and Signs

The key indicators of primary sclerosing cholangitis are jaundice, intermittent fevers, pruritus (itching of the skin), and fatigue. Because these symptoms occur in many different illnesses, physicians must rule out other causes. PSC can lead to GALLSTONES, CHOLANGITIS, and cholangiocarcinoma (cancer of the gallbladder). Ulcerative colitis that is associated with PSC may lead to colon cancer.

### Diagnosis and Treatment

Primary sclerosing cholangitis is diagnosed through the injection of dye into the bile ducts, followed by X rays known as endoscopic retrograde cholangiopancreatography (ERCP). The magnetic resonance imaging (MRI) scan is a valuable adjunct.

The treatment primarily deals with symptoms; for example, patients are given antibiotics to treat infections and/or medications to control itching. They may also take vitamin supplements if they are deficient in vitamins. The most common vitamin deficiencies of primary sclerosing cholangitis patients are of vitamins A, D, and K.

Some physicians treat patients with ursodiol, which is also used to treat PRIMARY BILIARY CIRRHOSIS patients; however, the efficacy of this medicine in improving outcome has not been proved in primary sclerosing cholangitis.

If the bile ducts are severely blocked, an ERCP with PAPILLOTOMY and even surgery may be indicated. If patients experience LIVER FAILURE, the only cure is LIVER TRANSPLANTATION.

For further information on primary sclerosing cholangitis, contact the following organization:

American Liver Foundation
75 Maiden Lane
Suite 603
New York, NY 10038
(800) 465-4837 (toll-free)
http://www.liverfoundation.org

See also CIRRHOSIS; LIVER.

Kaplan, Marshall M., M.D. "Toward Better Treatment of Primary Sclerosing Cholangitis." *New England Journal of Medicine* 336, no. 10 (March 6, 1997): 719–721.

**proctitis**   An irritation and inflammation of the rectum, which may be caused by an infection, drugs, or radiation therapy. Proctitis also occurs as a component of ULCERATIVE COLITIS in 95 percent of those who have that condition. Individuals who have proctitis have gastrointestinal bleeding and rectal pain. The treatment depends upon the cause.

See also PRIMARY BILIARY CIRRHOSIS.

**progressive familial intrahepatic cholestasis**   Inherited disorder that is characterized by defects in bile secretion that often appear in infancy or early childhood and are associated with growth failure and severe liver disease.

Progressive familial intrahepatic cholestasis type I, also known as Byler disease or Greenland familial cholestasis, is associated with a defect on chromosome 18q21. Another form is progressive familial intrahepatic cholestasis type II, which occurs primarily in families in Europe and the Middle East. It is caused by a defect in chromosome 2q24. In addition, a third form, progressive familial intrahepatic cholestasis type III, appears to be caused by mutations in a protein that is known as multidrug resistance protein-3-P-glycoprotein (PGY-3 or MDR-3). Physicians can treat the symptoms of familial intrahepatic cholestasis, but there is little else that they can do.

Another form of familial intrahepatic cholestasis is benign recurrent intrahepatic cholestasis (BRIC). This condition manifests itself in adolescence or early adulthood, with episodic symptoms and signs of poor appetite, itching, weight loss, and malabsorption. The episodes may last weeks to months, followed by complete normalization. There is no specific treatment for BRIC, and treatment is directed to the symptoms. Liver transplantation is not undertaken because the disease is episodic and nonprogressive in nature.

See also CHOLESTASIS; LIVER; LIVER FAILURE; LIVER TRANSPLANTATION.

**prokinetics**   A class of prescribed medications that was formerly popular in the use of treating patients with gastroesophageal reflux disease (GERD). These drugs are also known as promotility medications because they speed stomach emptying and/or transit through the gut. The drugs are useful for those who have GASTROPARESIS and intestinal pseudoobstruction.

In 2000 cisapride (Propulsid), a very popular medication, was virtually withdrawn from the market in the United States by the Food and Drug Administration (FDA) because some patients who used cisapride became sick or died of cardiac ailments. On a restricted basis, physicians may currently continue to prescribe cisapride to some who do not respond to other medications; however, patients who have heart problems cannot take this drug; nor should those who are taking some antibiotics or antidepressants because of problems with adverse drug reactions. Cisapride is widely available outside the United States.

The other primary prokinetic drug is metoclopramide (Reglan). Because metoclopramide has many side effects, especially on the brain, many physicians avoid prescribing this drug whenever possible. Domperidone, another prokinetic drug, is sold in some pharmacies where it is compounded by the pharmacist. It is like metoclopramide, but without many of its side effects on the brain. Erythromycin, in addition to its antibiotic function, has prokinetic activity. However, its effects are short-lived, lasting no more than a few weeks.

See also ACID REFLUX; GAS-BLOAT SYNDROME; HYPEREMESIS GRAVIDARUM; PROTON PUMP INHIBITORS.

Minocha, Anil, M.D., and Christine Adamec. *How to Stop Heartburn: Simple Ways to Heal Heartburn and Acid Reflux.* New York: John Wiley & Sons, 2001.

**prostaglandins**    Specialized products of arachidonic acid metabolism that are synthesized in many tissues of the body and that have a short half-life. They act locally close to the site of production in a variety of ways. There are various kinds of prostaglandins with different functions, such as prostaglandin $D_2$ ($PGD_2$) and $PGE_2$, that act as short-term hormones close to the area where they are synthesized. They are not stored; instead, they are released on an as-needed basis.

Prostaglandins are involved in regulating the kidney function, blood pressure, the production of blood clots, the functioning of the uterus and ovaries, and the generation or inhibition of pain and inflammation. They are also involved in erectile function.

NONSTEROIDAL ANTI-INFLAMMATORY DRUGS (NSAIDs) inhibit the production of prostaglandins, thus reducing inflammation; however, they also often cause damage to the gastric mucosa. Cyclooxygenase-2 (COX-2) inhibitor medications such as rofecoxib (Vioxx) and valdecoxib (Bextra) were developed to decrease inflammation and at the same time reduce toxicity to the gastrointestinal system. COX-2 inhibitors may cause some harm to the stomach, although usually less than is caused by an NSAID.

See also PAIN.

**proton pump inhibitors**    A class of medications that are given to people who suffer from chronic heartburn, also known as GASTROESOPHAGEAL REFLUX DISEASE, and/or to patients who have stomach or duodenal ulcers. Drugs in this class are more potent inhibitors of stomach acid than are the histamine-2 receptor blockers such as rantidine (Zantac) or cimetidine (Tagamet). The reduced acid secretion in the stomach due to these drugs allows time for healing. Proton pump inhibitors (PPIs) are also prescribed for individuals who have ZOLLINGER–ELLISON SYNDROME. As of this writing, the available PPIs include omeprazole (Prilosec), lansoprazole (Prevacid), rabeprazole (Aciphex), pantoprazole (Protonix), and esomeprazole (Nexium). Prilosec is also available over the counter.

See also ACID REFLUX; NONSTEROIDAL ANTI-INFLAMMATORY DRUGS; ULCERS, PEPTIC.

**pruritus ani**    Itching in the anal area that may be caused by poor personal hygiene or by parasites, for example, worms such as *Enterobius* (pinworms). Other causes include ALCOHOLISM, HEMORRHOIDS, and DIABETES MELLITUS.

See also PARASITIC INFECTIONS.

**pseudolithiasis, biliary**    Biliary sludge and small stones that are caused by the continued use of high doses of medications such as ceftriaxone (Rocephin) that are prescribed for severe infections. The drug is excreted in bile and when saturated, it precipitates out of the bile, appearing as tiny gallstones on an ultrasound. Patients may have abdominal pain and signs of cholestasis, although no underlying gallbladder disease is present. Discontinuation of the medication causes the pseudolithiasis to resolve within two months or so.

**pyloroplasty**    Surgery to dilate (widen) the opening that lies between the small intestine and the stomach, so that the stomach contents can move more easily from the stomach into the small intestine. Pyloroplasty is used as part of the treatment for ulcers as well as for pyloric obstruction.

**pylorus**    The opening from the stomach to the duodenum (upper part of the small intestine).

**radiation injury**    Damage to the body that occurs as a result of radiation therapy for cancer or radiation from another source. Radiation can harm the digestive system, causing problems with the colon and other parts of the gastrointestinal tract. Digestive symptoms may appear several years after radiation exposure. Patients who have radiation enteritis may experience diarrhea and gastrointestinal bleeding, as well as strictures. They may also have esophageal strictures that cause swallowing problems or intestinal strictures that cause bowel obstructions.

**radiation therapy**    Radiotherapy that is given to individuals who have digestive cancers (and other forms of cancer), in an attempt to destroy cancer cells. In some cases, the cancer may be too far advanced for the patient to be cured, but radiation therapy may prevent the cancer from spreading farther for some period, thus extending the individual's life by months or even by years and/or improving his or her quality of life. Sometimes radiation is also given to alleviate pain. Radiation therapy may also be used to shrink an otherwise nonresectable tumor to a resectable one in order to attempt curative surgery. Radiation treatments are overseen by radiation oncologists.

Depending on the type of cancer, some patients may receive implanted radiation therapy, whereas others need to go to a facility three or four times a week for several weeks to receive treatment from equipment that beams the radiation directly at the body part that is cancerous.

In some cases, patients may receive chemotherapy (cancer-killing drugs) at the same time as they are having radiation treatments. In other cases, chemotherapy is used separately.

See also CANCER; RADIATION INJURY.

**rectal prolapse**    The slippage of the rectum. It may be occult (hidden) or may be visible external to the anus. Patients who have rectal prolapse may report pain, difficulty with defecation, and bleeding. The treatment of symptomatic rectal prolapse is surgery.

**Roux-en-Y stasis syndrome**    A condition that may occur after gastric surgery, which includes chronic nausea, vomiting, and abdominal pain along with a bloated feeling, especially one that occurs after eating meals.

In Roux-en-Y stasis syndrome, motility is slowed in the stomach as well as in the small intestine, resulting in stasis of food. Treatment is difficult. The Roux limb, which is less than 45 centimeters in size, reduces the probability of occurrence of this disorder. Patients who have predominant gastric stasis may improve after a subtotal GASTRECTOMY. Medical treatment for Roux-en-Y stasis syndrome involves hydration (provision of fluids) and treatment with antiemetics such as promethazine (Phenergan) and ondansetron (Zofran), as well as with prokinetic agents, such as metoclopramide (Reglan) and domperidone (Motilium).

In one study, reported in 1998 in *Archives of Surgery,* patients who had severe symptoms of Roux-en-Y stasis syndrome improved significantly with intravenous administration of erythromycin, which, in addition to its antibiotic effect, has prokinetic action.

Petrakis, John, M.D., et al. "Enhancement of Gastric Emptying of Solids by Erythromycin in Patients with Roux-en-Y Gastrojejunostomy." *Archives of Surgery* 133, no. 7 (July 1998): 709–714.

**rumination syndrome**   A behavioral disorder that is an effortless regurgitation of recently eaten food, which is then followed by the patient's rechewing and then reswallowing the food. No nausea or retching is involved. It is unclear by what mechanism the food is regurgitated.

The behavior usually occurs at every meal. Although rumination is usually seen only in some developmentally disabled children or among subjects who have psychiatric problems, it may also occur in some patients without such problems. Patients report that the food tastes good and is just like the food that was swallowed. The patient experiences no nausea, although belching may precede the rumination. Some patients spit out the ruminated food, and others reswallow it.

This behavioral disorder is treated with reassurance, behavioral therapy, and explanations to the patient and to the family as well.

See also BELCHING; NAUSEA AND VOMITING.

**saliva/salivary problems**    Saliva is the substance that is formed in the mouth, especially when a person eats, and helps to lubricate as well as partially break down food. Saliva is secreted by the salivary glands. There are three major salivary glands: the parotid, submandibular, and sublingual glands. Causes of insufficient salivation include Sjögren's syndrome, anxiety, and use of many different antidepressant drugs, anticholinergic medications (phenothiazines), and diuretics.

**Salmonella**    Bacteria that can cause minor to life-threatening illnesses in children and adults. The infection that *Salmonella* organisms cause is called salmonellosis. *Salmonella* organisms are the most common cause of FOOD-BORNE ILLNESSES in the world and are often spread in contaminated food that was prepared by people who did not wash their hands after using the toilet. In the United States, *Salmonella* species account for $1 billion in both direct and indirect medical costs. According to the Centers for Disease Control and Prevention (CDC), there were 39,574 cases of *Salmonella* infection diagnosed in the United States in 2000.

In addition to being spread by individuals who prepared food that they contaminated, *Salmonella* organisms are also transmitted by individuals who are handling infected pet reptiles, especially turtles, lizards, and snakes.

Typhoid fever is also caused by a form of *Salmonella (S. typhi)*, but this form of bacteria is rarely found in the United States, Canada, and other developed countries. It is usually spread by contaminated water, especially after natural disasters such as earthquakes or floods, when the normal water systems are disrupted and the sewer systems overflow.

### Symptoms of Salmonellosis

The most frequently occurring symptoms of a *Salmonella* infection are as follows:

- Diarrhea
- Headache
- Fever
- Possible nausea and vomiting

In general, the symptoms of infection begin within one to three days. Sometimes diarrhea caused by salmonellosis is very severe, and the patient is hospitalized and given intravenous fluid in order to prevent DEHYDRATION.

### Diagnosis and Treatment

The physician may suspect a *Salmonella* infection on the basis of symptoms and may order an analysis of the stools to confirm the diagnosis. Blood cultures may be done. Most people recover without any medications within five to seven days. However, if doctors believe that the infection has spread to the blood, antibiotics are prescribed, because such infection can be dangerous and sometimes even fatal.

### Long-Term Effects

In some cases of *Salmonella* infection, the bacteria may cause the development of a chronic condition that is known as Reiter's syndrome, which can lead to arthritis, painful urination due to urethritis and painful red eye due to uveitis.

### Antibiotic-Resistant Salmonella Strains

Researchers have discovered that some *Salmonella* strains are resistant to antibiotics; for that reason, it is increasingly important that government agencies be vigilant and that consumers follow simple techniques that can help prevent the transmission of *Salmonella* infections.

### Preventing **Salmonella** *Infections*

Although it is not possible to wipe out all *Salmonella* bacteria, many infections can be prevented through simple actions. Examples of good preventive actions against *Salmonella* infection are the following:

- Washing hands immediately after handling reptiles
- Washing hands immediately after handling raw poultry or raw eggs
- Washing food surfaces that have had contact with uncooked poultry or eggs
- Cooking eggs and poultry thoroughly
- Drinking only pasteurized milk
- Avoiding foods that include raw eggs, such as found in raw cookie dough and homemade salad dressing

See also CONTAMINATED FOOD OR WATER.

David G. White, et al. "The Isolation of Antibiotic-Resistant *Salmonella* from Retail Ground Meats." *New England Journal of Medicine* 345, no. 16 (October 18, 2001): 1,147–1,154.

**sarcoidosis**    A systemwide disease with symptoms that are similar to those that are found among TUBERCULOSIS patients. In contrast to that of tuberculosis, the cause of sarcoidosis is unknown. It is not an infection, although some experts believe that sarcoidosis may be environmentally triggered by an exposure to antigens or metal dusts. No single genetic or environmental cause has been established to date for sarcoidosis, despite extensive investigations.

### Symptoms and Signs

The symptoms and signs of sarcoidosis depend on the organ involved, and there may be no symptoms or mild to severe symptoms. Sarcoidosis causes skin lesions and lymph node enlargements and fibrosis of the lungs. Fever, weight loss, joint pains, and lack of appetite are common problems. Many patients have an enlarged liver. The disease can also affect the eyes, causing cataracts, glaucoma, blurred vision, and abnormal amounts of tears, caused by ophthalmic lesions produced by the disease. Sarcoidosis may also lead to blindness.

A variety of skin rashes may also occur. In addition, the heart and brain may be involved. Some patients experience excessive absorption of calcium, which may ultimately lead to kidney failure.

The key symptoms are fatigue, fever, weight loss, and lack of appetite. Most patients also have chronic respiratory symptoms as well.

### Risk Factors

Most people diagnosed with sarcoidosis are younger than age 40. The disease is more commonly found among American blacks, and to a lesser extent, among Northern Europeans. In the United States, the incidence is about 35.5 per 100,000 blacks. Among whites in the United States, the incidence is about 10.9 per 100,000. Experts estimate the lifetime risk of sarcoidosis for blacks at 2.4 percent and at less than 1 percent (0.85) percent for whites. The symptoms are also often more severe among blacks who have the disease. There are no known gender differences in the incidence of sarcoidosis.

There appears to be a genetic risk for the disease because sarcoidosis occurs more commonly in identical twins than in fraternal twins. In addition, family members of people who have sarcoidosis have a higher risk of development of the disease. There appear to be racial disparities among people who are at risk for development of sarcoidosis; for example, when sarcoidosis is identified in a black family, as many as 19 percent of other members are diagnosed with the disease. When it is found in a white family, only about 5 percent of other members have sarcoidosis.

### Diagnosis and Treatment

During the physical examination, and with laboratory as well as imaging studies, the physician notes changes to the lungs, skin, heart, liver, and eyes. The chest X-ray finding is abnormal in 90 percent of patients with sarcoidosis. An ophthalmologic examination reveals eye changes that have been caused by sarcoidosis.

Sarcoidosis is definitively diagnosed with a biopsy. Chest X rays are also indirectly needed for diagnosis. Tuberculosis and fungal infections should be excluded as part of the diagnosis.

Patients who have few or no symptoms do not require any treatment. Most symptomatic patients with widespread involvement, including of the heart, brain, and eyes, as well as those who have hypercalcemia and respiratory problems, are treated with corticosteroid drugs such as prednisone. Some patients who are not responding to prednisone are treated with methotrexate. Some patients, especially those who have disfiguring skin conditions, are treated with antimalarial agents such as hydroxychloroquine.

Some sarcoidosis patients are very ill and may require lung or heart transplantation.

Newman, Lee S., et al. "Sarcoidosis," *New England Journal of Medicine* 336, no. 17 (April 24, 1997): 1,224–1,234.

**Schilling test**   A laboratory test used for detecting a cobalamin (vitamin $B_{12}$) deficiency that is caused by the decreased absorption of this vitamin, as seen in PERNICIOUS ANEMIA and in MALABSORPTION SYNDROME. The test is performed by oral administration of radiolabeled cyano-cobalamin followed by an intramuscular injection of cobalamin. A 24-hour urine sample is then collected. A low percent excretion of radiolabeled cobalamin suggests cobalamin malabsorption, due to pernicious anemia or other causes of intestinal malabsorption.

**scleroderma**   A condition that affects the connective tissues as well as the nerves and muscles, causing a hardening and tightening of the skin and affecting the digestive system as well. It may cause difficulty in swallowing (dysphagia), large diverticula (pockets in the small intestine and the colon), slow gut movements leading to constipation, and other medical problems. Scleroderma can affect organs throughout the body. For example, it can impair the esophagus, causing not only dysphagia but also gastroesophageal reflux disease (GERD). Some scientists

estimate that as many as 165,000 people in the United States have systemic scleroderma.

The disease can also cause swollen puffy skin as well as contractures of the hands, wrists and elbows. Men who have scleroderma may experience erectile dysfunction.

Scleroderma may be an autoimmune disorder, although researchers are not certain of the cause of this condition. There is a complex yet poorly understood interplay among immunological events, fibrogenic fibroblast cells, and the blood vessels in various parts of the body. The most common sign is thick and hardened skin, particularly on the face. Sometimes cosmetics can conceal scleroderma.

### Risk Factors

Scleroderma is much more commonly found among women than among men; women have scleroderma at about seven to 12 times the rate of men, according to the National Institutes of Health. It is more commonly found among people of European descent and is found infrequently among African Americans.

### Diagnosis and Treatment

Scleroderma diagnosis is based on the signs and symptoms of the patient, in addition to the results of blood and imaging studies. The symptoms are treated by physicians who are specialists in the field; for example, gastroenterologists treat dysphagia, GERD, gastroparesis, intestinal pseudoobstruction, constipation and fecal incontinence, and rheumatologists treat problems with the joints or muscles. A dermatologist may be consulted for skin problems. Scleroderma can also affect the heart and kidneys, and thus referrals to a cardiologist and nephrologist may also be needed.

Scleroderma patients who have gastrointestinal problems are often advised to eat small and frequent meals and to avoid fatty foods. They are also advised to raise the head of their bed to prevent the problems associated with gastroesophageal reflux disease. Patients may need antibiotics to treat small-intestine bacterial overgrowths that cause diarrhea and malabsorption syndrome.

For further information, contact the following organizations:

National Institute of Arthritis and Musculoskeletal and Skin Diseases Information Clearinghouse
1 AMS Circle
Bethesda, MD 20892
(877) 226-4267 (toll-free) or (301) 495-4484
http://www.niams.nih.gov

American Academy of Dermatology
P.O. Box 4014
Schaumburg, IL 60168
(847) 330-0230
http://www.aad.org

American College of Rheumatology
1800 Century Place
Suite 250
Atlanta, GA 30345
(404) 63-3777
http://www.rheumatology.org

Arthritis Foundation
1330 West Peachtree Street
Atlanta, GA 30309
(800) 283-7800 (toll-free) or (404) 872-7100
http://www.arthritis.org

Scleroderma Foundation
12 Kent Way, Number 101
Byfield, MA 01922
(800) 722-HOPE (toll-free) or (978) 463-5843
http://www.scleroderma.org

Scleroderma Research Foundation
2320 Bath Street
Suite 315
Santa Barbara, CA 93105
(800) 441-2873 (toll-free) or (805) 563-9133
http://www.srfcure.org

See also ACID REFLUX; CREST SYNDROME; DIVERTIC-ULOSIS; DYSPHAGIA; GASTROESOPHAGEAL REFLUX DISEASE; PRIMARY BILIARY CIRRHOSIS; SKIN DISEASES AND DIGESTIVE SYSTEM.

**secretin**    A natural hormone that causes the release of pancreatic juice. In physiologic doses, this hormone also inhibits stomach acidity and motility. In pharmacologic doses, secretin increases gastrointestinal motility as well as bile flow to the intestines.

Secretin has also been artificially synthesized and is used in some procedures done on patients for digestive problems. It is used for the diagnosis of PANCREATIC INSUFFICIENCY as well as of a pancreatic tumor that is known as gastrinoma or ZOLLINGER–ELLISON SYNDROME.

At one point, parents of children who had autism, a severe psychiatric disorder, believed that infusions of secretin would improve the children's condition. This belief was based on anecdotal findings that some autistic children improved after abdominal surgery in which secretin was used by physicians. Subsequent studies have proved that secretin is neither a cure nor a treatment for children or adults who have autism.

Sandler, Adrian D., M.D., et al. "Lack of Benefit of a Single Dose of Synthetic Human Secretin in the Treatment of Autism and Pervasive Development Disorder." *New England Journal of Medicine* 341, no. 24 (December 9, 1999): 1,801–1,806.

**selenium**    A trace mineral in the human body that is also an antioxidant (cancer fighter). Selenium is needed for healthy functioning of the thyroid gland and the immune system. Selenium is found in the soil and has a high concentration in northern Nebraska and North and South Dakota, where many residents have the highest concentrations of selenium in the United States. For adults, the recommended requirement of selenium is 70 micrograms per day for men and 55 micrograms per day for women.

Foods that are rich in selenium include the following:

• Brazil nuts

• Canned tuna

• Beef or calf liver

• Cod cooked in dry heat

• Enriched boiled noodles

• Oven roasted turkey breast

• Enriched elbow macaroni

• Spaghetti with meat sauce

## Deficiency of Selenium

Most people in the United States and Canada are not deficient in selenium. In some parts of China and Russia, selenium deficiency is very common. There are no obvious specific symptoms or signs of a selenium deficiency; however, such a deficiency can be detected by a blood test for selenium levels.

Patients who are deficient in selenium may have arthritis, decreased immune function, heart failure, and increased susceptibility to cancer. In China, patients deficient in selenium may have Keshan disease, which causes cardiac dysfunction. It can be prevented but not cured by selenium supplements. There is a direct correlation between selenium deficiency and a reduction in CD4 cell counts (the lower the count, the lower the immune function) in patients infected with the human immunodeficiency virus (HIV).

Other people who are at risk for development of a selenium deficiency include the following categories of individuals:

- People relying solely on intravenous (IV) nutrition because their digestive system is malfunctioning (selenium can be added to the IV drip). Newer trace-element solutions for total parenteral nutrition (TPN) contain selenium
- People who have had serious gastrointestinal surgery, such as having half or more of their small intestine removed
- People who have Crohn's disease

## Excessive Levels of Selenium

It is also possible to have too much selenium in the body. Selonisis occurs when selenium is consumed in high doses of greater than 900 micrograms per day. This condition is extremely rare, and the only reported cases have occurred in people who were taking selenium supplements that included an excessive level of selenium, the result of a mistake by the selenium seller. The Institute of Medicine has reported that the maximal amount of selenium that any adult should take is 400 micrograms per day; the usual supplemental dose is fifty to 200 micrograms per day.

The key symptoms of selenium excess are as follows:

- Hair loss
- Skin rash
- Gastrointestinal upset
- Mild nerve damage
- White blotchy fingernails
- Altered mental status

See also ALTERNATIVE MEDICINE; ANTIOXIDANTS.

**Shigella**   Common bacteria that cause dysentery in humans worldwide. In the United States alone, there are about 450,000 cases of shigellosis (infection with *Shigella* organisms) each year. There is a high risk of outbreaks of shigellosis in some facilities, such as day care centers and psychiatric institutions.

## Transmission of **Shigella**

The bacteria may be spread by person-to-person contact or in contaminated food prepared by food workers who did not wash their hands after using the toilet. The bacteria can also be spread through other means, such as swimming in a pool or lake contaminated by the bacteria passed through fecal contamination or by drinking contaminated water. The most common form of *Shigella* bacteria in the United States, Canada, and other developed countries is *Shigella sonnei,* which is also written as *S. sonnei.*

## Symptoms of Shigellosis

The severity of symptoms varies. Symptoms usually occur one to seven days after the person is infected; once they have begun, symptoms may last as long as five to seven days. The most common symptoms of shigellosis are as follows:

- Fever
- Bloody or watery diarrhea (about 10 stools, but there may be as many as 100 or more per day)
- Nausea and vomiting
- Abdominal pain
- Tiredness and weakness

### Diagnosis and Treatment

*Shigella* infection is usually suspected because of a patient's symptoms. The diagnosis is confirmed with results of stool tests. The illness resolves in about seven days in most cases; thus, doctors often just advise patients to wait for the body to recover on its own. Physicians prescribe antibiotics for patients with severe symptoms, as well as for food handlers, health care workers, elderly people, and immune-suppressed individuals. Antibiotics such as trimethoprim sulfamethoxazole (Bactrim) or ciprofloxacin (Cipro) may be prescribed.

### Effects of Shigellosis

Most people recover completely from a *Shigella* infection; however, some individuals have bowel problems for months afterward. Shigellosis may cause severe complications such as PROCTITIS (inflammation of the rectum), bowel obstruction or PERFORATION, BACTEREMIA (bacterial spread to the blood), MALNUTRITION, DEHYDRATION, and seizures. In some cases, these complications may be life-threatening.

In other cases, such as with infection with *S. flexneri*, the condition may worsen and Reiter's syndrome, a medical problem that may lead to chronic arthritis and to painful urination (urethritis) may develop.

### Prevention of Shigellosis

To prevent *Shigella* infection, the following steps are recommended:

- Individuals should drink only water they know is safe. Any unreliable water should be chlorinated.

- Anyone who prepares food should wash the hands with soap after using the toilet or changing a baby's diapers.

- People who prepare food should wash their hands with soap before preparing food (even if they have not just used the toilet).

- Strict refrigeration and proper cooking of food are important.

- Children should be trained to wash their hands after using the toilet, to lower the risk of their spreading disease to themselves and others.

- Swimmers should avoid swallowing swimming pool, pond, or lake water, which may be contaminated with *Shigella* organisms.

See also CONTAMINATED FOOD OR WATER; FOOD-BORNE ILLNESSES; PARASITIC INFECTIONS; TRAVEL.

Keene, William E., et al. "A Swimming-Associated Outbreak of Hemorrhagic Colitis Caused by *Escherichia coli* 0157:H7 and *Shigella sonnei*." *New England Journal of Medicine* 331, no. 9 (September 1, 1994): 579–584.

**short bowel syndrome**  A malabsorption condition in which the patient has difficulty absorbing nutrients after a large part of the small intestine has been removed as a treatment for CROHN'S DISEASE, CANCER, enterocolitis, or other medical conditions. It is also known as short gut syndrome.

Some signs and symptoms of short bowel syndrome are diarrhea, unintended weight loss, and weakness. Patients who have extensive short bowel removal need PARENTERAL NUTRITION. Small intestinal transplantation is an option, especially for patients who are not candidates for receiving long-term parenteral nutrition.

**sigmoidoscopy**  A procedure in which the rectum and the lower part of the colon is internally examined with a sigmoidoscope. A sigmoidoscope is a flexible tube, measuring about 65 centimeters. This procedure is performed to detect the presence of colorectal cancer, POLYPS, and other diseases and abnormalities. The procedure is usually performed after the rectum and lower colon have been evacuated with a couple of enemas given about 30 minutes to an hour before the procedure. Whereas sigmoidoscopy examines only a part of a colon, COLONOSCOPY, a much more comprehensive procedure, inspects the entire colon.

See also CANCER, COLORECTAL.

**signs and symptoms**  Possible indicators of disease or disorder. Signs are visible or measurable indicators of disease that a doctor can note, such as pallor, above-normal body temperature, or blood pressure that is high or low. Symptoms are problems that patients report, such as pain, weakness, bleeding, and heartburn.

See also PAIN.

**skin diseases and digestive system**   Some skin disorders and infections can cause minor or long-standing harm to the digestive system; for example, staphylococcal infection can cause nausea and vomiting and may worsen in rare cases. CELIAC SPRUE is associated with dermatitis herpetiformis; hyperpigmentation of skin is seen in WHIPPLE'S DISEASE. Pemphigus vulgaris may involve the esophagus, causing dysphagia (difficulty in swallowing food) and odynophagia (painful swallowing). Pyoderma gangrenosum and ERYTHEMA NODOSUM may be seen in INFLAMMATORY BOWEL DISEASE. HEPATITIS C is associated with porphyria cutanea tarda and mixed CRYOGLOBULINEMIA.

See also SCLERODERMA; *STAPHYLOCOCCUS.*

**sleep**   A period of unconsciousness during which the body relaxes, dreams, and replenishes itself. Sleep is important for the individual's overall well-being. A lack of sleep can moderately or severely affect digestion, as well as affecting other body processes.

Sometimes medical problems prevent sleep or impair an individual from obtaining sufficient sleep; for example, individuals who have GASTROESOPHAGEAL REFLUX DISEASE may have troubled sleep. Pain and irritation due to ulcers or DIARRHEA caused by INFLAMMATORY BOWEL DISEASE may waken a person in the middle of the night, thus preventing or impairing normal sleep. Sleep patterns are also often disturbed among IRRITABLE BOWEL SYNDROME (IBS) patients.

See also ULCERS, PEPTIC.

**small intestine**   A key organ in the digestive system, where most of the digestion and absorption of nutrients and fluids occur. The small intestine starts at the pylorus and includes the duodenum, the jejunum, and the ileum. It ends at the ileocecal valve, where the ileum opens into the cecum, the first part of the large intestine (colon).

**smoking**   Inhalation of tobacco smoke, usually through cigarettes, but also through cigars or pipes. Smoking is extremely harmful to the body over the long term. Many people start smoking as adolescents because their friends smoke and/or they think smoking impresses others. Then they become addicted to the nicotine in tobacco and find stopping smoking extremely difficult. According to the National Center for Health Statistics, 80 percent of all smokers smoke every day.

Whereas smoking was once believed to enhance digestion, researchers have subsequently discovered that smoking seriously impedes digestion, and this habit can also cause many chronic and long-term serious digestive diseases and cancers. The Centers for Disease Control and Prevention (CDC) estimates that about 440,000 deaths in the United States each year can be directly attributed to smoking.

### *Risk Factors for Smokers*

According to a report that was released by the National Center for Health Statistics in 2003 on cigarette smoking among adults in 1997–98, about 24 percent of all adults who are 18 and older in the United States are smokers. Men are slightly more likely to smoke than women: about 28 percent of men in the United States smoke, versus 22 percent of women.

In considering racial differences among those who smoke, about 25 percent of white adults smoke and about 26 percent of black non Hispanics do. Among Hispanic adults, about 19 percent are smokers. Asians and Pacific Islanders are the least likely to smoke: about 14 percent are smokers.

Marital status also has an impact on whether people smoke: for example, 21 percent of married adults in the United States smoke, versus 36 percent of adults who are either divorced or separated and 40 percent of adults who live with a partner to whom they are not married.

Generally, smokers are less educated than nonsmokers, and the incidence of cigarette smoking steadily declines with education. About 34 percent of adults who have less than a high school diploma smoke, compared to only 8 percent with a master's degree, doctorate, or medical degree. Among women, about 30 percent with less than a high school diploma smoke, compared to about 8 percent who have an advanced degree.

An individual's income level is also directly related to whether he or she smokes. Men with an income below the poverty level are nearly twice as likely to smoke (38 percent) as men in the highest-income group (20 percent). Income clearly affects whether women smoke as well: about 31 percent of women with income below the poverty level smoke, compared to 16 percent at the highest income level.

### Health Problems Caused or Worsened by Smoking

A large number of cases of oral and lung cancer are attributable to smoking. Smoking is also linked to anal cancer, bladder cancer, esophageal cancer, pancreatic cancer, and cervical cancer. It may also contribute to colorectal cancer and kidney cancer.

Smoking does not cause DIABETES MELLITUS, but it makes controlling the disease much more difficult. Smoking also worsens GASTROPARESIS, or slowed stomach emptying. Smoking increases the risk for development of cardiovascular disease. In addition, healing in CROHN'S DISEASE patients is difficult for those who continue to smoke.

The harmful effects of active smoking (smoking by an individual) can also be documented in cases of passive smoking (being in the presence of another person who smokes). Paradoxically, however, smoking apparently has a preventive or beneficial effect on ULCERATIVE COLITIS. In fact, when used as a medication, nicotine has been shown to be of therapeutic benefit in this disorder.

### Smoking Cessation Methods

Physicians urge their patients to stop smoking immediately, regardless of their health status. It is even more imperative for ill patients to stop smoking. Some patients are successful with nicotine replacement drugs, in the form of oral tablets and skin patches. Nasal sprays and inhalers are being tested. The goal is to start at one dose of nicotine and gradually taper. The risk of complications is higher if the patient continues to smoke while also using nicotine patches.

Some patients use bupropion (Zyban), a drug that helps suppress the desire for nicotine in some individuals. Alternative methods of quitting smoking include acupuncture and hypnotherapy.

A major problem that many smokers face, in addition to their own addiction, is that they may associate frequently with other smokers among their family members and friends. These other individuals may refrain from urging the smoker to continue smoking, but when he or she observes constant smoking, quitting becomes much more difficult. In addition, many smokers associate certain cues with smoking, such as smoking after a meal. Asking to be seated in the nonsmoking section of a restaurant may help to break that association, and choosing to eat at a different time or changing the place at home where the food is consumed may help extinguish other smoking cues.

See also CANCER, ANAL; CANCER, ESOPHAGEAL; CANCER, ORAL; CANCER, PANCREATIC.

Blackwell, D. L., J. G. Collins, and R. Coles. "Summary Health Statistics for U.S. Adults: National Health Interview Survey, 1997." National Center for Health Statistics. *Vital Health Statistics* 10, no. 205 (2002).

Schoenborn, Charlotte A., Jackline A. Vickerie, and Patricia M. Barnes. Division of Health Interview Statistics. "Cigarette Smoking Behavior of Adults: United States, 1997–1998." *Advance Data from Vital and Health Statistics* no. 331 (February 7, 2003).

**Society of Gastroenterology Nurses and Associates (SGNA)**  Professional organization of more than 6,500 nurses, technicians, and other nonphysician personnel who work in the field of gastroenterology including endoscopic procedures. For further information, contact the SGNA at

401 North Michigan Avenue
Chicago, IL 60611
(800) 245-7462 (toll-free)
http://www.sgna.org

**sphincter**  Specialized muscle tissue that allows for opening and closing. The lower esophageal sphincter is a muscle that allows opening between the esophagus and the stomach. There is also a sphincter between the stomach and duodenum (the pyloric sphincter or just the pylorus). The sphincter of Oddi involves the confluence of the common bile duct and the pancreatic duct as they enter the wall of the duodenum. An anal sphincter, which is made up of internal and external anal components, allows regulation of defecation.

**spleen**  An organ that participates in cellular immunity and generating antibodies to attack infectious invaders. It is a reservoir for blood elements like white blood cells and platelets, while it also works to clean the blood of unwanted particulate matter, such as bacteria and senescent blood elements.

***Staphylococcus***  Ubiquitous bacteria that are even found on the skin and anterior nares of healthy adults, it may be spread in food by preparers who fail to wash their hands. "Staph" infections can cause severe nausea and vomiting and abdominal cramps within one to six hours of consuming infected food. Fever and diarrhea may also occur in a small number of cases. In most cases of *Staphylococcus* infection, patients recover within two to three days.

    *Staphylococcus* infections can be prevented by infected people's washing their hands before preparing food. Since most people infected with *Staphylococcus* bacteria do not know that they are infected, everyone should wash their hands before food preparation, to be on the safe side.

    It should also be noted that *Staphylococcus* infections can occur in the blood (bacteremia), the heart (endocarditis), and prosthetic joints. Staphylococcal scalding skin syndrome is a deadly disease, which is treated with methicillin or vancomycin. Another severe illness that is caused by *Staphylococcus* bacteria is staphylococcal toxic shock syndrome.

    See also CONTAMINATED FOOD OR WATER; FOOD-BORNE ILLNESSES; SKIN DISEASES AND DIGESTIVE SYSTEM.

**steatorrhea**  High levels of fat that are found in the stool due to malabsorption, which may indicate the presence of a disease, such as chronic PANCRE-ATITIS, CELIAC SPRUE, WHIPPLE'S DISEASE, small intestinal bacterial overgrowth, or ZOLLINGER-ELLISON SYNDROME.

**steroids**  Drugs that are prescribed for some illnesses characterized by excessive or uncontrolled inflammation, such as CROHN'S DISEASE, ULCERATIVE COLITIS, autoimmune hepatitis, and rheumatoid arthritis. They can also be used in the form of enemas, topical ointments and creams to treat such problems as colitis, hemorrhoids, pruritus ani and anal FISSURES. The long-term use of steroids has serious side effects, including a change in the body shape and structure (such as the development of a plump and moonlike face), osteoporosis, DIABETES MELLITUS, and immunosuppression. Thus, physicians taper the dose of the steroid to the lowest possible level as soon as possible, since the side effects are both dose- and duration-related. Steroids are also synthesized inside the body.

**stomach**  Key organ of the digestive system, lying between the esophagus and the small intestine. Digestion of proteins begins in the stomach. The stomach breaks food down into small particles about one to two millimeters in size before allowing them to proceed to the small intestine for further digestion and absorption. Hydrochloric acid produced in the stomach kills many infectious organisms that are consumed with food. There are a wide variety of diseases and disorders that can occur in the stomach, such as ulcers, CANCER, and GASTROPARESIS (slow stomach emptying).

    See also CANCER, STOMACH; ULCERS, PEPTIC.

**stomach cancer**  See CANCER, STOMACH.

**stress**  Emotional or psychological strain. Stress can greatly affect digestion, slowing it down. Some people who are under stress may have diarrhea. In addition, people who are experiencing severe stress often engage in either overeating, which may lead to obesity, or undereating. Often stress does not cause diseases (such as GASTROESOPHAGEAL REFLUX

DISEASE, ulcers, or many other digestive disorders) but considerably exacerbates already-existing ailments. Relaxation therapy or hypnotherapy may be helpful to alleviate stress. Some patients improve with psychotherapy. Therapists should understand that the painful condition may improve but may not completely resolve with therapy alone.

Another form of stress is the physical stress of a severe illness that occurs among patients who are admitted to the intensive care units of hospitals, such as patients who have a serious head injury, severe burns, and so forth. In such cases, ulcers in the stomach may occur, and they may bleed. Such stress-induced ulcers can be prevented by use of acid blocking medications (such as ranitidine [Zantac] or famotidine [Pepcid]) by individuals who are at high risk for development of such ulcers.

See also ULCERS, PEPTIC.

**stricture**    An abnormal narrowing of the lumen in the hollow tube of the digestive system. It is also called stenosis especially when the narrow-

ing involves the junction of two different parts of the digestive tube; for example, pyloric stenosis is a narrowing of the pylorus between the stomach and the duodenum. In the esophagus a stricture may develop as a result of long-standing ACID REFLUX, and this stricture may cause difficulty with swallowing. A stricture may develop in the intestines as a result of CROHN'S DISEASE or RADIATION THERAPY.

Strictures may be minor and asymptomatic or may cause pain and even completely block the hollow tube of the digestive tract. Strictures can be treated by dilation during endoscopy or by surgery called stricturoplasty. In another surgical option the narrowed segment is excised and the normal lumens are hooked back at both ends.

**surgery**    A minor or major procedure that usually involves cutting of the skin to reach the affected organ. Surgery may be performed to remove harmful or diseased body parts, such as an inflamed gallbladder, or to remove cancerous tissue from organs that have been affected by disease, for example, cancer of the colon.

**taste impairments** Difficulties or inabilities to taste normal flavors. A total loss of taste (ageusia) is rare. Taste is important for enjoying food, but it is also a gatekeeper to what is consumed. It is also a protective factor in some cases; for example, spoiled food or milk tastes unpleasant and, thus, people who have normal taste capacity do not eat or drink it.

Hypogeusia is a below-average ability to detect tastes. It may be caused by illness or by medications. Dysgeusia is taste distortion or phantom taste (tasting of something that is not present). Aliageusia is an unpleasant taste of food or fluids that are normally pleasant.

Aging affects the sensation of taste, and many elderly people have impaired ability to taste, which may affect their appetite and even cause weight loss. Other causes of taste dysfunctions are infections, acid reflux, gastritis, and exposure to chemicals such as mercury, copper, zinc, chromium, and lead. Some medications can affect the ability to taste such as the antibacterial drug ciprofloxacin (Cipro) and some blood pressure and chemotherapy drugs. Lithium can cause dysgeusia. Irradiation in head and neck surgery may impair the ability to taste.

See also APPETITE.

**thrombosis, mesenteric venous** A blood clot in the veins of the intestines, which is the cause of 5 to 15 percent of the incidences of mesenteric ISCHEMIA. This form of thrombosis may be a mild, chronic, or severe acute problem. In the most extreme case, a mesenteric venous thrombosis can cause intestinal gangrene. It can also recur. Mesenteric venous thrombosis may be an acute, subacute, or chronic venous thrombosis.

Sometimes this medical problem is caused by another illness or by a medication or another known cause, and if so, it is said to be secondary mesenteric venous thrombosis. If the cause is unknown, it is deemed to be a primary mesenteric venous thrombosis. A cause can be determined in about 75 to 90 percent of patients who have a mesenteric venous thrombosis.

If the mesenteric venous thrombosis worsens, it can lead to PERITONITIS, a life-threatening condition requiring hospitalization.

Some common causes of a mesenteric venous thrombosis are the following:

- Inherited blood clotting disorders
- Cancer
- Portal hypertension
- Oral contraceptive use

### Symptoms and Signs

Mesenteric venous thrombosis patients may or may not have abdominal pain, depending on the severity and chronicity of their condition. If pain is present, it is usually concentrated in the middle part of the abdomen. Other symptoms and signs which may occur include the following:

- Nausea and vomiting
- Loss of appetite
- Diarrhea
- Presence of either frank or occult blood in the stools

### Diagnosis and Treatment

Laboratory tests and plain X rays do not aid the physician in his or her diagnosis of mesenteric venous thrombosis. Computed tomography (CT) is the preferred test to identify this medical problem; CT scan can accurately pinpoint the presence of mesenteric venous thrombosis in the majority of cases. Angiography may be performed; it also allows for the administration of vasodilator drugs, if needed.

Once the condition has been diagnosed, patients with acute cases may be treated with clot-busting drugs (thrombolytics), followed by anticoagulants such as warfarin (Coumadin). This therapy may last six months or longer or it may be lifelong for some patients, such as those who have an inherited disorder that has led to mesenteric venous thrombosis. Some patients also require surgery, with or without bowel resection, particularly if bowel infarction is suspected or if they have PERITONITIS. The underlying cause of the thrombosis, such as an abdominal infection or cancer, should also be treated. The prognosis is good for most patients, with the exception of those who have cancer.

See also ISCHEMIA.

Kumar, Shaji, M.D., Michael G. Sarr, M.D., and Patrick S. Kamath, M.D. "Mesenteric Venous Thrombosis." *New England Journal of Medicine* 345, no. 23 (December 6, 2001): 1,683–1,688.

**thrush**    A yeast infection that often occurs in the mouth and is more common among infants and small children than in people of other ages. Thrush is common among immune-suppressed individuals, such as acquired immunodeficiency syndrome (AIDS) patients. The chronic use of antibiotics may sometimes cause thrush. Medications such as nystatin can usually clear up minor infections. In more serious cases, stronger drugs like Diflucan may be needed. Some physicians may recommend the use of probiotics.

See also ANTIBIOTICS; *LACTOBACILLUS;* YEAST.

**thyroid disease**    Generally either an excessively low or excessively high level of circulating thyroid hormone, which affects the entire metabolism and directly affects a person's energy level, appetite, mood state, and many other aspects of an individ-

ual's life. However, thyroid disease may be seen in the presence of normal levels of thyroid hormone.

Many thyroid diseases are autoimmune disorders; for example, Hashimoto's thyroiditis is an autoimmune disorder that causes hypothyroidism, and Graves' disease is an autoimmune disorder that causes hyperthyroidism. In both of these diseases, the individual may have a visibly enlarged gland (goiter). However, the symptoms and signs of thyroid disease, especially when it is mild, may not be clearly detectable to the layperson or even to a physician. Instead, abnormal thyroid levels are often found through a blood test of a patient's thyroid stimulating hormone (TSH) level. The TSH is a test often administered as part of a general physical examination for employment, life or disability insurance, or another purpose, such as excluding thyroid disease as a cause of constipation.

Other thyroid diseases include thyroid cancer and thyroid nodules that may be benign or cancerous.

In general, women have a greater risk for development of thyroid diseases than men. Outside the United States and Canada, shortages of iodine in the diet can sometimes cause thyroid disease. Exposure to excessive radiation of the neck or head may also induce thyroid disease.

### Symptoms and Signs
People who are low in thyroid hormone level (hypothyroid) may be sluggish, have a puffy face and dry skin, and become cold (cold intolerance) very readily. They experience constipation and may have unexplained weight gain. In contrast, hyperthyroidism patients are more active, may have diarrhea, and may sometimes even seem manic.

Individuals with hyperthyroidism often experience heat intolerance and heavy sweating, moist skin, and unexplained weight loss despite a normal or even high appetite. Paradoxically, however, some individuals who have hypothyroidism may lose weight and some patients who have hyperthyroidism may gain weight. Symptoms and signs of thyroid disease also vary with age; for example, the symptoms and signs are far more subtle in elderly individuals than they are among younger or middle-aged adults.

## Diagnosis and Treatment

The physician diagnoses thyroid disease on the basis of the patient's symptoms and signs as well as on thyroid hormone blood levels. Thyroid hormone levels are easily tested with the TSH blood test, which has a normal range of about 0.3 to 3.0 mU/l (milliunits per liter) as indicated by 2003 guidelines of the Amercian Academy of Clinical Endocrinologists (AACE).

In this test, *above-normal* blood levels indicate hypothyroidism. (One might think that high levels indicate hyperthyroidism, but the reverse is actually true). Thus, TSH greater than 3.0 indicates hypothyroidism. The higher the value, the more severe the degree of hyperthyroidism; consequently, a level of 10.0 indicates a more severe hypothyroid condition than one of 4.0. Conversely, *below*-normal blood levels, levels less than 0.3, indicate hyperthyroidism.

Low levels of thyroid hormone can be treated with supplemental dosages of thyroid hormone. Usually physicians start a patient at a low dosage of thyroid medication and then retest the patient two to four weeks later to see whether his or her level is in the normal range. If the patient is still hypothyroid, the physician increases the dosage.

If the patient's levels of thyroid hormone are excessively high, physicians may administer medication to decrease the levels. Sometimes radiation is used to destroy the thyroid gland. President George H. W. Bush received radioactive iodine for treatment of his hyperthyroidism. In some cases, a partial thyroidectomy is indicated.

**travel**  Many people experience digestive diseases while away from their home, especially when they travel to other countries, or travelers may be diagnosed with such illnesses after their return home. Most people recover from these illnesses, although some individuals become chronically ill, and others become extremely ill and die.

Diarrhea is the most common form of digestive disease that travelers experience, and it is so common that "traveler's diarrhea" is a universally recognized problem. Interestingly, when people from other countries visit the United States and Canada, they may have diarrhea as well, although to a lesser degree. One underlying problem is the difference in water, and sometimes the difference in food is a factor as well. Another potential problem is that people may be infected by microbes that are unusual in their country of origin and thus have inadequate immunities to these particular germs. Most traveler's diarrhea is short-lived. Medications such as ciprofloxacin (Cipro) help relieve it. Prophylactic antibiotics for travel abroad are not routinely recommended.

Travelers to foreign countries may also be susceptible to infection with viral hepatitis (hepatitis A) caused by conditions of poor sanitation. CHOLERA may also be seen as part of epidemics in overcrowded conditions when the sanitation system breaks down, for example, where there are floods, large fairs, and so forth.

See also CONTAMINATED FOOD OR WATER; DIARRHEA; FOOD-BORNE ILLNESSES; HEPATITIS; PASTEURIZATION.

Ryan, Edward T., M.D., and Kevin C. Kain, M.D. "Health Advice and Immunizations for Travelers." *New England Journal of Medicine* 342, no. 23 (June 8, 2000):1,716–1,725.

Ryan, Edward T., M.D., Mary E. Wison, M.D., and Kevin C. Kain, M.D. "Illness after International Travel." *New England Journal of Medicine* 347, no. 7 (August 15, 2002): 505–516.

**trichinosis**  An infection with *Trichinella* species, the parasite that can be ingested in the cyst form by eating infected uncooked or undercooked pork, sausage, wild game, or other contaminated foods. Several species are recognized to infect humans, and *T. spiralis* is the most common.

In his 2001 article in *Archives of Internal Medicine*, Jan V. Hirschmann speculates that the famous composer Mozart died of a trichinosis infection in 1791. Trichinosis, said Hirschmann, caused death within weeks of infection in past centuries, and caused "fever, rashes, and edema without dyspnea [shortness of breath]. Limb pain and swelling from muscle inflammation and vascular damage are common, prominent findings." According to Hirschmann, Mozart apparently ate pork 44 days before he became ill.

In the United States today, trichinosis is very rare, primarily because of laws on meat packing and food preparation as well as public education on the necessity of cooking meats such as pork. (No one should eat pork as a sushi dish.) According to the Centers for Disease Control and Prevention (CDC), from 1991 to 1996, only about 38 cases of infection occurred each year in the entire country.

### The Course of the Infection

When humans eat infected meat containing the encysted larvae of the worms, the gastric acid and pepsin in the digestive system cause the larvae to be released. They then enter the small intestine and mature into adulthood.

After about a week, the fertilized female worms release their larvae. The adult worms burrow through the intestinal wall and enter the bloodstream. They then spread in the body and attach themselves to the muscles of the host. Sometimes the parasite does not encyst. This is especially likely with *Trichinella pseudospiralis*. During the muscle phase, symptoms include muscle pain, fatigue, and weakness that may last months to years, especially with *T. pseudospiralis*. Other symptoms may include skin rash, cough, shortness of breath, difficulty in swallowing, and headaches.

### Symptoms and Signs of Infection

Trichinosis patients exhibit some symptoms and signs that are common to many other digestive diseases and disorders, including the following:

- Diarrhea
- Nausea and vomiting
- Fatigue
- Fever
- Abdominal pain
- Headaches
- Aching joints
- Pruritus (itching skin)
- Hemorrhages
- Swelling of the eyes
- Muscle pain
- Weakness
- Difficulty in swallowing
- Cough

The abdominal symptoms caused by trichinosis infection usually occur within a day or two after the patient is infected. Other symptoms may appear within two weeks to two months of the time of infection. Some patients have mild symptoms and others are severely ill, depending on the number of worms ingested in the contaminated meat. The heart and brain may also be involved.

### Diagnosis and Treatment

Some patients who have traveled to other countries and eaten uncooked or undercooked meat may contract trichinosis. Physicians should ask patients who have digestive symptoms about their travel to other countries in the past year or so. If the doctor suspects trichinosis, he or she orders laboratory tests; for example, tests reveal an eosinophil count that is high. Serologic tests for antibody levels are reliable, but they may not yield positive findings for at least three weeks after infection. A muscle biopsy is the test of choice for trichinosis.

Most patients have spontaneous resolution of their problems and do not require treatment. For patients who have symptoms, especially symptoms involving the heart, respiratory muscles, or central nervous system, corticosteroids such as prednisone and drugs such as mebendazole or albendazole are generally prescribed.

### Prevention

To prevent potential trichinosis infection, all meat should be thoroughly cooked. Even the meat that is fed to pigs or other animals should be cooked, to prevent contamination from animal to human. Microwaving or marinating infected meat does not kill the worms. Instead, the meat must be cooked until either the meat juices run clear or the internal temperature of the meat is 77°C. Smoking or salting meat does not kill the worms.

See also PARASITIC INFECTIONS.

Hirschmann, Jan V., M.D. "What Killed Mozart?" *Archives of Internal Medicine* 161 (June 11, 2001): 1,381–1,389.

**tropical sprue**   A digestive disorder that is characterized by intestinal abnormalities as well as by a reduction in carbohydrate-digesting enzymes. This causes an impaired carbohydrate digestion plus the malabsorption of all types of nutrients from ingested foods. Tropical sprue affects people who live in Central America, Asia, and the West Indies, as well as travelers to these areas. In most patients, anemia develops as a result of tropical sprue. The cause of tropical sprue is unknown but is presumed to be infectious in origin.

Patients who have tropical sprue have such symptoms as diarrhea, cramps, fatigue, and weight loss. Physicians diagnose tropical sprue on the basis of medical history as well as information about areas where patients have lived or traveled to an endemic area (an area where tropical sprue is known to occur). Rarely, the disease may not manifest for months to years after traveling back from an endemic area. The stools are checked to exclude other infections, such as AMEBIASIS or GIARDIASIS. Laboratory test results show macrocytic anemia. Other illness such as ACQUIRED IMMUNODEFICIENCY SYNDROME should be excluded as the cause of patients' complaints. Although the finding is nonspecific, a small intestinal biopsy is performed to confirm the diagnosis of tropical sprue.

Patients with anemia due to tropical sprue are treated with the administration of vitamin $B_{12}$ and folic acid. Folic acid administration improves most symptoms, although intestinal abnormalities may persist. Prescribing broad-spectrum antibiotics, such as tetracycline taken for three to six months and given in combination with folic acid, is an effective treatment, although 20 percent of patients may experience relapse.

See also CELIAC SPRUE.

**trypsin**   A digestive enzyme that is released in the pancreatic juice and that digests the proteins in food. Serum trypsin levels are elevated in patients who have acute PANCREATITIS; however, the trypsin level is not routinely tested in diagnosing pancreatitis. The immunoreactive trypsin test is used for the diagnosis of cystic fibrosis, in cases when sweat test and genetic test findings are inconclusive. Pancreatic enzyme supplements include trypsin for the treatment of MALABSORPTION SYNDROME caused by PANCREATIC INSUFFICIENCY.

**tuberculosis**   A chronic infection of *Mycobacterium tuberculosis* that has seen a resurgence in recent years in the United States and in other countries, particularly among some groups of institutionalized people, such as elderly adults who live in nursing homes. Tuberculosis is a serious public health problem. According to the Centers for Disease Control and Prevention (CDC) there were 16,337 cases of tuberculosis diagnosed in the United States in 2000. In the United States, about half of all new cases of tuberculosis are diagnosed among people who were born in other countries.

Tuberculosis kills nearly 2 million per year worldwide, making it the second leading cause of death that resulted from infection, just after the human immunodeficiency virus (HIV). An estimated 1.7 billion people in the world are believed to be infected with tuberculosis.

An airborne disease, tuberculosis (TB) is contracted by contact with people who have active symptoms, especially coughing and sneezing. A chance encounter with a person who has TB is unlikely to cause tuberculosis; however, frequent contacts, such as the contacts that family members or hospital workers experience, significantly raise the risk of contracting tuberculosis.

Most people with tuberculosis have an inactive form of the disease, and only an estimated one in 10 patients infected with tuberculosis has an active and symptomatic form of the disease. As a result, many people who have tuberculosis never know that they have it, unless they are tested for it.

### Risk Factors

The World Health Organization reports that globally more men contract tuberculosis than women, although it is a severe disease for both genders. According to the National Institute of Allergy and Infectious Diseases in the United Sates, tuberculosis is a worse problem among some racial groups in the United States; for example, 54 percent of the active cases of tuberculosis in 1999 were among blacks and Hispanics and 20 percent of active cases were among Asians.

People who have been recently exposed to tuberculosis, as well as other groups, including the following, are at risk and should be tested for tuberculosis:

- Employees of health care facilities that treat tuberculosis patients
- Immigrants from countries with a high rate of tuberculosis
- People who have HIV
- People who have kidney failure
- Patients on immunosuppressive therapy
- Patients who are malnourished

### Symptoms of Tuberculosis

People who have an active form of tuberculosis may have a chronic cough and may cough up blood. In addition, they may be fatigued, lose their appetite, and lose weight. They may also experience night sweats and fevers. Many patients, especially those who are in the early stages of the disease or have an inactive form of TB, have no symptoms at all.

Digestive involvement in tuberculosis may take the form of tuberculous peritonitis, ileocecal tuberculosis, or tuberculosis of the lymph nodes in the abdomen that surround the gut.

### Testing for TB

A skin test, the purified protein derivative (PPD) test, is usually used to check for tuberculosis and evaluated 48 to 72 hours later. It is a screening test that yields both false positive and false negative findings.

To determine whether a patient actually has tuberculosis, a chest X ray is needed, along with a complete medical history. Serial sputum examinations are done to check for tuberculosis involving the lungs. In patients who have tuberculosis that involves the digestive system, the chest X ray and sputum tests may have negative results.

### Tuberculosis in Children

According to S. Jody Heymann and colleagues in a 2000 article in *Pediatrics*, programs to control tuberculosis have not worked as well among populations of children as among adults. The assumption has been that treating adults would benefit children. But infected children themselves need treatment. In addition, some children face high risks of development of TB, such as children infected with HIV or children in the United States born to parents from other countries. They also argue that treatment of infected children offers major advantages: "A 5% increase in the number of children who enter treatment leads to a 25% decline in the number of TB cases among children and a 16% decline in the number of TB deaths after 10 years."

### Treatment of Tuberculosis

If the patient's TB skin test result is positive, but active TB is not confirmed, patients may be given preventive medications to lower the risk of tuberculosis. These patients are treated with the drug isoniazid for six to nine months. Unfortunately, hepatitis is a common side effect of this drug, and the risk increases with age. Patients taking isoniazid must also completely abstain from using all alcohol, to prevent damage to the liver.

Patients who have active TB take a combination of three to four medications, such as isoniazid, rifampin, pyrazinamide, and ethambutol.

If the tuberculosis is drug resistant, then the physician may treat the patient with a four-drug combination.

One problem with treating tuberculosis is that patients may be resistant to taking medication, in part because of potential side effects. Some public health departments provide the medication and watch the patient take the drug to make sure it is taken.

Acquired immunodeficiency syndrome (AIDS) patients can contract an opportunistic form of tuberculosis caused by *Mycobacterium avium intracellulare* (MAI), which can be widespread in the body, including in the liver. Treatment of MAI is unsatisfactory.

For further information, contact the following organization:

National Institute of Allergy and Infectious
   Diseases
Building 31, Room 7A-50
31 Center Drives MSC 2520
Bethesda, MD 20892
http://www.niaid.nih.gov

Heymann, S. Jody, M.D., et al. "Pediatric Tuberculosis: What Needs to Be Done to Decrease Morbidity and Mortality." *Pediatrics* 106, no. 1 (July 2000): 1

Jasmer, Robert M., M.D., Payam Nahid, M.D., and Philip C. Hopewell, M.D. "Latent Tuberculosis Infection." *New England Journal of Medicine* 347, no. 23 (December 5, 2002): 1,860–1,866.

Khan, Kamran, M.D., et al. "Global Drug-Resistance Patterns and the Management of Latent Tuberculosis Infection in Immigrants to the United States." *New England Journal of Medicine* 347, no. 23 (December 5, 2002): 1,850–1,859.

Schaaf, H. Simon, et al. "Evaluation of Young Children in Contact with Adult Multidrug-Resistant Pulmonary Tuberculosis: A 30-Month Follow-Up." *Pediatrics* 109, no. 5 (May 2002): 765–771.

Small, Peter M., M.D., and Paula I. Fujiwara, M.D. "Management of Tuberculosis in the United States." *New England Journal of Medicine* 345, no. 3 (July 19, 2001): 189–200.

**ulcerative colitis**   A chronic disease that causes sores and inflammation of the colon. Ulcerative colitis is one of the two medical problems that constitute inflammatory bowel disease (IBD); the other is Crohn's disease. (Patients must have only one of these diseases to have IBD. Both do not occur simultaneously although the type of IBD may be indeterminate in 10 to 15 percent of the cases.)

The inflammation in the rectum/colon causes it to bleed and to empty frequently; bowel movements are more frequent than is normal and are usually loose, bloody stools.

The cause of ulcerative colitis is unknown; it may be linked to an immune system abnormality. It is not caused by a food allergy or sensitivity, although foods may trigger symptoms. Stress does not cause ulcerative colitis but may worsen the symptoms of the condition.

Ulcerative colitis increases the risk for development of colorectal cancer, and as a result, patients who have long-standing disease need periodic colonoscopy to look for any early signs of cancer. The frequency of the colonoscopy is determined by the patient's physician but may be every one to two years or more often.

### Risk Factors

People of any age can have ulcerative colitis, but the illness is more commonly found among people between the ages of 15 and 40. According to the National Institutes of Health, both men and women can have ulcerative colitis. One study, reported in a 2001 issue of the *New England Journal of Medicine,* found that people who had appendectomy before age 20 had a significantly reduced risk of later development of ulcerative colitis; the reason for the reduced risk is not known. Several other studies, including one by Minocha (1997), have shown similar results in the United States.

### Symptoms and Signs

Most patients have bloody diarrhea and abdominal pain, often on the left side. Other signs and symptoms that may occur are as follows:

- Loss of appetite and unintended weight loss
- Fatigue
- Fecal incontinence (accidents)
- Rectal bleeding
- Loss of nutrients and body fluids
- Constipation instead of diarrhea among patients who have PROCTITIS only

Ulcerative colitis may cause or be associated with other medical problems, such as arthritis, liver disease, osteoporosis (low bone density), ANEMIA, PRIMARY SCLEROSING CHOLANGITIS, and pyoderma gangrenosum.

### Diagnosis and Treatment

The physician takes a complete medical history and performs a physical examination. Laboratory tests such as complete blood count are frequently ordered to test for anemia or for a high white blood cell count indicating infection and/or inflammation.

The doctor also frequently orders testing of a stool sample, particularly for bloody diarrhea, in order to rule out infection as the cause of the diarrhea. In addition, a colonoscopy with biopsy is required to establish a diagnosis, so that a visual inspection of the colon can be made and the doctor can check for ulcers or inflammation.

Some patients have relatively mild symptoms, whereas ulcerative colitis is a severe and disabling condition for others. Some patients experience spontaneous (even without medications) remission of ulcerative colitis for periods lasting months or years, although no one knows why the disease eventually recurs.

Ulcerative colitis is different from Crohn's disease, but differentiating them in a patient can be difficult in about 15 percent of the cases; such cases are labeled indeterminate colitis. The perinuclear antineutrophil cytoplasmic antibody (pANCA) is seen in about two-thirds of patients with ulcerative colitis and about 10 to 20 percent of patients with Crohn's disease. In contrast, the anti-*Saccharomyces cereviciae* antibody (ASCA) is positive in about two-thirds of patients with Crohn's disease and about 10 percent of patients with ulcerative colitis. Using the two tests in combination may distinguish ulcerative colitis from Crohn's disease in patients with indeterminate colitis.

In general, according to Ghosh and colleagues in 2000 in *British Medical Journal,* ulcerative colitis patients are not smokers (or are former smokers), whereas Crohn's disease patients usually smoke. Ulcerative colitis patients usually do not have osteopenia (low bone density) when they are diagnosed, in contrast to patients who have Crohn's disease. In ulcerative colitis, the problem is usually restricted to the colon; in Crohn's disease, any part of the entire gut (the esophagus, the stomach, the small intestine, the colon, rectum and anal canal) may be affected.

There are other differences: ulcerative colitis patients usually do not have strictures or fistulas in the bowel and granulomas on biopsy and their presence suggests the diagnosis of Crohn's disease. The rectum is almost always involved in ulcerative colitis (95 percent of the cases) but is rarely involved in Crohn's disease (5 percent of cases).

Antibiotics usually do not help patients who have ulcerative colitis, although they may improve the condition of patients who have Crohn's disease. Ulcerative colitis patients are cured of illness by surgery to remove the colon and rectum, whereas Crohn's disease frequently recurs after surgery.

**Lifestyle changes** Physicians may ask people who have ulcerative colitis to keep a food diary to help determine whether particular foods trigger a worsening of the illness. For many people with ulcerative colitis, spicy foods or the lactose in milk can exacerbate illness; other foods may be the cause for others. If specific foods that aggravate the condition can be identified, patients can actively avoid them.

Some patients may need psychological support, including from mental health professionals, because the disease may seem to overpower their life. Patients who seek help from mental health professionals should be sure to work only with psychologists or psychiatrists who understand the medical aspect of ulcerative colitis and recognize that although stress can make the condition worse, it does not cause it. Thus, psychological counseling alone cannot cure ulcerative colitis, although it may help patients to learn to accept their condition and deal better with stress.

Interestingly, however, in the cotton top tamarin monkey, an animal model of ulcerative colitis, colitis rarely occurs when the animal lives freely in the jungle, and in most cases occurs in animals that are in captivity. The stress of captivity may be involved.

**Medications can help** Many ulcerative colitis patients are treated with drugs such as sulfasalazine (Azulfidine) which combines a sulfonamide (sulfapyridine) and aminosalicylate (ASA). Other patients are given drugs in the form of 5-aminosalicylic acid (5-ASA) without the sulfonamide (mesalamine [Asacol or Pentasa]). Some patients are treated with corticosteroids, such as prednisone or hydrocortisone, which may be given as a pill, intravenously or in an enema. Doctors may hesitate to prescribe corticosteroids for an extended period because of the many side effects they can cause, such as hypertension, increase of facial hair, change in body shape and structure, osteoporosis, weight gain, and mood swings.

**Surgery sometimes is necessary** If ulcerative colitis is very severe, causing severe bleeding and/or extreme weight loss, physicians may decide that the best treatment for an individual patient is surgical removal of the colon and rectum in order to achieve a cure. According to the National Institutes of Health, up to 40 percent of all patients with ulcerative colitis eventually need surgery because of severe bleeding, colonic rupture, or other serious conditions caused by the disorder. A colectomy is also performed if cancer or a precancerous lesion is found during a colonoscopy.

The surgery requires the creation of a stoma, an opening to the outside, through which the fecal contents pass into a pouch that the patient empties regularly. Presently, many surgeons create a reservoir (artificial rectum) from the small intestine and hook it up to the anal canal so that the patient can have continued bowel movements instead of an ileostomy.

For further information on ulcerative colitis, contact the following organizations:

Crohn's and Colitis Foundation of America
386 Park Avenue South
New York, NY 10016
(800) 932-2423 (toll-free) or (212) 685-3440
http://www.ccfa.org

National Digestive Diseases Information
   Clearinghouse
National Institutes of Health
9000 Rockville Pike
Bethesda, MD 20892
(800) 891-5389 (toll-free) or (301) 654-3810
http://www.niddk.nih.gov

United Ostomy Association, Inc.
19772 MacArthur Boulevard
Suite 200
Irvine, CA 92612
(800) 826-0826 (toll-free) or (949) 660-8624
http://www.uoa.org

See also APPENDICITIS; CANCER, COLORECTAL; COLITIS; COLONOSCOPY; CROHN'S DISEASE; ERYTHEMA NODOSUM; FISH OIL; INFLAMMATORY BOWEL DISEASE; PROCTITIS.

Andersson, Roland E., M.D. et al. "Appendectomy and Protection against Ulcerative Colitis." *New England Journal of Medicine* 344, no. 11 (March 15, 2001): 808–814.
Ghosh, Subrata, Alan Shand, and Anne Ferguson. "Ulcerative Colitis." *British Medical Journal* 320 (April 22, 2000): 1,119–1,123.
Minocha, Anil, and C. A. Raczkowski. "Role of Appendectomy and Tonsillectomy in Pathogenesis of Ulcerative Colitis." *Digestive Disease Sciences* 42 (1997): 1,567–1,569.

**ulcer, peptic**   A break of the lining of the stomach or duodenum that causes mild, moderate, or severe pain. Some ulcers are painless, especially among patients who are taking nonsteroidal anti-inflammatory drugs (NSAIDs) or steroids. An ulcer may occur in the stomach (gastric ulcer) or the duodenum (duodenal ulcer). According to statistics released by the National Center for Health Statistics in 2002, as of 1997, 9 percent of all adults in the United States older than age 18, or about 17.7 million Americans, will be diagnosed with a peptic ulcer at some point in time.

If an ulcer becomes very severe, it can produce bleeding, and ulcers constitute about 50 percent of all the causes of cases of upper gastrointestinal bleeding. In addition to causing possibly life-threatening bleeding in the most extreme case, an ulcer can be life-threatening when it is perforated and food, acid and bacteria from the stomach or duodenum are spilled into the peritoneum. Patients who have perforation need both emergency hospitalization and surgery.

According to the National Institute on Diabetes and Digestive and Kidney Diseases (NIDDK) in the United States, about 40,000 people in the United States have surgery for problems caused by ulcer. The NIDDK also reports that about 6,000 people die each year in the United States of complications related to the presence of an ulcer.

### Causes of Ulcers

Most peptic ulcers (about 60 to 90 percent) are caused by *Helicobacter pylori* bacteria; some ulcers are caused by medications, particularly NSAIDs given to treat arthritis and other chronic ailments. *H. pylori* is seen more often with duodenal ulcers than with gastric ulcers. Complicated ulcers (with bleeding and perforation) are more likely to be caused by NSAIDs.

For about a century and until the early 1990s, most physicians throughout the world believed that ulcers were caused by increased acid, stress or diet and, consequently, urged patients to relax and prevent stress and/or to change their diet. In 1982, the Australian physicians Marshall and Warren insisted that *H. pylori* was the cause of most cases of gastritis and ulcers. They were ridiculed for years and finally proved right. The presence of HP results in production of increased gastric acid in patients with duodenal ulcers. Paradoxically, in some cases HP may cause decreased gastric acidity.

*Age may matter* Some studies have shown that when only the population of patients who are age 65 and older are considered, medications are responsible for up to 50 percent of peptic ulcers. In one study, reported in a 2001 issue of the *Journal of the American Medical Association,* when elderly patients were screened for *H. pylori* and if positive, treated, there was no reduction in the rate of repeat hospitalizations for ulcers. In contrast, patients who took NSAIDs and were counseled that the drugs could cause ulcers *did* have a decreased subsequent rate of hospitalization. The researchers concluded that NSAIDs play a large role in the development of peptic ulcers among older individuals.

*Effects of stress are present* Stress, although it does not cause ulcer, may worsen the symptoms of an existing ulcer. Smoking also exacerbates ulcer symptoms.

Some physicians point out that in some extreme cases of stress, such as in war, earthquake, or another severe event, the event has been followed by an increase in the incidence of peptic ulcers in the population affected by the event. Physicians emphasize that although stress does not usually cause ulcers, stress may cause or exacerbate ulcer symptoms in some cases. In fact, hypnotherapy has been shown to be an effective remedy in the prevention of relapse of peptic ulcer disease, although it is not widely accepted or recommended.

*Other diseases can increase the risk for ulcers* It is also true that some illnesses, such as ZOLLINGER–ELLISON SYNDROME, may cause ulcers among some patients who are diagnosed with this disease.

### Risk Factors

Some studies have shown a higher incidence of ulcers among men; for example, in the Finnish Twin Cohort, which studied thousands of twins who were born before 1958, the incidence of ulcers was 6.2 percent among men and only 2.8 percent among women. However, other studies have indicated virtually no gender difference in individuals who are at risk for development of peptic ulcers. The Finnish Twin Cohort study also found other factors among patients that increased their risk for development of ulcers, including high stress, as well as smoking among men and long-term use of analgesics (painkillers) among women.

In the United States, as indicated by information provided in 2002 by the National Center for Health Statistics for 1997, the numbers of men and women with peptic or stomach ulcers are nearly equal: 8,882,000 males and 8,816,000 females. However, considering the percentage of population alone, in the United States men are slightly more likely to have ulcers than women: 9.5 percent of males age 18 and above had ulcer in 1997 compared to 8.7 percent of women.

Older people have a greater risk of development of ulcers than younger people. According to National Center for Health Statistics data, 14.1 percent of people ages 65 to 74 years had ulcer and the percentage of ulcer incidence increased slightly to 14.4 percent of those 75 and older. In contrast, only about 6 percent of individuals 18 to 44 years had ulcer. Middle-aged people faced an increased risk: 11.5 percent of individuals in this group have ulcer.

In considering race and ethnicity, whites represent the largest percentage of people with ulcer, or 9.8 percent, compared to 8.4 percent of blacks and only 5.8 percent of Hispanics. The reasons for these racial and ethnic differences are unknown.

Looking at different geographic locations in the United States, the largest percentage of people who have ulcer are located in the South: 10.5 percent of adults. The smallest percentage of people who have ulcer are found in the Northeast: 7.1 percent. The reasons for these differing percentages are unknown.

### Symptoms and Signs of Ulcers

The key symptom of an ulcer is pain in the upper abdominal area, which is often said to be gnawing pain. Other indicators of a peptic ulcer are as follows:

- Nausea and/or vomiting
- Loss of appetite
- Unintended weight loss
- Upper abdominal pain that occurs two to three hours after eating a meal when the stomach is empty, in the case of duodenal ulcer
- Upper abdominal pain that occurs in the night, when the stomach is empty, in the case of a duodenal ulcer
- Upper abdominal pain that occurs shortly after eating, causing a fear of eating, as found with a gastric ulcer
- Pain that is relieved by eating and/or by use of antacids

Patients who experience gastrointestinal bleeding may feel weak and lethargic and sometimes may even pass out. If gastrointestinal bleeding is severe, blood may appear in the patient's vomit or stools. Patients may bleed without a prior history of any significant abdominal pain or discomfort.

It is also true that ulcers may be totally silent. In addition, the predictability of whether a person has an ulcer on solely clinical grounds is poor.

**Emergency symptoms** Some symptoms and signs are emergency indicators that the patient needs to see a physician as soon as possible, without delay. The reason for the urgency is that these symptoms may indicate perforation, bleeding, or an obstruction of the stomach. These symptoms include the following:

- Black, tarry stools
- Sudden sharp and persistent pain in the stomach that is worse with movement
- Vomit that includes blood or has a coffee grounds appearance
- Weakness and dizziness
- Persistent vomiting, especially vomiting of undigested food ingested several hours or a day earlier
- Weight loss

### Refractory ulcers

Some patients have ulcer that is not responsive to the usual treatments. A study of risk factors associated with refractory peptic ulcers (ulcers resistant to treatment) was reported in 1995 in *Gastroenterology*. The researchers found that the risk factors for refractory ulcers included an earlier onset of development of ulcer, a longer history of symptoms caused by the ulcer, and more frequent incidences of relapses from the ulcer. In addition, the patients who had a refractory ulcer were more likely to smoke during the refractory period, and presumably the smoking caused an impairment of the healing process.

About 40 percent of the patients were abusing nonsteroidal anti-inflammatory drugs (NSAIDs) or analgesics: this one factor alone accounted for the greatest risk for development of a refractory ulcer.

### Diagnosis and Treatment

An ulcer is diagnosed on the basis of a patient's symptoms and the findings of the physical examination, along with the results of such tests as an upper gastrointestinal series (barium X ray) and/or an esophagogastroduodenoscopy (EGD). Clinically distinguishing gastric from duodenal ulcer often yields an inaccurate diagnosis. In addition, less than 25 percent of patients who have classic symptoms of ulcer disease are found to have an ulcer when they have endoscopy (EGD) or upper gastrointestinal X ray.

If an ulcer is seen on an upper gastrointestinal barium X ray, doctors may still use EGD, especially in the case of gastric ulcer, in order to take a biopsy specimen during the procedure, in order to make sure that there is no cancer. In some cases, as of obstruction or perforation, a computed tomography (CT) scan or magnetic resonance imaging (MRI) scan may be indicated.

Once an ulcer has been identified, the patient is usually given acid blocking medications so that the damaged tissue can have a chance to heal. Common histamine-2 blockers include cimetidine (Tagamet), ranitidine (Zantac), famotidine (Pepcid), and nizatidine (Axid). Common proton pump inhibitors (PPIs) that physicians may prescribe include omeprazole (Prilosec), pantoprazole (Protonix), rabeprazole (Aciphex), lansoprazole

(Prevacid), and esomeprazole (Nexium). Some physicians also treat their peptic ulcer patients with mucosal protective drugs such as sucralfate (Carafate), which are as effective as H-2 blockers. PPIs are superior to H2 blockers in their efficacy.

Rarely, ulcer patients require surgery, particularly in cases of complicated ulcers (with perforation, obstruction, and bleeding) and of ulcers that are refractory (do not respond) to medical treatment.

**When H. pylori *may be causing the ulcer***
When a patient is found to have an ulcer through EGD or physicians suspect that *H. pylori* is causing the ulcerlike symptoms, they can test for *H. pylori* with BREATH TESTS, a stool test, or blood tests. Doctors can also take tissue samples during an endoscopy to test for the presence of *H. pylori*. If tests identify that *H. pylori* is present, then physicians use antibiotic treatment to eradicate the bacteria. *H. pylori* is a very resistant organism, and multiple antibiotics are required.

Usually a three-drug regimen for two weeks is recommended to eradicate *H. pylori*. Most medication regimens have either metronidazole (Flagyl) or clarithromycin (Biaxin) or both. "Dosepaks" such as Prevpac and Helidac enhance compliance. (A dosepak includes two or more medications in one package, with days and times marked appropriately and in order, to help patients remember to take all their medicine.) PPIs also have actions against *H. pylori* and are part of many regimens, including Prevpac.

**When NSAIDs *may be the cause***   When physicians know that patients are taking nonsteroidal anti-inflammatory drugs (NSAIDs) for medical problems, they may assume that an ulcer was caused by the NSAID and treat the patient accordingly. In addition to prescribing acid blocking medication to heal the ulcer, they may choose to reduce the dosage of the NSAID or try another medication like a COX-2 inhibitor that is less harmful to the stomach and/or the duodenum. The risks of NSAIDs causing a bleeding peptic ulcer increases with the use of corticosteroids or anticoagulants, a history of peptic disease, and older age.

Another course of action is to continue the NSAID and at the same time prescribe preventive antiulcer medications for those who are at risk for development of ulcers. In research reported in 2002 in the *Archives of Internal Medicine,* the researchers studied 537 patients who did not have *H. pylori* but were long-term NSAID users and also had peptic ulcers in the past, as verified through endoscopies. The patients took their NSAID medication. One group of subjects were given misoprostol four times a day. Another group was given 15 mg of lansoprazole (Prevacid), a proton pump inhibitor medication, once a day, and a third group was given a higher dosage of lansoprazole (30 mg). The fourth group was given a placebo (no medication). The subjects were later evaluated on whether an ulcer developed after eight weeks and after 12 weeks.

The researchers found that the patients who took the misoprostol had the lowest incidence of ulcers (93 percent), followed by those who took proton pump inhibitors. In contrast, 82 percent of the patients taking 30 mg of lansoprazole were ulcer-free and 80 percent of those taking 15 mg of lansoprazole had no ulcer at the end of the study. Among the placebo group, 51 percent were ulcer-free; thus, in almost half of the patients ulcers developed.

It would initially seem evident that misoprostol is the best ulcer preventive. However, misoprostol has many side effects, such as abdominal pain and diarrhea, and thus, there is less compliance in using medication among patients; for example, more than 90 percent of those in the placebo group and the lansoprazole group took their medication as directed, compared to only 73 percent of patients in the misoprostol group. When those factors were considered, misoprostol and the proton pump inhibitor performed about the same in preventing the development of ulcers.

**Considering *cyclooxygenase-2 (COX-2) inhibitors***
Another class of anti-inflammatory medication are the COX-2 inhibitors, which include medications such as rofecoxib (Vioxx). Rofecoxib has been tested to determine whether it is less likely to cause peptic ulcers than NSAIDs among patients who need to reduce the inflammation of arthritis. According to information reported in 1999 in the *Journal of the American Medical Association,* arthritis patients who were treated with rofecoxib had a significantly lower risk of development of peptic

ulcers than patients taking the classic NSAIDs such as ibuprofen, diclofenac, or nabumetone. (However, the risk is not 0, and some patients have ulcers when taking COX-2 inhibitor medications.) Valdecoxib (Bextra) is another COX-2 inhibitor that is prescribed by physicians.

It should be noted that if patients have bleeding ulcer caused by NSAIDs, the medication is usually stopped immediately. In fact, it is best that such patients stop taking NSAIDs permanently. Alternatively, if they must continue to take an NSAID, they are preferably treated with COX-2 inhibitors and/or have adjunctive treatment with misoprostol or a PPI medication.

***If surgery is needed*** Sometimes the ulcer is so severe (refractory or complicated) that surgery must be performed. The type of surgery depends upon the nature of the problem, for example, whether it is bleeding, perforation, or obstruction or a medically refractory ulcer. Surgeons may perform a VAGOTOMY, in which the vagus nerve is severed to reduce acid secretion. In other cases, surgeons may need to perform an antrectomy of the last part of the stomach that is involved in acid secretion.

A third type of surgery that may be performed is the pyloroplasty, which enables the surgeon to dilate the opening to the small intestine. Gastrojejunostomy, hooking up of the stomach through a new surgically created opening to the distant part of the small bowel (the jejunum), is also frequently performed. The operation to treat the ulcer frequently involves various combinations of the aforementioned surgical techniques.

See also CANCER, STOMACH; BLEEDING, GASTROINTESTINAL; GASTRECTOMY; GASTRITIS; *HELICOBACTER PYLORI*; HISTAMINE-2 INHIBITORS; MULTIPLE ENDOCRINE NEOPLASIA (MEN); NONSTEROIDAL ANTI-INFLAMMATORY DRUGS; PANCREATITIS; PROTON PUMP INHIBITORS; VAGOTOMY.

Blackwell, D. L., J. G. Collins, and R. Coles. "Summary Health Statistics for U.S. Adults: National Health Interview Survey, 1997." National Center for Health Statistics. *Vital Health Statistics* 10, no. 205, (2002).

Brock, Jane, M.D., M.S.P.H. "Process of Care and Outcomes for Elderly Patients Hospitalized with Peptic Ulcer Disease: Results from a Quality Improvement Project." *Journal of the American Medical Association* 286, no. 16 (October 24/31, 2001): 1,985–1,993.

Colgan, S. M., E. B. Faragher, and P. J. Whorwell. "Controlled Trial of Hypnotherapy in Relapse Prevention of Duodenal Ulceration." *Lancet* (June 11, 1988): 1,299–1,300.

El-Serag, Hashem B., M.D., et al. "Prevention of Complicated Ulcer Disease among Chronic Users of Nonsteroidal Anti-inflammatory Drugs: The Use of a Nomogram in Cost-Effectiveness Analysis." *Archives of Internal Medicine* 162 (October 14, 2002): 2,105–2,110.

Graham, David Y., M.D., et al. "Ulcer Prevention in Long-Term Users of Nonsteroidal Anti-inflammatory Drugs." *Archives of Internal Medicine* 162 (January 28, 2002): 169–175.

Laine, Loren, and Walter L. Peterson. "Bleeding Peptic Ulcer." *New England Journal of Medicine* 331, no. 11 (September 15, 1994): 717–727.

Lanas, A. I., et al. "Risk Factors Associated with Refractory Peptic Ulcers." *Gastroenterology* 109, no. 4 (1995): 1,124–1,133.

Langman, Michael J., M.D. "Adverse Upper Gastrointestinal Effects of Rofecoxib Compared with NSAIDs." *Journal of the American Medical Association* 282, no. 20 (November 24, 1999): 1,929–1,933.

Levenstein, Susan, M.D., et al. "Stress and Peptic Ulcer Disease." *Journal of the American Medical Association* 281, no. 1 (January 6, 1999): 10–11.

Minocha, Anil, M.D., and Christine Adamec. *How to Stop Heartburn: Simple Ways to Heal Heartburn and Acid Reflux.* New York: John Wiley & Sons, 2001.

Räihä, Ismo, M.D., et al. "Lifestyle, Stress, and Genes in Peptic Ulcer Disease: A Nationwide Twin Cohort Study." *Archives of Internal Medicine* 158 (April 13, 1998): 698–704.

**ultrasound** An imaging procedure that uses sound waves to provide a view of internal organs. The procedure may be performed from outside the body, by touching a sensor to the body, or the sensor may be attached to a scope, such as an endoscope, to provide an internal view.

Ultrasound is used to diagnose inflammation, cancer spread, or other abnormalities of the digestive organs, such as the liver, pancreas, gallbladder, and stomach, as well as other abdominal organs, such as the ovaries and the uterus. It may also be used with procedures that are performed by gastroenterologists or surgeons, such as the endoscopic ultrasound, wherein the ultrasound sensor is attached to the endoscope, which is then passed into the digestive tract, for example, into the stomach or the rectum, and images are then obtained from a closer distance. While an ultrasound from outside the body is risk-free, the endoscopic ultrasound is associated with significant risk for complications.

Ultrasound is also used to monitor the fetus during pregnancy and to check the heart and blood vessels.

See also IMAGING TESTS.

**upper gastrointestinal X ray**    A common diagnostic procedure in which the esophagus, stomach, and duodenum are all imaged after a person drinks contrast dye (such as barium) so that a physician can detect medical problems such as ULCERS, STRICTURE, CANCER, and other diseases and conditions.

**vagotomy**   A procedure that cuts the vagus nerve, which partly controls the production of stomach acid. This surgery causes the stomach to produce less acid. The procedure is used in surgical treatment of ulcers. Vagotomy may result in disordered stomach emptying of food.

See also ULCERS, PEPTIC.

**vasculitis, small vessel**   Inflammation of the blood vessel walls, a condition that can lead to a variety of illnesses in various parts of the body, including the digestive system. Vasculitis may cause a decreased blood supply to the intestines, resulting in abdominal pain and a lack of appetite.

Various forms of vasculitis are recognized. CHURG–STRAUSS SYNDROME is a form of small-vessel vasculitis first described in 1951. Mixed CRYOGLOBU-LINEMIA is another example of small-vessel vasculitis.

Medications may cause vasculitis, particularly drugs such as penicillamine, hydralazine, quinolones, minocycline and sulfonamides.

In the early stages of vasculitis, patients may experience flulike symptoms of aches and pains in their joints and fever. Different vessels may be affected, including vessels in the gut, the kidneys, and the respiratory tract. Patients may also have skin lesions and nodules.

Jennette, J. Charles, M.D., and Ronald J. Falk, M.D. "Small-Vessel Vasculitis." *New England Journal of Medicine* 337, no. 21 (November 20, 1997): 1,512–1,523.

**vitamin deficiencies/excesses**   An imbalance of levels of vitamins in the body, including a lack of needed vitamins as well as an excessive or even toxic level of vitamins (hypervitaminosis).

### Vitamin A and Carotenoids

Vitamin A affects vision. It also helps the body to maintain the lining of the intestinal tract, the eyes, the urinary tract, and the respiratory tract. In addition, vitamin A is involved in the immune system in fighting off infections. Carotenoids are provitamins that are easily converted to vitamin A. Although there are numerous carotenoids, beta-carotene is the most active and many others serve as antioxidants. Foods that contain vitamin A or provitamin A carotenoids include eggs, whole milk, liver, cheddar cheese, carrots, green vegetables, and orange fruits. Many prepared foods are also fortified with vitamin A.

*Deficiencies of vitamin A*   Few people in the United States have a deficiency of vitamin A, but many children in poor countries suffer from dietary deprivation and lack a sufficient store of vitamin A; that lack can cause blindness. In the United States, night blindness is an early indicator of a deficiency of vitamin A. Sometimes vitamin A deficiency can develop as a result of celiac sprue, cystic fibrosis, and intestinal infections.

Alcoholism can cause vitamin A deficiency, and vegetarians who do not eat eggs or dairy products may experience vitamin A deficiency. Deficiencies in vitamin A translate into difficulty in fighting infection.

Some doctors in the United States are concerned by subclinical (slightly low, so that patients do not have symptoms) levels of vitamins, especially among growing children. Children at particular risk for subclinically low levels of vitamin A include the following groups:

- Poor children, including those living at or below the poverty level

- Children who have immigrated from countries where there are known deficiencies of vitamin A
- Children who have been diagnosed with disease of the liver, pancreas, or intestines
- Children who have difficulty in digesting or absorbing fat
- Children who have received inadequate health care

*Hypervitaminosis vitamin A*   It is also possible to have too much vitamin A, and excessive levels of vitamin A can cause increased pressure in the brain, vomiting, and yellowing of skin. Babies born to pregnant women who have overly high levels of vitamin A can have birth defects.

Hypervitaminosis vitamin A can occur in a short period (days) if a person ingests an excessive amount of this vitamin. The key signs of toxic levels of vitamin A include the following:

- Headache
- Weakness
- Joint pains
- Nausea and vomiting
- Blurred vision
- Poor muscle coordination

Because these signs and symptoms are also characteristic of many other diseases, the physician must obtain a complete medical history. Patients should cooperate by reporting all drugs that they take, especially over-the-counter vitamins or herbal preparations.

### Vitamin B$_6$

The human body needs vitamin B$_6$ for a variety of functions, including maintaining red blood cells, assisting function of both the immune system and the nervous system, and converting tryptophan (a natural amino acid) into serotonin. It is also needed to maintain normal blood sugar (glucose) levels. Vitamin B$_6$ is used as a treatment for the nausea and vomiting of pregnancy.

Vitamin B$_6$ is found in beans, cereals, fish, meats, poultry, and some fruits and vegetables. Good sources of vitamin B$_6$ are potatoes, bananas, chicken breast, lean pork loin, cooked rainbow trout, sunflower seeds, canned tuna, avocado, creamy peanut butter, and lima beans.

*Deficiencies of vitamin B$_6$*   Most people in the United States and other developed countries are not deficient in vitamin B$_6$. However, some older individuals, particularly those age 65 and older, may have low levels of this vitamin, primarily because of poor diet. Individuals at risk include those who have malabsorption syndrome, alcoholics, and women who are using oral contraceptives.

Physical indicators of a deficiency of vitamin B$_6$ include the following signs and symptoms:

- Sore tongue (glossitis)
- Skin inflammation (dermatitis)
- Depression
- Confusion
- Convulsions
- Anemia

Because these signs can indicate many other medical problems, patients must be evaluated by their physician. If a deficiency is diagnosed, individuals may be given supplements.

*Vitamin B$_6$ hypervitaminosis*   It is also possible to have excessive levels of vitamin B$_6$. The recommended daily allowance (RDA) of vitamin B$_6$ is 2 mg/day for adult males and 1.6 mg/day for adult females. Adults should avoid taking more than 100 mg of this vitamin per day. Toxicity occurs when doses of 250 mg per day or more are taken for several months, and can cause patients to suffer dizziness and nerve damage, creating problems related to walking and various sensations of touch, pain, and temperature. Most patients who are taking supplemental vitamin B$_6$ improve, but may not recover completely, when they stop using it.

In the past, some health books have recommended that people who have carpal tunnel syndrome take supplements of vitamin B$_6$. Data related to whether vitamin B$_6$ can help improve carpal tunnel syndrome or asthma are controversial, and some individuals have experienced nerve damage (neuropathy) after taking high doses of this vitamin.

Some women who have premenstrual syndrome have taken vitamin $B_6$ to alleviate symptoms, but there is limited clinical evidence that this vitamin improves symptoms, particularly among patients who have depression. There is evidence that high doses are toxic to women who have taken the vitamin for this purpose.

### Vitamin $B_{12}$

Vitamin $B_{12}$ is important for the nerve cells and the blood. Foods that are high in vitamin $B_{12}$ include the following: cooked liver, fortified breakfast cereals, cooked rainbow trout, cooked beef, cooked haddock, breaded or fried clams, breaded or fried oysters, canned white tuna, milk, and yogurt.

***Deficiencies in vitamin $B_{12}$*** Deficiencies of vitamin $B_{12}$ are rare, because it is stored in the liver and the stores can last up to 10 years. The most common deficiency of vitamin $B_{12}$ is due to pernicious anemia, in which a substance normally produced in the stomach and needed for absorption of vitamin $B_{12}$ (intrinsic factor) is absent. People who have pernicious anemia need intramuscular shots of this vitamin throughout their life. For others deficient in $B_{12}$, oral, sublingual or nasal administration may be undertaken, especially after the $B_{12}$ levels have normalized with parenteral administration.

People who have digestive disorders may also have a deficiency of vitamin $B_{12}$, such as those who have celiac sprue or a chronic inflammation of the stomach or small intestine called CROHN'S DISEASE. People who have had gastric surgery may also become deficient in vitamin $B_{12}$.

Sometimes older people (individuals who are age 65 and older) have a deficiency of vitamin $B_{12}$. Vegetarians who avoid fish, eggs, or milk can also have deficiency. People who are deficient in this vitamin may need to take supplements and increase their intake of foods that are rich in vitamin $B_{12}$.

Experts report that most people are not harmed by high doses of this vitamin; however, people should consult their physician before adding vitamin $B_{12}$ supplements to their diet.

### Vitamin E

Vitamin E is a powerful antioxidant, or cancer fighter, in the body. It protects against free radicals that can harm the cells. Vitamin E is found in green leafy vegetables, nuts, and vegetable oils. Some foods that are high in vitamin E are wheat germ oil, almonds, safflower oil, turnip greens, mangoes, peanuts, and broccoli.

***Deficiencies of vitamin E*** Vitamin E deficiencies are rare in people worldwide. They can develop when people have disorders of fat metabolism. It has also been found in very low birth weight infants, weighing three-and-a-half pounds or less at birth. Others who may be deficient in vitamin E include those who have the following:

- Cystic fibrosis
- Crohn's disease
- Some forms of chronic liver disease
- Pancreatic insufficiency

Some people have a rare hereditary fat metabolism disorder that is called abetalipoproteinemia, which makes their body unable to absorb adequate amounts of vitamin E or fat. They need prescribed vitamin E supplements. Ataxia with vitamin E deficiency (AVED) is a genetic defect in the alpha-tocopherol transfer protein (A-TTP).

A person deficient in vitamin E may experience muscle weakness, impaired vision, drooping eyelids, speech difficulty, and other neurological problems. He or she also has abnormal breakdown of red blood cells.

***Excessive levels of vitamin E*** Clinical studies have not tested the effects of very high doses of vitamin E, which generally are not recommended. Doses up to 800 IU per day appear to be safe. High doses, especially in excess of 1200 IU per day, may cause bleeding problems because high doses of vitamin E supplements may interfere with the absorption of vitamin K, which is needed for synthesis of clotting factors. As a result, anyone taking blood thinner drugs should not also take high doses of vitamin E. In addition, no one should take vitamin E supplements (or any other supplements) without checking with his or her physician to make sure that such supplements will not be harmful. Other symptoms of toxicity include diarrhea and headache.

The recommended intake of vitamin E in adults is 10 mg per day for men and 8 mg per day for women. The Institute of Medicine, a Washington, D.C., organization that performs studies for federal government agencies, has set an upper level of vitamin E at 1,000 mg of supplemental alpha-tocopherol per day.

### Vitamin D

Vitamin D helps the body to maintain normal levels of calcium and phosphorus. The body uses sunshine to make vitamin D and obtains it from foods that are consumed. Many foods are fortified with vitamin D. Foods high in vitamin D include cod liver oil, cooked salmon, cooked mackerel, sardines, eels, and milk (nonfat, reduced fat, or whole milk).

**Deficiencies of vitamin D**   People can become deficient in vitamin D if they have little or no sunlight exposure. In some people the body cannot absorb vitamin D from the gastrointestinal tract. Sometimes the kidney is unable to produce 1, 25 (OH)2-vitamin D. The most commonly known deficiencies of vitamin D are rickets and osteomalacia. Rickets is a childhood disease caused by a vitamin D deficiency, which causes weak bones and skeletal abnormalities. Osteomalacia, which causes muscle and bone weakness, is the disease in adults caused by vitamin D deficiency.

People older than age 50 have a greater risk of being deficient in vitamin D than do younger individuals, and consequently, they may need to take supplemental vitamin D. People who may become deficient in vitamin D include the following groups:

- People who have Crohn's disease
- Individuals who have kidney disease
- People who have celiac sprue
- Individuals who have liver disease
- People who have pancreatic enzyme deficiency
- Elderly individuals

**Hypervitaminosis vitamin D**   It is also possible to have too much vitamin D. It is almost impossible to have toxic levels of vitamin D through diet alone. Most people who have an excessively high level are taking supplements. Vitamin D excess can cause the following problems:

- Nausea and vomiting
- Constipation
- Increased thirst and urination
- Itching
- Weakness
- Poor appetite
- Weight loss
- Mental confusion

The treatment of hypervitaminosis of vitamin D employs discontinuation of vitamin D, a low-calcium diet, and acidification of urine. Sometimes corticosteroids (such as prednisone) are prescribed.

For further information, contact:

Office of Dietary Supplements
National Institutes of Health
6100 Executive Boulevard
Room 3B01, MSC 7517
Bethesda, MD 20892
(301) 435-2920
http://dietary-supplements.info.nih.gov

See also ANEMIA; IRON; MAGNESIUM; SELENIUM.

**walking**   Simple ambulation of the body. Many experts consider walking one of the best exercises, and it is an exercise that even most sedentary people can perform with ease.

See also EXERCISE.

**watermelon stomach**   A rare condition of upper gastrointestinal bleeding that causes the stomach lining to have a characteristic endoscopic appearance of parallel red sores that form stripes similar to the striped pattern that is found on a watermelon. The condition is also known as gastric antral vascular ectasia (GAVE). Most who have watermelon stomach are elderly females (older than 65 or 70 years old). Watermelon stomach is a form of a malformation of blood vessels. Bleeding may be slow occult (microscopic) or overt; if it is untreated, the condition can lead to anemia and even vomiting of blood. Sometimes watermelon stomach is also associated with cirrhosis or scleroderma.

| A SAMPLE WALKING PROGRAM | | | | |
|---|---|---|---|---|
| | Warmup | Exercising | Cool Down | Total Time |
| **Week 1** | | | | |
| Session A | Walk 5 min | Then walk briskly 5 min | Then walk more slowly 5 min | 15 min |
| Session B | Repeat above pattern | | | |
| Session C | Repeat above pattern | | | |

Continue with at least three exercise sessions during each week of the program.

| | | | | |
|---|---|---|---|---|
| **Week 2** | Walk 5 min | Walk briskly 7 min | Walk 5 min | 17 min |
| **Week 3** | Walk 5 min | Walk briskly 9 min | Walk 5 min | 19 min |
| **Week 4** | Walk 5 min | Walk briskly 11 min | Walk 5 min | 21 min |
| **Week 5** | Walk 5 min | Walk briskly 13 min | Walk 5 min | 23 min |
| **Week 6** | Walk 5 min | Walk briskly 15 min | Walk 5 min | 25 min |
| **Week 7** | Walk 5 min | Walk briskly 18 min | Walk 5 min | 28 min |
| **Week 8** | Walk 5 min | Walk briskly 20 min | Walk 5 min | 30 min |
| **Week 9** | Walk 5 min | Walk briskly 23 min | Walk 5 min | 33 min |
| **Week 10** | Walk 5 min | Walk briskly 26 min | Walk 5 min | 36 min |
| **Week 11** | Walk 5 min | Walk briskly 28 min | Walk 5 min | 38 min |
| **Week 12** | Walk 5 min | Walk briskly 30 min | Walk 5 min | 40 min |
| **Week 13 on:** | | | | |

Gradually increase your brisk walking time from 30 to 60 minutes, three or four times a week. Remember that your goal is to get the benefits you are seeking and enjoy your activity.

**Walking Tips**
- Hold your head up and keep your back straight.
- Bend your elbows as you swing your arms.
- Take long, easy strides.

GAVE is formally diagnosed with an endoscopy. In addition, when GAVE is present, the patient's stool specimens may test positive for occult bleeding. Occasionally, patients need blood transfusions. Patients who have watermelon stomach may be treated with cautery or laser therapy, and most need repeated procedures over time. Surgery may be needed for refractory cases. Some patients have been treated with female hormone replacement therapy (estrogen/progesterone).

See also ENDOSCOPY; OCCULT GASTROINTESTINAL BLEEDING; STOMACH.

**Wernicke's encephalopathy**  A condition that constitutes a medical emergency, which is caused by a severe deficiency of thiamine (vitamin $B_1$), along with a continued intake of carbohydrates. It is also often brought on by chronic ALCOHOLISM. The condition was named after Carl Wernicke, a German neurologist.

Patients who are on prolonged vitamin-free intravenous nutrition, as after surgery, or who are engaging in fad diets are also at risk for development of Wernicke's encephalopathy. This condition is also called cerebral BERIBERI; it is precipitated by an acute deficiency as well as the acute or already chronic deficiency of thiamine. Typically, it occurs when glucose is administered to an alcoholic who is already deficient in thiamine, further depleting the body of thiamine.

Wernicke's encephalopathy causes a malfunction of the central nervous system, leading to balance disorder, severe confusion, and disorders of the eye movements. It may progress to coma and death.

Treatment requires intravenous or intramuscular administration of thiamine for prolonged periods. Recovery is not always complete; some symptoms start to improve within a few hours of treatment, and others may take a few months to improve. Wernicke's encephalopathy can be fatal.

See also VITAMIN DEFICIENCIES/EXCESSES.

O'Brien, Robert, Morris Chafetz, M.D., and Sidney Cohen, M.D., eds. *The Encyclopedia of Understanding Alcohol and Other Drugs.* New York: Facts On File, 1999.

**Whipple's disease**  An extremely rare systemwide bacterial infection that was first described in the medical literature in 1907 by a medical missionary, George Whipple. (About 30 cases per year are reported worldwide.) The disease is caused by the bacterium *Tropheryma whippelii.* These bacteria invade the gut wall, blood vessels, colon, liver, brain, heart, lung, synovium, kidney, bone marrow, and skin. When found, the disease has usually been diagnosed in middle-aged or older men.

Despite considerable difficulty, scientists were able to culture this infection; its cultivation was reported in 2000 in the *New England Journal of Medicine.*

### Symptoms

The most common symptoms found among patients with Whipple's disease are

- Chronic weight loss
- Arthralgias (joint pains)
- Abdominal pain
- Diarrhea
- Anemia
- Hyperpigmentation
- Abnormal rhythmic movements of the eyes and jaws

Other symptoms that have been seen in some patients with Whipple's disease include the following:

- Hypotension (low blood pressure)
- Fever
- Swollen lymph nodes
- Shortness of breath

Patients may also exhibit a wasting away, or CACHEXIA, such as occurs in other diseases, such as ACQUIRED IMMUNODEFICIENCY SYNDROME and in advanced stages of cancer.

### Diagnosis and Treatment

Because it is so rare, and the symptoms are so diverse and nonspecific, physicians may initially have difficulty in diagnosing Whipple's disease.

However, the diagnosis can be easily made by a microscopic view of a biopsy tissue sample from the small intestine. Special tests using polymerase chain reaction (PCR) may be able to identify the infection in the future.

Most Whipple's disease patients are treated with long-term antibiotics for a year or more, though they start to feel better within a few days. The disease relapses after discontinuation of treatment in 17 to 35 percent of cases.

For further information, contact the following organizations:

Association for Neuro-Metabolic Diseases
5223 Brookfield Lane
Sylvania, OH 43560
(419) 885-1497

National Digestive Diseases Information
    Clearinghouse
2 Information Way
Bethesda, MD 20892
(301) 654-3810 or (800) 891-5389 (toll-free)
www.niddk.nih.gov

Raoult, Didier, M.D., et al. "Cultivation of the Bacillus of Whipple's Disease." *New England Journal of Medicine* 342, no. 9 (March 2, 2000): 620–625.
Swartz, Morton N., M.D. "Whipple's Disease—Past, Present, and Future," *New England Journal of Medicine* 342, no. 9 (March 2, 2000): 648–650.

**Whipple procedure**   Major surgery that is performed on an individual, usually diagnosed with pancreatic cancer, in an attempt to prolong life. (Pancreatic cancer has a low survival rate.) This procedure has no relation to Whipple's disease and may be done for diseases other than pancreatic cancer.

**Wilson's disease**   An unusual genetic disease in which the body retains toxically high levels of copper, primarily in the liver and brain; it is also known as hepatolenticular degeneration.

The neurologist Samual A. Kinnier Wilson first described the disease in 1912, and it was subsequently named after him. Wilson's disease is found among men and women in all racial and ethnic groups. The symptoms are usually first identified in childhood or adolescence but may be missed altogether.

Experts estimate that Wilson's disease occurs in about one in 100,000 births, although it may be underdiagnosed. Some experts believe that the true incidence is actually one in 30,000 births.

The cause of Wilson's disease is a genetic defect found on protein chromosome 13.

### Symptoms and Signs

Some Wilson's disease patients may appear healthy; their illness draws attention when they are found to have abnormal liver test results on routine testing. Children and adolescents who have Wilson's disease usually have liver problems, whereas adults experience neuropsychiatric disorders, such as tremors, rigidity, difficulty with speaking and walking, and drooling.

A classic sign of Wilson's disease is found in the eye: a rusty brown ring in the cornea that is caused by the accumulation of copper. This sign, called the Kayser-Fleischer ring, is usually seen by an ophthalmologist, using a procedure called a slit lamp examination. Rarely, the sign may be visible to the naked eye. However, this sign may not be present, especially in an early stage of the disease. Another problem is that observing it may be difficult to impossible in a routine physical examination of individuals who have brown eyes.

Other symptoms of hepatic disease found in the stages of Wilson's disease include the following:

• Appetite loss
• Dark urine
• Jaundice

As the disease progresses, indicators of advanced disease are found. Some symptoms of neuropsychiatric problems are:

• Slurred speech
• Tremors
• Double vision
• Dysphagia (difficulty with swallowing)
• Weakness

- Tremors
- Spastic movements

Some Wilson's disease patients may present for the first time with a life-threatening fulminant hepatic failure; such patients require liver transplantation on an emergency basis.

### Diagnosis and Treatment

Wilson's disease can be a very difficult disease to diagnose, because it can mimic the symptoms of cirrhosis and hepatitis due to different causes, as well as a wide variety of diseases of the brain, liver, blood, and kidneys (such as kidney stones). In addition, some individuals diagnosed with schizophrenia, a severe psychiatric disease, may actually have Wilson's disease. Patients who have psychotic disorders should be screened for Wilson's disease, because medications given to treat psychosis may worsen the illness and not resolve the psychotic behavior.

If Wilson's disease is diagnosed in the early stages, patients can be treated with medications called chelators, which combine with metals and decrease copper accumulation in the body. Treatment is aimed at removing the excess copper and preventing it from reaccumulating. Thus, people who have Wilson's disease must take these drugs for the rest of their life; those who stop treatment may worsen rapidly.

The most commonly used chelator is D-penicillamine. If a patient is unable to tolerate this drug, trientine is an alternate option. For the prevention of reaccumulation, lower doses of these chelators or, alternatively, zinc may be used. If the disease is diagnosed in a later stage, patients who have severe liver damage may need a liver transplantation in order to save their life.

For further information, contact these organizations:

American Liver Foundation
75 Maiden Lane
New York, NY 10038
(212) 668-1000
http://www.liverfoundation.org

National Center for the Study of Wilson's Disease
432 West 58th Street
Suite 614
New York, NY 10019
(212) 523-8717

Wilson's Disease Association
1802 Brookside Drive
Wooster, OH 44691
(800) 399-0266
http://www.wilsonsdisease.org

See also HEMOCHROMATOSIS; LIVER; LIVER ENZYMES/FUNCTION TESTS; LIVER TRANSPLANTATION.

**women and digestive diseases**   Although both men and women have a variety of digestive diseases and disorders, women are more likely to have some illnesses, such as GALLSTONES, gallbladder cancer, HIRSCHSPRUNG'S DISEASE, IRRITABLE BOWEL SYNDROME (IBS), PRIMARY BILIARY CIRRHOSIS, and WATERMELON STOMACH. In contrast, men have a much greater risk of development of KAPOSI'S SARCOMA than women (15 men to one woman). Men also have a higher risk of cirrhosis of the liver, esophageal cancer, liver cancer, stomach cancer, alcoholic pancreatitis, and HEPATOCELLUCLAR CARCINOMA.

**World Health Organization (WHO)**   An international health organization that was established in 1948 by the United Nations to study common diseases throughout the world and to offer reports and recommendations. WHO is governed by 192 member states worldwide.

For further information on WHO, contact the organization at

WHO Headquarters
Avenue Appia 20
1211 Geneva 27
Switzerland
+ 41 22 791 21 11
http://www.who.int

**yeast**    See *CANDIDA;* THRUSH.

**yo-yo dieting**    The process of frequently gaining and losing significant amounts of weight (20 pounds or more in a short period, such as a month or less). It is also known as weight cycling. Some experts believe that individuals who repeatedly gain and lose large amounts of weight are at risk for development of some illnesses, such as gallbladder disease, hypertension, and high cholesterol levels. That conclusion is controversial, and firm data about the harmful effects of yo-yo dieting are lacking.

Obese individuals should try to lose weight; a slow, steady weight loss of several pounds per month is recommended by most physicians. Rapid weight loss can cause development of GALLSTONES as well as NONALCOHOLIC STEATOHEPATITIS/NONALCOHOLIC FATTY LIVER DISEASE.

See also DIET DRUGS; OBESITY.

**Zenker's diverticulum**  A pouch that forms in the upper esophagus as a result of a restrictive myopathy of the muscles of the pharynx, resulting in disordered motility of the upper esophageal sphincter. (More than one diverticulum are *diverticula*.) A second diverticulum is present in 1 to 2 percent of all cases.

Named after Albert Zenker, a German physician and pathologist who described the problem in 1877, these diverticula constitute about two-thirds of all esophageal diverticula. Men are two to three times more likely to have Zenker's diverticula, and generally they are found among elderly individuals, age 70 years and older.

### Signs and Symptoms

Zenker's diverticulum does not always cause symptoms or signs. It can result in bad breath (halitosis) as well as regurgitation of food. The regurgitation can be frightening because it is more likely to occur when the patient is lying down and can lead to aspiration and pneumonia in some patients. Zenker's diverticulum patients may also experience difficulty with swallowing (dysphagia). Some patients report a bad taste in the mouth and a feeling of something stuck in the throat. Patients may also have neck pain, and some experience weight loss. Zenker's diverticulum can even cause cancer in the pouch. An ulcer in the diverticulum and bleeding due to retained medications such as aspirin may occur.

### Diagnosis and Treatment

Physicians identify Zenker's diverticulum through barium swallow. Some physicians use manometry to measure esophageal pressures. Physicians may also use an upper endoscopy.

Patients who have symptomatic Zenker's diverticula usually need surgery. Procedures using an endoscope may be performed in some centers.

See also MECKEL'S DIVERTICULUM.

Overbeck, J. J. van. "Pathogenesis and Methods of Treatments of Zenker's Diverticulum," *Otology, Rhinology, Laryngology* 112, no. 7 (July 2003): 583–593.

**zinc**  An essential mineral that is involved in more than 100 enzyme systems and that helps promote numerous important biochemical reactions in the human body. The body contains about 2 to 3.0 grams of zinc. Zinc is also important in providing support to the immune system, healing wounds, and maintaining the senses of smell and taste. Zinc is essential for normal growth during childhood and adolescence and for fetal growth during pregnancy.

Foods that are high in zinc include the following items: shellfish, oysters, whole-grain cereals, lean cooked beef shank (leg meat), lean cooked beef chuck, lean cooked pork shoulder, roasted chicken leg meat, and legumes. Zinc supplementation is useful in treating WILSON'S DISEASE, in which there is an overload of copper. Zinc prevents copper absorption and/or promotes copper excretion into the feces, and hence is useful for treatment of Wilson's disease.

### Deficiencies of Zinc

In most cases, a person's daily diet provides sufficient amounts of zinc. (The recommended allowance for adults is 15 mg per day for men and 12 mg per day for women.) Some people have a zinc deficiency. People who are at most risk for a zinc deficiency include the following groups:

- Vegetarians
- Elderly people
- Individuals who have liver disease
- Alcoholics
- People who have Crohn's disease or short bowel syndrome
- People who have chronic diarrhea
- Patients on total parenteral nutrition without adequate zinc supplementation

Pharmacologic doses of zinc supplementation may help increase linear growth and weight gain in infants and enhance immune function of the elderly; they are also beneficial in cases of preterm labor, premature birth, prolonged labor, intrapartum hemorrhage and low sperm counts. Before anyone takes a zinc supplement, he or she should consult a physician to ensure that it is really necessary.

Signs of a zinc deficiency include the following:

- Impaired taste
- Impaired immunity
- Skin rash
- Impaired wound healing
- Delayed growth of a child
- Loss of hair
- Diarrhea
- Sterility and impotence
- Appetite loss
- Night blindness

### Toxic Levels of Zinc

It is possible for individuals to take too much zinc. It is virtually impossible to attain toxic levels in the diet, but a zinc overdose may occur when people take zinc supplements in excessive amounts. Excessive levels of zinc may cause nausea and vomiting and may impair important metabolic functions in the body. In addition, they may lead to copper deficiency.

See also VITAMIN DEFICIENCIES/EXCESSES.

**Zollinger-Ellison syndrome**    A medical condition that is characterized by digestive problems, such as peptic ulcers, diarrhea, and abdominal pain. This syndrome was first described by Doctors Zollinger and Ellison in 1955.

Individuals who have Zollinger-Ellison syndrome have tumors (called gastrinomas) that secrete a hormone called gastrin, which in turn leads to the excessive secretion of digestive acid (hydrochloric acid). Tumors may be single or multiple and are frequently present in the gastrinoma triangle which is bordered by the head of the pancreas and duodenum, but they may also occur in the stomach, bones, ovaries, liver, heart or abdominal lymph nodes. The gastrinoma may be benign or cancerous (localized or metastatic), with an associated spread to other organs, such as the liver and the bones. About one-third of the tumors are metastatic at the time of diagnosis. In about 25 percent of cases, the disease is associated with multiple endocrine neoplasia type 1 (MEN-1), a genetic syndrome that is characterized by tumors of the pituitary and parathyroid glands, in addition to the gastrinomas frequently seen in the pancreas.

### Risk Factors

Zollinger-Ellison syndrome usually is diagnosed when an individual is between 20 and 50 years, although it may also be seen in children as well as elderly adults.

### Symptoms of Zollinger-Ellison Syndrome

Symptoms of this medical condition include abdominal pain, diarrhea, and high amounts of fat found in the patient's stool (steatorrhea). As many as 90 percent of these patients have peptic ulcer disease.

### Diagnosis and Treatment

Patients are suspected to have Zollinger-Ellison syndrome on the basis of symptoms of abdominal pain and/or diarrhea, with the associated finding of atypical peptic ulcer disease and/or MALABSORPTION SYNDROME. However, less than 1 percent of peptic ulcer patients have Zollinger-Ellison syndrome.

Once this medical problem is suspected, the physician orders testing of serum level of the hormone gastrin in a fasting state, which may be complemented by testing after stimulation injection of secretin, another hormone. Hydrochloric acid levels of the stomach can also be measured;

they are abnormally high among Zollinger-Ellison syndrome patients.

After the diagnosis, the physician orders tests such as radionuclide somatostatin scan and/or computed tomography (CT) scan to localize the gastrinoma. An endoscopic ultrasound is also helpful.

Acid suppression with proton pump inhibitor medications is required for these patients, in order to suppress the effects and complications of excess acid secretion. In sporadic cases, the tumor is usually a single one, and there is no spread to distant organs such as the liver or bones, surgery is the treatment of choice. In individuals who have metastatic disease (in which the cancer has spread), chemotherapy may be employed. Palliative surgery (to relieve pain) may also be chosen by the physician. Surgery is not recommended in patients with gastrinoma as part of MEN.

Wynbrandt, James, and Mark D. Ludman. *The Encyclopedia of Genetic Disorders and Birth Defects.* 2d ed. New York: Facts On File, 2000.

# APPENDIXES

# APPENDIX I
## IMPORTANT ORGANIZATIONS

**AARP**
601 E Street NW
Washington, DC 20049
(202) 434-2277 or (888) 687-2277
http://www.aarp.org

**Administration on Aging**
Department of Health and Human Services
200 Independence Avenue SW
Washington, DC 20201
(202) 619-0724
http://www.aoa.gov

**Agency for Healthcare Research & Quality
(AHRQ)**
Publications Clearinghouse
540 Gaither Rd.
Rockville, MD 20850
(301) 427-1364
http://www.ahrq.gov

**Alcoholics Anonymous**
Grand Central Station
P.O. Box 459
New York, NY 10163
http://www.alcoholics-anonymous.org

**Alliance for Aging Research**
2021 K Street NW
Suite 305
Washington, DC 20006
(202) 293-2856
http://www.agingresearch.org

**Alpha-1 Foundation**
2937 Southwest 27th Avenue
Suite 302
Miami, FL 33133

(877) 2-CURE-A1
http://www.alphaone.org

**American Academy of Allergy, Asthma and
Immunology**
611 East Wells Street
Milwaukee, WI 53202
(414) 272-6071
(800) 822-2762 (toll-free)
http://www.aaaai.org

**American Academy of Family Physicians
(AAFP)**
11400 Tomahawk Creek Parkway
Leawood, KS 66211
(800) 274-2237 (toll-free)

**American Academy of Ophthalmology**
P.O. Box 7424
San Francisco, CA 94120
(415) 561-8500
http://www.aao.org

**American Academy of Pediatrics**
141 Northwest Point Boulevard
Elk Grove Village, IL 60007
(847) 434-4000
http://www.aap.org

**American Anorexia Bulimia Association**
165 West 46 Street, #1108
New York, NY 10036
(212) 575-6200

**American Association for the Study of Liver
Diseases (AASLD)**
1729 King Street
Suite 200

Alexandria, VA 22314
(703) 299-9766
http://www.aasld.org

**American Association of Clinical
     Endocrinologists**
1000 Riverside Avenue
Suite 205
Jacksonville, FL 32304
(904) 353-7878
http://www.aace.com

**American Association for Diabetes
     Educators**
100 West Monroe Street, 4th floor
Chicago, IL 60603
(800) 338-3633
http://www.aadenet.org

**American Association for Higher Education**
One Dupont Circle
Suite 360
Washington, DC 20036
(202) 293-6440
http://www.aahe.org

**American Association of Poison Control
     Centers**
3201 New Mexico Avenue
Suite 330
Washington, DC 20016
(202) 362-7217
http://www.aapcc.org
*Note: The organization provides nonemergency
     information on poisoning.*

**American Autoimmune Related Diseases
     Association**
22100 Gratiot Avenue
East Detroit, MI 48021
(586) 776-3900
http://www.aarda.org

**American Bar Association**
Commission on Mental and Physical Disability
     Law
740 Fifteenth Street NW
Washington, DC 20005
(202) 666-1570
http://www.abanet.org/disability

**American Behçet's Disease Association**
P.O. Box 19952
Amarillo, TX 79114
(800) 723-4238 (toll-free)
http://www.behcets.com

**American Board of Medical Specialties**
47 Perimeter Center East
Suite 500
Atlanta, GA 36346
(800) 776-2378

**American Board of Pediatric Surgery**
1601 Dolores Street
San Francisco, CA 94110
(415) 826-3200

**American Cancer Society**
1599 Clifton Road NE
Atlanta, GA 30329
(800) 277-2345 or (404) 320-3333
http://www.cancer.org

**American Celiac Society**
59 Crystal Avenue
West Orange, NJ 07052
(973) 325-8837

**American Chronic Pain Association**
P.O. Box 850
Rocklin, CA 95677
(916) 632-0922
http://www.theacpa.org

**American College of Gastroenterology**
P.O. Box 3099
Alexandria, VA 22302
(703) 820-7400
http://www.acg.gi.org

**American College of Physicians, American
     Society of Internal Medicine (ACP-ASIM)**
190 North Independence Mall West
Philadelphia, PA 19106
(800) 523-1546 or (215) 351-2400
http://www.acponline.org

**American College of Sports Medicine**
P.O. Box 1440
Indianapolis, IN 46206
(317) 637-9200
http://www.ascm.org/sportsmed

## American College of Surgeons (ACS)

633 North Saint Clair Street
Chicago, IL 60611
(312) 202-5000
http://www.facs.org

## American Diabetes Association (ADA)

1701 North Beauregard Street
Alexandria, VA 22311
(800) 232-3472 or (703) 549-1500
http://www.diabetes.org/

## American Dietetic Association

216 West Jackson Boulevard
Chicago, IL 60606
(312) 899-0040
http://www.eatright.org

## American Gastroenterological Association (AGA)

National Office
4930 Del Ray Avenue
Bethesda, MD 20814
(301) 654-2055
http://www.gastro.org

## American Heart Association/American Stroke Association

7272 Greenville Avenue
Dallas, TX 75231
800-AHA-USAI (242-8721) (toll-free)
http://www.americanheart.org

## American Hemochromatosis Society

4044 W. Lake Mary Blvd., Unit 104
Lake Mary, FL 32746
(888) 655-IRON (toll-free)
http:/www.americanhs.org

## American Hospital Association (AHA)

One North Franklin
Chicago, IL 60606
(312) 422-3000
http://www.aha.org

## American Institute for Cancer Research

1759 R Street NW
Washington, DC 20009
(202) 328-7744 or (800) 843-8114
http://www.aicr.org

## American Liver Foundation

75 Maiden Lane
Suite 603
New York, NY 10038
(800) 465-4837 (toll-free) or (212) 668-1000
http://www.liverfoundation.org

## American Lung Association

1740 Broadway
New York, NY 10019
(212) 315-08700
http://www.lungusa.org

## American Medical Association

515 North State Street
Chicago, IL 60610
(312) 464-5000
http://www.ama-assn.org

## American Menopause Foundation

350 Fifth Avenue
Suite 2822
New York, NY 10118
(212) 714-2398
http://www.americanmenopause.org

## American Motility Society

c/o Dr. Dhung Owyang
Gastroenterology Division
University of Michigan Medical Center
3912 Taubman Center
P.O. Box 0362
Ann Arbor, MI 48109
(734) 936-4785

## American Nurses Association

600 Maryland Avenue SW
Suite 100 West
Washington, DC 20024
(800) 274-4ANA
http:/www.nursingworld.org

## American Obesity Association

1250 24th Street NW
Suite 300
Washington, DC 20037
(202) 776-7711
http://www.obesity.org

## American Pancreatic Association

c/o Howard A. Reber, M.D.

UCLA School of Medicine
10833 LeConte Avenue
72-259 CHS
Los Angeles, CA 90095
(310) 825-4976

**American Pharmaceutical Association**
2215 Constitution Avenue NW
Washington, DC 20037
(202) 628-4410
http://www.aphanet.org

**American Psychiatric Association**
1400 K Street NW
Washington, DC 20005
(202) 682-6000
http://www.psych.org

**American Psychological Association**
750 First Street NE
Washington, DC 20002
(202) 336-5500
http://www.apa.org

**American Society for Bariatric Surgery**
7328 West University Avenue
Suite F
Gainesville, FL 32607
(353) 331-4900
http://www.asbs.org

**American Society of Bariatric Physicians**
5453 East Evans Place
Denver, CO 80222
(303) 770-2526
http://www.asbp.org

**American Society for Gastrointestinal Endoscopy (ASGE)**
1520 Kensington Rd.
Suite 202
Oak Brook, IL 60523
http://www.asge.org

**American Society for Parenteral and Enteral Nutrition (ASPEN)**
8630 Fenton Street
Suite 412
Silver Spring, MD 20910
(301) 587-6315
http://www.nutritioncare.org

**American Society of Abdominal Surgeons**
675 Main Street
Melrose, MA 02176
(781) 665-6102
http://www.abdominalsurg.org

**American Society of Colon and Rectal Surgeons (ASCRS)**
85 West Algonquin Road
Suite 550
Arlington Heights, IL 60005
(847) 290-9184
http://www.fascrs.org

**American Society of Human Genetics**
9650 Rockville Pike
Bethesda, MD 20814
(301) 571-1825
http://www.faseb.org/genetics

**American Thyroid Association**
Montefiore Medical Center
111 East 210th Street, Room 311
Bronx, NY 10467
(718) 882-6047
http://www.thyroid. org

**Anorexia Nervosa and Related Eating Disorders, Inc.**
P.O. Box 5102
Eugene, OR 97405
(503) 334-1144

**Association of American Indian Physicians**
1235 Sovereign Row
Suite C-9
Oklahoma City, OK 73108
(405) 946-7651

**Association of Asian Pacific Community Health Organizations**
1440 Broadway, #510
Oakland, CA 94612
(510) 272-9536
http://www.aapcho.org

**Association of Gastrointestinal Motility Disorders, Inc.**
11 North Street
Lexington, MA 02420
(781) 861-3874
http://www.agmd-gimotility.org

**Cancer Research Foundation of America**
1600 Duke Street
Suite 110
Alexandria, VA 22314
(703) 836-4412 or (800) 227-2732
http://www.preventcancer.org

**Celiac Disease Foundation**
13251 Ventura Boulevard, #1
Studio City, CA 91604
(818) 990-2354
http://www.celiac.org

**Celiac Sprue Association USA**
P.O. Box 31700
Omaha, NE 68131
(800) CSA-4CSA
http://www.csaceliacs.org

**Centers for Disease Control and Prevention (CDC)**
1600 Clifton Road NE
Atlanta, GA 30333
(404) 371-5900
http://www.cdc.gov

**Centers for Medicare and Medicaid Services (formerly the Health Care Financing Administration)**
6325 Security Boulevard
Baltimore, MD 21207
(410) 786-3000
http://www.hcfa.gov

**Colorectal Cancer Network**
P.O. Box 182
Kensington, MD 20895
(301) 879-1500
http://www.colorectal-cancer.net

**Crohn's & Colitis Foundation of America**
386 Park Avenue South, 17th Floor
New York, NY 10016
(800) 932-2423 (toll-free) or (212) 685-3440
http://www.ccfa.org

**Cushing's Support and Research Foundation, Inc.**
65 East India Row, 22B
Boston, MA 02110
(617) 723-3824

**Cyclic Vomiting Syndrome Association**
3585 Cedar Hill Road NW
Canal Winchester, OH 43110
(614) 837-2586
http://www.cvsaonline.org

**The Cystic Fibrosis Foundation**
6931 Arlington Road
Bethesda, MD 20814
(301) 951-4422 or (800) FIGHT CF
http://www.cff.org

**Department of Veterans Affairs (VA)**
Office of Public Affairs
810 Vermont Avenue NW
Washington, DC 20420
(800) 827-1000 (toll-free)
(800) 829-4833 (tty)
http://www.va.gov

**Diabetes Action Research and Education Foundation**
426 C Street NE
Washington, DC 20002
(202) 333-4520
http://www.diabetesaction.org

**Diabetes Exercise and Sports Association**
1647 West Bethany Home Road, #B
Phoenix, AX 85015
(800) 898-4322 (toll-free)
http://www.diabetes-exercise.org

**Digestive Disease National Coalition**
507 Capitol Court NE
Suite 200
Washington, DC 20002
(202) 544-7497
http://www.ddnc.org

**Disability Rights Education and Defense Fund, Inc.**
221 Sixth Street
Berkeley, CA 94710
(510) 644-2555 or (800) 466-4232

**Eating Disorder Referral and Information Center**
2923 Sandy Pointe
Suite 6
Del Mar, CA 92014

(858) 792-7463
http://www.edreferral.com

**Family Caregiver Alliance**
690 Market Street
Suite 600
San Francisco, CA 94104
(415) 434-3388
http://www.caregiver.org

**Food Allergy & Anaphylaxis Network**
11781 Lee Jackson Highway
Suite 160
Fairfax, VA 22033
(800) 929-4040
http://www.foodallergy.org

**Food and Drug Administration (FDA)**
5600 Fishers Lane
Rockville, MD 20857
(888) 463-6332 (toll-free)
http://www.fda.org

**Food and Nutrition Information Center**
National Agricultural Library/USDA
10301 Baltimore Boulevard
Room 304
Beltsville, MD 20705
(301) 504-5719

**Gastro-Intestinal Research Foundation**
70 East Lake Street
Suite 1015
Chicago, IL 60601
(312) 332-1350
http://www.girf.org

**The Genetic Alliance**
4301 Connecticut Avenue NW
Suite 404
Washington, DC 20008
(202) 966-5557
http://www.geneticalliance.org

**Gluten Intolerance Group of North America**
15110 Tenth Avenue SW
Suite A
Seattle, WA 98166
(206) 246-6652
http://www.gluten.net

**Hemochromatosis Foundation, Inc.**
P.O. Box 8569
Albany, NY 12208
(518) 489-0972
http://www.hemochromatosis.org

**Hepatitis B Coalition/Immunization Action Coalition**
1573 Selby Avenue
Suite 234
St. Paul, MN 55104
(651) 647-9009
http://www.immunize.org

**Hepatitis B Foundation**
700 East Bulter Avenue
Doylestown, PA 18901
(215) 489-4900
http://www.hepb.org

**Hepatitis Foundation International**
504 Blick Drive
Silver Spring, MD 20904
(800) 891-0707 or (301) 622-4200
http://www.hepfi.org

**Human Growth Foundation**
7777 Leesburg Pike
Suite 202 South
Falls Church, VA 22043
(703) 883-1773
http://www.hgfound.org

**Huntington's Disease Society of America**
158 West 29th Street, 7th Floor
New York, NY 10001
(800) 345-HDSA
http://www.hdsa.org

**Hypoglycemia Support Foundation**
3822 NW 122nd Terrace
Sunrise, FL 33323
(954) 742-3098
http://www.hypoglycemia.org

**Institute of Medicine**
The National Academies
500 Fifth Street NW
Washington, DC 20001
(202) 334-2169
http://www.ion.edu/iomhome.nsf

**International Association for Medical Assistance to Travelers**
417 Center Street
Lewiston, NY 14092
(716) 754-4883

**International Diabetic Athletes Association**
1647 West Bethany Home Road, #B
Phoenix, AZ 85015
(800) 898-4322
http://www.diabetes-exercise.org

**International Foundation for Functional Gastrointestinal Disorders, Inc.**
P.O. Box 170864
Milwaukee, WI 53217
(888) 964-2001 (toll-free) or (414) 964-1799
http://www.iffgd.org

**Intestinal Disease Foundation**
Landmarks Building
Suite 525
One Station Squire
Pittsburgh, PA 15219
(877) 587-9606 (toll-free) or (412) 261-5888
http://www.intestinalfoundation.org

**Iron Overload Diseases Association, Inc.**
433 Westward Drive
North Palm Beach, FL 33408
(561) 840-8512
http://www.ironoverload.org

**Joslin Diabetes Center**
One Joslin Place
Boston, MA 02215
(617) 732-2415
http://www.joslin.harvard.edu

**Juvenile Diabetes Research Foundation (JDF) International**
120 Wall Street, 19th Floor
New York, NY 10005
(800) 533-2873
http://www.jdf.org

**Medic Alert Foundation**
P.O. Box 109
Turlock, CA 95831
(209) 668-3331
http://www.medicalalert.org

**National Alliance for Hispanic Health**
1501 Sixteenth Street NW
Washington, DC 20036
(202) 387-5000
http://www.hispanichealth.org

**National Arthritis and Musculoskeletal and Skin Diseases Information Clearinghouse**
One AMS Circle
Bethesda, MD 20892
(301) 495-4484

**National Association of Anorexia Nervosa and Associated Disorders**
P.O. Box 7
Highland Park, IL 60035
(847) 831-3438
http://www.anad.org

**National Association of Nutrition and Aging Service Programs**
1101 Vermont Avenue NW
Suite 1001
Washington, DC 20005
(202) 682-6899
http://www.nanasp.org

**National Cancer Institute**
Division of Cancer Epidemiology and Genetics
6120 Executive Boulevard, MSC-7234
Executive Plaza South, 7th Floor
Rockville, MD 20852
(301) 496-1691

**National Center for Complementary and Alternative Medicine Clearinghouse**
P.O. Box 8281
Silver Spring, MD 20907
(888) 644-6226 (toll-free)
http://www.nccam.nih.gov

**National Center for Health Statistics**
6525 Belcrest Road, Room 1064
Hyattsville, MD 20782
http://www.cdc.gov/nchs

**National Center for the Study of Wilson's Disease**
432 West 58th Street
Suite 614
New York, NY 10091
(212) 523-8717

**National Chronic Pain Outreach Association**
P.O. Box 274
Millboro, CA 24460
(540) 997-5004

**National Clearinghouse for Alcohol and Drug Information**
11426 Rockville Pike
Suite 200
Rockville, MD 20852
(800) 729-6686 (toll-free)
http://www.health.org

**National Coalition for Cancer Survivorship (NCCS)**
1010 Wayne Avenue
Suite 770
Silver Spring, MD 20910
(877) 622-7937 (toll-free)
www.cansearch.org

**National Council on Aging**
409 Third Street NW
Second Floor
Washington, DC 20024
(202) 479-1200 or (800) 424-9046

**National Council on Alcoholism and Drug Dependence (NCADD)**
20 Exchange Place
Suite 2902
New York, NY 10005
(800) NCA-CALL or (212) 269-7797
http://www.ncadd.org

**National Diabetes Information Clearinghouse**
1 Information Way
Bethesda, MD 20892
(301) 654-3327
http://www.niddk.nih.gov/health/diabetes.ndic.htm

**National Digestive Diseases Information Clearinghouse**
2 Information Way
Bethesda, MD 20892
(800) 891-5389 (toll-free)
www.niddk.nih.gov/health/digest/nddic.htm

**National Easter Seal Society**
230 West Monroe Street
Suite 1800

Chicago, IL 60606
(800) 221-6827 (toll-free)
http://www.easter-seals.org

**National Eating Disorders Organization**
603 Stewart Street
Suite 803
Seattle, WA 98101
(206) 382-3587
http://www.edap.org

**National Family Caregivers Association**
10400 Connecticut Avenue
Suite 500
Kensington, MD 20895
(301) 942-6430
http://www.nfcacares.org

**National Health Information Center (NHIC)**
Office of Disease Prevention and Health Promotion (ODPHP)
Department of Health and Human Services
P.O. Box 1133
Washington, DC 20013
(800) 336-4797 (toll-free)
http://www.health.gov/NHIC

**National Heart, Lung and Blood Institute Information Center**
P.O. Box 30105
Bethesda, MD 20824
(301) 592-8573
http://www.nhlbi.nih.gov/health/public/heart/index.htm

**National Information Center for Children and Youth with Disabilities**
P.O. Box 1492
Washington, DC 20013
(800) 695-0285
http://www.nichcy.org

**National Institutes of Allergy and Infectious Diseases**
Building 31, Room 7A-50
31 Center Drive, MSC 2520
Bethesda, MD 20892

**National Institute of Diabetes and Digestive and Kidney Diseases**
National Institutes of Health

Building 31, Room 9A04
31 Center Drive
MSC 2560
Bethesda, MD 20892
(301) 496-3583
http://www.niddk.nih.gov

### National Institutes of Health (NIH)
P.O. Box 8218
Silver Spring, MD 20907
(888) 644-6226 (toll-free)
http://www.nccam.nih.gov

### National Institute on Aging
Building 31, Room 5C27
31 Center Drive
MSC 2292
Bethesda, MD 20892
(301) 496-1752
http://www.nih.gov/nia

### National Institute of Mental Health (NIMH)
Public Inquiries
6001 Executive Boulevard
Room 8184, MSC 9663
Bethesda, MD 20892
(301) 443-4513
http://www.nimh.nih.gov

### National Kidney Foundation, Inc.
30 East 33rd Street
New York, NY 10016
(800) 622-9010 or (212) 889-2210 (toll-free)
http://www.kidney.org

### National Oral Health Information Clearinghouse
1 NOHIC Way
Bethesda, MD 20892
(301) 402-3500
http://www.nohic.nidcr.nih.gov

### National Organization for Rare Disorders (NORD)
P.O. Box 8923
New Fairfield, CT 06812
(203) 746-6518
http://www.rarediseases.org

### National Rehabilitation Information Center
1010 Wayne Avenue

Suite 800
Silver Spring, MD 20910
(800) 346-2742 (toll-free)
http://www.naric.com

### National Women's Health Network
514 10th Street NW
Suite 400
Washington, DC 20004
(202) 347-1140
http://www.womenshealthnetwork.org

### Nevus Outreach, Inc.
1601 Madison Blvd.
Bartlesville, OK 74006
(918) 331-0595
http://www.nevus.org

### North American Menopause Society (NAMS)
P.O. Box 94527
Cleveland, OH 44101
(440) 442-7550
www.menopause.org

### North American Society for Pediatric Gastroenterology, Hepatology, and Nutrition
P.O. Box 6
Flourtown, PA 19031
(215) 233-0808
http://www.naspghan.org

### Office of Dietary Supplements
National Institutes of Health
6100 Executive Boulevard
Room 3B01, MSC 7517
Bethesda, MD 20892
(301) 435-2920
http://dietary-supplements.info.nih.gov

### Office of Minority Health Resource Center
P.O. Box 37337
Washington, DC 20013
(800) 444-6472 (toll-free)
http://www.omhrc.gov

### Oley Foundation for Home Parenteral and Enteral Nutrition (HomePEN)
214 Hun Memorial, MC-28
Albany Medical Center
Albany, NY 12208

(800) 776-OLEY (toll-free) or (518) 262-5079
http://www.oley.org

## Organization of Chinese Americans
1001 Connecticut Avenue NW
Suite 601
Washington, DC 20036
(202) 223-5500

## Overeaters Anonymous
6075 Zenith Street NE
Rio Rancho, NM 87124
(505) 891-2664

## Pancreatic Cancer Action Network
2221 Rosecrans Ave.
Suite 131
El Segundo, CA 90245
http://www.pancan.org

## Pediatric/Adolescent Gastroesophageal Reflux Association (PAGER)
P.O. Box 1153
Germantown, MD 20875
(301) 601-9541 (East Coast)
(760) 747-5001 (West Coast)

## Pediatric Crohn's & Colitis Association
P.O. Box 188
Newton, MA 02468
(617) 489-5854
http://www.pcca.hypermart.net

## President's Council on Physical Fitness and Sports
701 Pennsylvania Avenue NW
Suite 250
Washington, DC 20004
(202) 272-3421
http://www.surgeongeneral.gov

## Reach Out for Youth with Ileitis and Colitis, Inc.
84 Northgate Circle
Melville, NY 11747
(631) 293-3102
http://www.reachoutforyouth.org

## Scleroderma Foundation
12 Kent Way, Number 101
Byfield, MA 01922

(800) 722-HOPE or (978) 463-5843 (toll-free)
http://www.scleroderma.org

## Scleroderma Research Foundation
2320 Bath Street
Suite 315
Santa Barbara, CA 93105
(800) 441-2873 (toll-free) or (805) 563-9133
http://www.srfcure.org

## Shape Up America
4500 Connecticut Avenue
Washington, DC 20008
(202) 244-3560
http://www.shapeup.org

## Social Security Administration (SSA)
Office of Public Inquiries
6401 Security Boulevard
Baltimore, MD 21235
(800) 772-1213 (toll-free)
http://www.ssa.gov

## Society for Surgery of the Alimentary Tract
900 Cummings Center
Suite 221-U
Beverly, MA 01915
(978) 927-8330
http://www.ssat.com

## Society for Neuroscience
11 Dupont Circle NW
Suite 500
Washington, DC 20036
(202) 462-6688
http://www.sfn.org

## Society of American Gastrointestinal Endoscopic Surgeons (SAGES)
2716 Ocean Park Boulevard
Suite 3000
Santa Monica, CA 90405
(310) 314-2404
http://www.sages.org

## Society of Gastroenterology Nurses and Associates, Inc. (SGNA)
401 North Michigan Avenue
Chicago, IL 60611

(800) 245-SGNA (toll-free) or (312) 321-5165
http://www.sgna.org

## Substance Abuse and Mental Health Services Administration (SAMHSA)
Department of Health and Human Services
5600 Fishers Lane
Rockville, MD 20857
(800) 729-6686 (toll-free)
(800) 487-4889 (tty)

## TEF-Vater International
15301 Grey Fox Road
Upper Marlboro, MD 20772
(301) 952-6837
http://www.tefvater.org

## Thyroid Foundation of America, Inc.
Ruth Sleeper Hall, Room 350
40 Parkman Street
Boston, MA 02114
(617) 726-8500 or (800) 832-8321 (toll-free)
http://www.tsh.org

## TOPS Club (Take Pounds Off Sensibly)
P.O. Box 07360
Milwaukee, WI 53207
(414) 482-4620

## Transplant Recipient International Organization
1000 Sixteenth Street NW
Washington, DC 10036
(202) 293-0980
http://www.transweb.org

## United Network for Organ Sharing
1100 Boulders Parkway
Suite 500
P.O. Box 13770
Richmond, VA 23225
(804) 330-8500
http://www.unos.org

## United Ostomy Association, Inc.
19772 MacArthur Boulevard
Suite 200

Irvine, CA 92612
(800) 826-0826 (toll-free) or (949) 660-8624
http://www.wocn.org

## United States Department of Agriculture
Food Safety and Inspection Service
1400 Independence Avenue SW, Room 2932-S
Washington, DC 20250
(800) 256-7072 (toll-free)
http://www.fsis.usda.gov

## Veterans Health Administration
810 Vermont Avenue NW
Washington, DC 20420
(202) 273-8490

## Weight-Control Information Network (WIN)
1 WIN Way
Bethesda, MD 20892
(877) 946-4627 (toll-free)
http://www.niddk.nih.gov/health/nutrit/nutrit.htm

## Weight Watchers International
175 Crossways Park West
Woodbury, NY 11797
(800) 651-6000 (toll-free)

## Wilson's Disease Association
1802 Brookside Drive
Wooster, OH 44691
(800) 399-0266 (toll-free)
http://www.wilsonsdisease.org

## WHO Headquarters
Avenue Appia 20
1211 Geneva 27
Switzerland
+ 41 22 791 21 11
http://www.who.int

## Wound, Ostomy, and Continence Nurses Society
4700 West Lake Avenue
Glenview, IL 60025
(888) 224-9626 (toll-free)

# APPENDIX II
## STATE HEALTH DEPARTMENTS IN THE UNITED STATES

### ALABAMA

**Alabama Department of Public Health**
RSA Tower
201 Monroe Street
Suite 914
Montgomery, AL 36104
(334) 206-5300
http://www.adph.org

### ALASKA

**Department of Health and Social Services**
350 Main Street, Room 229
P.O. Box 110601
Juneau, AK 99811
(907) 465-3030
http://www.hss.state.ak.us

### ARIZONA

**Arizona Department of Health Services**
1740 West Adams
Phoenix, AZ 85007
(602) 542-1001
http://www.hs.state.az.us

### ARKANSAS

**Arkansas Department of Public Health**
4815 West Markham Street, Slot Y
Little Rock, AR 72205
(501) 661-2392
http://www.healthyarkansas.com

### CALIFORNIA

**California Department of Health Services**
P.O. Box 942732
Sacramento, CA 94234
(916) 445-4171

### COLORADO

**Colorado Department of Public Health and Environment**
4300 Cherry Creek Drive South
Denver, CO 80246
(303) 692-2035
http://www.cdphe.state.co.us

### CONNECTICUT

**Connecticut Department of Public Health**
410 Capitol Avenue
P.O. Box 340308
Hartford, CT 06134
(860) 609-8000

### DELAWARE

**Delaware Department of Health and Social Services**
Division of Public Health
1901 North DuPont Highway, Main Building
New Castle, DE 19720
(302) 255-9040
http://wwww.state.de.us/dhss/dph/index.htm

### DISTRICT OF COLUMBIA

**Department of Health**
825 North Capitol Street, NE
Washington, DC 20002
(202) 442-5999
http://schealth.dc.gov

### FLORIDA

**Florida Department of Health**
4052 Bald Cypress Way, Bin A07
Tallahassee, FL 32399
(850) 245-4245
http://apps3.doh.state.fl.us/IRM/DOHContacts

## GEORGIA

**Georgia Department of Human Resources**
Division of Public Health
2 Peachtree Street NW
Atlanta, GA 30303
(404) 657-2700
http://www.ph.dhr.state.ga.us

## HAWAII

**Hawaii State Department of Health**
1250 Punchbowl Street
Honolulu, HI 96813
(808) 586-4400

## IDAHO

**Idaho Department of Health & Welfare**
450 West State Street, Tenth Floor
Boise, ID 83720
(208) 334-5500
http://www2.state.id.us/dhw/index.htm

## ILLINOIS

**Illinois Department of Public Health**
535 West Jefferson Street
Springfield, IL 62761
(217) 782-4977
http://www.idph.state.il.us

## INDIANA

**Indiana State Department of Health**
2 North Meridian Street
Indianapolis, IN 46204
(317) 233-7424
http://www.state.in.us

## IOWA

**Iowa Department of Public Health**
Lucas State Office Building
Des Moines, IA 50319
(515) 281-5787
http://www.idph.state.ia.us

## KANSAS

**Kansas Department of Health and Environment**
Charles Curtis State Office Building
1000 Southwest Jackson
Topeka, KS 66612
(785) 296-1500
http://www.kdhe.state.ks.us

## KENTUCKY

**Kentucky Cabinet for Health Services, Department for Public Health**
275 East Main Street
Frankfort, KY 40621
(502) 564-3970
http://chs.state.ky.us

## LOUISIANA

**Louisiana Department of Health and Hospitals**
1201 Capitol Access Road
P.O. Box 629
Baton Rouge, LA 70821
(225) 342-9500
http://www.dhh.state.la.us

## MAINE

**Department of Human Services**
Maine Bureau of Health
11 State House Station
Key Plaza
286 Water Street
Augusta, ME 04333
(207) 287-8016
http://www.state.me.us/dhs

## MARYLAND

**Maryland Department of Health and Mental Hygiene**
201 West Preston Street
Suite 400
Baltimore, MD 21201
(410) 767-4055
http://www.dhmh.state.md.us

## MASSACHUSETTS

**Department of Public Health**
250 Washington Street
Boston, MA 02108
(617) 624-6000
http://www.state.ma.us/dph/dphhome.htm

## MICHIGAN

**Michigan Department of Community Health**
Lewis Cass Building, Sixth Floor
320 South Walnut Street
Lansing, MI 48913
(517) 373-3500

## MINNESOTA

**Minnesota Department of Health**
85 East Seventh Place
St. Paul, MN 55101
(651) 215-5800
http://www.health.state.mn.us

## MISSISSIPPI

**Mississippi State Department of Health**
570 East Woodrow Wilson Drive
Jackson, MS 39216
(601) 576-7400
http://www.msdh.state.ms.us/msdhssite

## MISSOURI

**Missouri Department of Health and Senior Services**
P.O. Box 570
Jefferson City, MO 65102
(573) 751-6400
http://www.health.state.mo.us

## MONTANA

**Department of Public Health & Human Services**
111 North Sanders
Helena, MT 59620
(406) 444-5622
http://www.dphhs.state.mt.us

## NEBRASKA

**Nebraska Health and Human Services**
P.O. Box 95044
Lincoln, NE 68509
(402) 471-2306
http://www.hhs.state.ne.us

## NEVADA

**Nevada Health Division**
505 East King Street
Suite 201
Carson City, NV 89701
(775) 684-4200

## NEW HAMPSHIRE

**New Hampshire Department of Health and Human Services**
Office of Community and Public Health
6 Hazen Drive
Concord, NH 03301
(603) 271-5926

## NEW JERSEY

**Department of Health and Senior Services**
P.O. Box 360
Trenton, NJ 08625
(609) 588-3500
http://www.state.nj.us/health

## NEW MEXICO

**New Mexico Department of Health**
1190 South Saint Francis Drive
P.O. Box 26110
Santa Fe, NM 87502
(505) 827-2613
http://www.health.state.nm.us

## NEW YORK

**New York State Department of Health**
Corning Tower
Empire State Plaza
Albany, NY 12237
http://www.health.state.ny.us

## NORTH CAROLINA

**Division of Public Health**
North Carolina Department of Health and Human Services
1915 Mail Service Center
Raleigh, NC 27699
(919) 733-7081
http://www.dhhs.state.nc.us/dph

## NORTH DAKOTA

**North Dakota Department of Health**
Health Resources Section
600 East Boulevard Avenue
Bismarck, ND 58505
(701) 328-2352
http://www.health.state.nd.us/ndhd

## OHIO

**Ohio Department of Health**
246 North Main Street
Columbus, OH 43216
http://www.odh.state.oh.us

### OKLAHOMA

**Oklahoma State Department of Health**
1000 Northeast Tenth Street
Oklahoma City, OK 73117
(405) 271-5600
http://www.health.state.ok.us

### OREGON

**Oregon Public Health Services**
800 NE Oregon Street
Portland, OR 97232
(503) 731-4000

### PENNSYLVANIA

**Pennsylvania Department of Health**
555 Walnut Street, 6th Floor
Harrisburg, PA 17101
(717) 783-2548
http://www.health.state.pa.us

### RHODE ISLAND

**Rhode Island Department of Health**
3 Capitol Hill
Providence, RI 02908
(401) 222-2231
http://www.health.state.ri.us

### SOUTH CAROLINA

**Department of Health and Human Service**
P.O. Box 8206
Columbia, SC 29202
(803) 898-2500

### SOUTH DAKOTA

**South Dakota Department of Health**
600 E. Capitol
Pierre, SD 57501
(605) 773-3361
http://www.state.sd.us/doh/index.htm

### TENNESSEE

**Tennessee Department of Health**
425 Fifth Avenue North
Cordell Hull Building, Third Floor
Nashville, TN 37247
(615) 741-3111
http://www2.state.tn.us/health

### TEXAS

**Texas Department of Health**
1100 West 49th Street
Austin, TX 78756
(512) 458-7111
http://www.tdh.state.tx.us

### UTAH

**Utah Department of Health**
P.O. Box 1010
Salt Lake City, UT 84114
(801) 538-6101
http://health.utah.gov

### VERMONT

**Vermont Department of Health**
108 Cherry Street
P.O. Box 70
Burlington, VT 05402
(802) 863-7200
http://www.healthyvermonters.info

### VIRGINIA

**Virginia Department of Health**
P.O. Box 2448
Richmond, VA 23218
(804) 786-1668
http://www.vdh.state.va.us

### WASHINGTON

**Department of Health**
1112 SE Quince Street
P.O. Box 47890
Olympia, WA 98504
(360) 236-3676
http://www.doh.wa.gov

### WEST VIRGINIA

**West Virginia Department of Health and Human Resources**
Bureau of Public Health
350 Capitol Street
Charleston, WV 25301
(304) 558-6421
http://www.wvdhr.org

**WISCONSIN**

**Department of Health and Family Services**
1 West Wilson Street
Madison, WI 53702
(608) 266-1865
www.dhfs.state.wi.us

**WYOMING**

**Wyoming Department of Health**
6101 Yellowstone Road
Cheyenne, WY 82002
(307) 777-3477
http:wdhfs.state.wy.us

# APPENDIX III
# IMPORTANT HEALTH ORGANIZATIONS IN CANADA

**Canadian Cancer Society**
National Office
10 Alcorn Avenue
Suite 200
Toronto, Ontario
M4V 3B1
(416) 961-7223
www.cancer.ca

**Canadian Celiac Association**
5170 Dixie Road
Suite 204
Mississauga, Ontario
L4W 1E3
(905) 507-6208
www.celiac.ca

**Canadian Cystic Fibrosis Foundation**
2221 Yonge Street
Suite 601
Toronto, Ontario
M4S 2B4
(416) 485-9149
http://www.cysticfibrosis.ca

**Canadian Diabetes Association**
National Office
15 Toronto Street
Suite 800
Toronto, Ontario
M5C 2E3
(800) BANTING (toll-free) or (416) 363-3373
http://www.diabetes.ca

**Canadian Liver Foundation**
2235 Sheppard Avenue East
Suite 1500
Toronto, Ontario
M2J 5B5
(416) 491-3353
http://www.liver.ca

**Canadian MedicAlert Foundation**
2005 Sheppard Avenue East
Suite 800
Toronto, Ontario
M2J 5B4
(800) 668-1507 (English) (toll-free)
(800) 668-6381 (French)

**Health Canada**
Brooke Claxton Building, Tunney's Pasture
P.L. 0906C
Ottawa, Ontario
K1A 0K9
(613) 957-2991
http://www.hc-sc.gc.ca/english

**Heart and Stroke Foundation of Canada**
222 Queen Street
Suite 1402
Ottawa, Ontario
K1P 5V9
(613) 569-4361
http://ww2.heartandstroke.ca

# APPENDIX IV
## GOVERNMENT HEALTH AGENCIES IN CANADA

Each province or territory in Canada manages its own health agency. The following is a list of government health agencies throughout Canada.

### ALBERTA

**Alberta Health Insurance Plan**
P.O. Box 1360
Edmonton, Alberta
T5J 2N3
(780) 427-1432
http://www.health.gov.ab.ca/talk/index.htm

### BRITISH COLUMBIA

**Ministry Office**
P.O. Box 9050 Stn. Provincial Government
Victoria, British Columbia
V8W 9E2
(250) 952-3456

### MANITOBA

**Manitoba Health**
300 Carlton Street
Winnipeg, Manitoba
R3B 3M9
(800) 392-1207 (toll-free) or (204) 786-7101

### NEW BRUNSWICK

**Department of Health and Wellness**
P.O. Box 5100
Fredericton, New Brunswick
E3B 5G8
(506) 453-2536
http://www.gnb.ca/0051/contacts-e.asp

### NEWFOUNDLAND

**Newfoundland Medical Care Plan**
P.O. Box 5000
20 High Street

Grand Falls-Windsor, Newfoundland
A2A 2Y4
(709) 292-4000

### NORTHWEST TERRITORIES

**Department of Health and Social Services**
Government of the Northwest Territories
Box 1320
Yellowknife, NT
Z1A 2L9
(867) 920-6173
http://www.hlthss.tov.nt.ca/Content/contact.htm

### NOVA SCOTIA

**Department of Health**
P.O. Box 488
Halifax, NS
B3J 2R8
(902) 424-3377
http://www.gov.ns.ca/heal/about.htm

### NUNAVUT

**Nunavik Regional Board of Health and Social Services**
C.P. 9000
Kuujjuaq (Quebec) JOM ICO
(819) 964-2222
http://www.rrsss17.gouv.qc.ca/en/main/aspx

### ONTARIO

**Ontario Ministry of Health and Long-Term Care**
80 Grosvenor Street, 11th Floor
Toronto, Ontario
M7A 1S2
(800) 268-1154 (toll-free) or (416) 314-5518
http://www.gov.on.ca/health/english/tools/
feedback.html

**PRINCE EDWARD ISLAND**

**Health and Social Services**
Jones Building, Second Floor
11 Kent Street
P.O. Box 2000
Charlottetown, PE
C1A 7N8
(902) 368-4900

**SASKATCHEWAN**

**Saskatchewan Health**
3475 Albert Street

Regina, Saskatchewan
S4S 6X6
(306) 787-3251

**YUKON**

**Health and Social Services**
Government of Yukon
Box 2703
Whitehorse, Yukon
Y1A 2C6
(867) 667-3673
http://www.hss.gov.yk.ca

# APPENDIX V
## POISON CONTROL CENTERS IN THE UNITED STATES

Individuals in the United States can call a nationwide toll-free number to be routed to their nearest poison control center. They may also call the poison control center number directly. Note: the poison control center number is usually included in the inside front of the telephone directory. Individuals can also call their local emergency number for immediate assistance. The emergency phone number for all centers is 800-222-1222. Some centers have TDD or TYY lines, and if so, those numbers are included.

### ALABAMA

**Alabama Poison Center**
2503 Phoenix Drive
Tuscaloosa, AL 35405
http://www.alapoisoncenter.org

**Regional Poison Control Center**
Children's Hospital
1600 Seventh Avenue South
Birmingham, AL 35233
http://www.chsys.org

### ARIZONA

**Arizona Poison & Drug Info Center**
Arizona Health Sciences Center, Room 1156
1501 North Campbell Avenue
Tucson, AZ 85724
http://www.pharmacy.arizona.edu/centers/apdic/
apdic.html

### ARKANSAS

**Arkansas Poison & Drug Information Center**
College of Pharmacy, University of Arkansas for
Medical Sciences
4301 West Markham, Mail Slot 522-2
Little Rock, AR 72205
(800) 641-3805 (TDD/TYY)

### CALIFORNIA

**California Poison Control System, Fresno/
Madera Division**
Children's Hospital Central California
9300 Valley Children's Place, MB 15
Madera, CA 93638
Poison Action Line: (800) 876-4766
(800) 972-3323 (TDD/TYY)
http://www.calpoison.org

**California Poison Control System,
Sacramento Division**
University of California Davis Medical Center
2315 Stockton Boulevard
Sacramento, CA 95817
(800) 972-3323 (TDD/TYY)
http://www.calpoison.org

**California Poison Control System, San
Francisco Division**
University of California, San Francisco
UCSF Box 1369
San Francisco, CA 94143
(800) 972-3323 (TDD/TYY)
http://www.calpoison.org

**California Poison Control System, San Diego
Division**
University of California, San Diego Medical Center
200 West Arbor Drive
San Diego, CA 92103
(800) 972-3323 (TDD/TYY)
http://www.calpoison.org

### COLORADO

**Rocky Mountain Poison & Drug Center**
1001 Yosemite Street
Suite 200
Denver, CO 80230
(303) 739-1127 (TDD/TYY)
http://www.RMPDC.org

## CONNECTICUT

**Connecticut Poison Control Center**
University of Connecticut Health Center
263 Farmington Avenue
Farmington, CT 06030
(866) 218-5372 (TTY/TDD)
http://poisoncontrol.uchc.edu

## DISTRICT OF COLUMBIA

**National Capital Poison Center**
3201 New Mexico Avenue, NW
Suite 310
Washington, DC 20016
http://www.poison.org

## FLORIDA

**Florida Poison Information Center, Jacksonville**
655 West Eighth Street
Jacksonville, FL 32209
http://www.fpicn.org

**Florida Poison Information Center, Miami**
University of Miami, Department of Pediatrics
P.O. Box 016960, Room 131
Miami, FL 33101
http://www.fpicn.org

**Florida Poison Information Center, Tampa**
Tampa General Hospital
P.O. Box 1289
Tampa, FL 33601
http://www.fpicn.org

## GEORGIA

**Georgia Poison Center**
Hughes Spalding Children's Hospital
Grady Health System
80 Jesse Hill Jr. Drive Southeast
P.O. Box 26066
Atlanta, GA 30303
(404) 616-9287 (TDD/TYY)
http://www.georgiapoisoncenter.org

## ILLINOIS

**Illinois Poison Center**
222 South Riverside Plaza
Suite 1900
Chicago, IL 60606
(312) 906-6185 (TDD/TYY)
http://www.mchc.org/ipc

## INDIANA

**Indiana Poison Center**
Methodist Hospital
Clarian Health Partners
1-65 at 21st Street
Indianapolis, IN 46206
(317) 962-2336 (TDD/TYY)
http://www.clarian.org/clinical/poisoncontrol

## IOWA

**Iowa Statewide Poison Control Center**
St. Luke's Regional Medical Center
2720 Stone Park Boulevard
Sioux City, IA 51104
http://www.iowapoison.org

## KANSAS

**Mid-America Poison Control Center**
University of Kansas Medical Center
3901 Rainbow Boulevard, Room B-400
Kansas City, KS 66160
(913) 588-6639 (TDD/TYY)

## KENTUCKY

**Kentucky Regional Poison Center**
Medical Towers South
Suite 847
234 East Gray Street
Louisville, KY 40202
http://www.krpc.com

## LOUISIANA

**Louisiana Drug and Poison Information Center**
University of Louisiana at Monroe
College of Pharmacy, Sugar Hall
Monroe, LA 71209
http://www.lapcc.org

## MAINE

**Northern New England Poison Center**
22 Bramhall Street
Portland, ME 04102
(877) 299-4447 (TDD/TYY)

## MARYLAND

**Maryland Poison Center**
University of Maryland at Baltimore

School of Pharmacy
20 North Pine Street, PH 772
Baltimore, MD 21201
(410) 706-1858 (TDD/TYY)
http://www.pharmacy.umaryland/edu/~mpc/

## MASSACHUSETTS

**Regional Center for Poison Control and Prevention Serving Massachusetts and Rhode Island**
300 Longwood Avenue
Boston, MA 02115
(888) 244-5313 (TDD/TYY)
http://maripoisoncenter.com

## MICHIGAN

**Children's Hospital of Michigan**
Regional Poison Control Center
4160 John R. Harper Professional Office Building
Suite 616
Detroit, MI 48201
(800) 356-3232 (TDD/TYY)
http://www.mitoxic.org

**DeVos Children's Hospital Regional Poison Center**
1300 Michigan NE
Suite 203
Grand Rapids, MI 49503
http://www.spectrum-health.org

## MINNESOTA

**Hennepin Regional Poison Center**
Hennepin County Medical Center
701 Park Avenue
Minneapolis, MN 55415
http://www.mnpoison.org

## MISSISSIPPI

**Mississippi Regional Poison Control Center**
University of Mississippi Medical Center
2500 North State Street
Jackson, MS 39216

## MISSOURI

**Missouri Regional Poison Center**
7980 Clayton Road
Suite 200

St. Louis, MO 63117
(314) 612-5705 (TDD/TYY)

## NEBRASKA

**The Poison Center**
Children's Hospital
8200 Dodge Street
Omaha, NE 68114
http://www.Poison-Center.org

## NEW HAMPSHIRE

**New Hampshire Poison Information Center**
Dartmouth-Hitchcock Medical Center
One Medical Center Drive
Lebanon, NH 03756
http://www.hitchcock.org

## NEW JERSEY

**New Jersey Poison Information and Education System**
65 Bergen Street
Newark, NJ 07107
800-222-1222
http://www.njpies.org

## NEW MEXICO

**New Mexico Poison & Drug Info Center**
MSC 09 5080
University of New Mexico
Albuquerque, NM 87131
http://hsc.unm.edu/pharmacy/poison

## NEW YORK

**Central New York Poison Center**
750 East Adams Street
Syracuse, NY 13210
http://www.cnypoison.org

**Finger Lakes Regional Poison & Drug Information Center**
University of Rochester Medical Center
601 Elmwood Avenue, Box 321
Rochester, NY 14642
(585) 273-3854 (TDD/TYY)
http://www.stronghealth.com/services/poison

**Long Island Regional Poison and Drug Information Center**
Winthrop University Hospital

259 First Street
Mineola, NY 11501
http://www.lirpdic.org

**New York City Poison Control Center**
New York City Department of Health
455 First Avenue, Room 123
P.O. Box 81
New York, NY 10016
(212) 688-9014 (TDD/TYY)
http://www.nyc.gov/health

**Western New York Poison Center**
Children's Hospital of Buffalo
219 Bryant Street
Buffalo, NY 14222
http://www.chob.edu/poison

### NORTH CAROLINA

**Carolinas Poison Center**
Carolinas Regional Medical Center
5000 Airport Center Parkway
Suite B
Charlotte, NC 28208
http://www.carolinas.org/services/poison

### OHIO

**Central Ohio Poison Center**
700 Children's Drive, Room L032
Columbus, OH 43205
(614) 228-2272 (TDD/TYY)
http://www.bepoisonsmart.com

**Cincinnati Drug & Poison Information Center**
3333 Burnet Avenue
Vernon Place, Third Floor
Cincinnati, OH 45229
http://www.cincinnatichildrens.org/dpic

**Greater Cleveland Poison Control Center**
11100 Euclid Avenue
Cleveland, OH 44106

### OKLAHOMA

**Oklahoma Poison Control Center**
Children's Hospital at Oklahoma University
    Medical Center
940 Northeast 13th Street, Room 3510
Oklahoma City, OK 73104
http://www.oklahomapoison.org

### OREGON

**Oregon Poison Center**
Oregon Health Sciences University
3181 Southwest San Jackson Park Road, CB550
Portland, OR 97201
http://www.oregonpoison.org

### PENNSYLVANIA

**Penn State Poison Center**
Pennsylvania State University
The Milton S. Hershey Medical Center
500 University Drive
MC H043
P.O. Box 850
Hershey, PA 17033
(717) 531-8335 (TDD/TYY)
http://www.pennstatepoisoncenter.com

**Pittsburgh Poison Center**
Children's Hospital of Pittsburgh
3705 Fifth Avenue
Pittsburgh, PA 15213
http://chp.edu/clinical/03a_poison.php

**Poison Control Center**
Children's Hospital of Philadelphia
34th and Civic Center Boulevard
Philadelphia, PA 19104
(215) 590-8789 (TDD/TYY)
http://poisoncontrol.chop.edu

### SOUTH CAROLINA

**Palmetto Poison Center**
College of Pharmacy
University of South Carolina
Columbia, SC 29208
http://www.pharmsc.edu/pps/pps.htm

### TENNESSEE

**Middle Tennessee Poison Center**
501 Oxford House
1161 21st Avenue South
Nashville, TN 37232
(615) 936-2047 (TDD/TYY)
http://www.poisonlifeline.org

**Southern Poison Center**
University of Tennessee
875 Monroe Avenue

Suite 104
Memphis, TN 38163

## TEXAS

**Central Texas Poison Center**
Scott and White Memorial Hospital
2401 South 31st Street
Temple, TX 76508
http://www.poisoncontrol.org

**North Texas Poison Center**
Texas Poison Center Network
Parkland Health and Hospital System
5201 Harry Hines Boulevard
Dallas, TX 75235

**Southeast Texas Poison Center**
The University of Texas Medical Branch
3112 Trauma Building
Galveston, TX 77555
(800) 764-7661 (TDD/TYY)
http://www.utmb.edu/setpc

**South Texas Poison Center**
The University of Texas Health Science Center, San Antonio
Department of Surgery, Mail Code 7849
7703 Floyd Curl Drive
San Antonio, TX 78229
http://www.uthscsa.edu/surgery/poisoncenter

**Texas Panhandle Poison Center**
1501 South Coulter
Amarillo, TX 79106
http://www.panhandlepoison.org

**West Texas Regional Poison Center**
Thomason Hospital
4815 Alameda Venue
El Paso, TX 79905
http://www.poisoncenter.org

## UTAH

**Utah Poison Control Center**
410 Chipeta Way
Suite 230
Salt Lake City, UT 84108
http://uuhsc.utah.edu/poison

## VIRGINIA

**Blue Ridge Poison Center**
1222 Jefferson Park Avenue
P.O. Box 800774
Charlottesville, VA 22903
http://hsc.virginia.edu/brpc

**Virginia Poison Center**
Medical College of Virginia Hospitals
Virginia Commonwealth University Health System
P.O. Box 980522
Richmond, VA 23298
http://www.vcu.edu/mcved

## WASHINGTON

**Washington Poison Center**
155 Northeast 100th Street
Suite 400
Seattle, WA 98125
(800) 572-0638 (TDD/TYY) (Washington state only)

## WEST VIRGINIA

**West Virginia Poison Center**
3110 MacCorkle Avenue Southeast
Charleston, WV 25304
(304) 388-9698 (TDD/TYY)

## WISCONSIN

**Children's Hospital of Wisconsin Poison Center**
P.O. Box 1997 Mail Station 677 A
Milwaukee, WI 53201
(414) 266-2542 (TDD/TYY)
http://www.chw.org/Emergency/emergency.htm

# APPENDIX VI
## EMERGENCY POISON CENTERS IN CANADA

This listing includes the key emergency poison information centers in Canada, by province.

### ALBERTA

**Poison and Drug Information Service**
Foothills Medical Centre
1403 29th Street, Northwest
Calgary, Alberta
T2N 2T9
(800) 332-1414 (emergency phone Alberta only)

### BRITISH COLUMBIA

**British Columbia Drug & Poison Information Centre**
1081 Burrard Street
Vancouver, British Columbia
V6Z 1Y6
(800) 567-8911 (Emergency Phone)

### NOVA SCOTIA

**IWK Regional Poison Centre**
IWK Health Centre
5850 University Avenue
P.O. Box 3070
Halifax, Nova Scotia
B3J 3G0
(800) 565-8161 (Emergency Phone)

### ONTARIO

**Ontario Regional Poison Centre**
Children's Hospital of Eastern Ontario
401 Smyth Road
Ottawa, Ontario
K1H 8LI
(800) 267-1373 (Emergency Phone)

### QUEBEC

**Quebec Poison Control Center**
Aile "L" 1er etage
1050 Chemin Sainte-Foy
Quebec
G1S 4L8
(800) 463-5060 (Emergency Phone)

# APPENDIX VII

## PERCENTAGES AND FREQUENCIES OF SELECTED DISEASES AND CONDITIONS AMONG PERSONS 18 YEARS OF AGE AND OLDER, IN THE UNITED STATES

FREQUENCIES OF SELECTED DISEASES AND CONDITIONS AMONG PERSONS 18 YEARS OF AGE AND OLDER, BY SELECTED CHARACTERISTICS: UNITED STATES, 1997

| Selected Characteristic | All Persons 18 Years of Age and Older | Diabetes[1] | Ulcers[1] | Liver Disease[2] |
|---|---|---|---|---|
| | Number in thousands[2] | | | |
| Total | 195,276 | 10,031 | 17,698 | 1,795 |
| **Sex** | | | | |
| Male | 93,680 | 4,528 | 8,882 | 975 |
| Female | 101,596 | 5,503 | 8,816 | 819 |
| **Age** | | | | |
| 18–44 years | 108,391 | 1,650 | 6,910 | 699 |
| 45–64 years | 54,878 | 4,181 | 6,261 | 697 |
| 65–74 years | 18,170 | 2,587 | 2,548 | 286 |
| 75 years and older | 13,837 | 1,613 | 1,979 | 113 |
| **Race and ethnicity[3]** | | | | |
| White non-Hispanic | 146,613 | 6,800 | 14,264 | 1,353 |
| Black non-Hispanic | 21,719 | 1,793 | 1,829 | 173 |
| Other non-Hispanic | 7,677 | 342 | 491 | 69 |
| Hispanic | 19,267 | 1,097 | 1,113 | 200 |
| **Poverty status[4]** | | | | |
| Poor | 19,915 | 1,473 | 2,183 | 399 |
| Near poor | 29,968 | 2,037 | 3,296 | 394 |
| Not poor | 109,832 | 4,309 | 9,659 | 750 |
| **Region** | | | | |
| Northeast | 39,518 | 2,167 | 2,799 | 329 |
| Midwest | 49,249 | 2,308 | 4,505 | 425 |
| South | 69,408 | 3,937 | 7,249 | 661 |
| West | 37,101 | 1,619 | 3,144 | 381 |
| **Sex and age** | Number in thousands[2] | | | |
| Male: | | | | |
| 18–44 years | 53,653 | 786 | 3,281 | 413 |
| 45–64 years | 26,556 | 2,013 | 3,347 | 416 |
| 65 years and older | 13,471 | 1,729 | 2,254 | 146 |
| Female: | | | | |
| 18–44 years | 54,738 | 863 | 3,629 | 286 |
| 45–64 years | 28,322 | 2,168 | 2,914 | 281 |
| 65 years and older | 18,536 | 2,471 | 2,273 | 252 |

*(continues)*

**FREQUENCIES OF SELECTED DISEASES AND CONDITIONS AMONG PERSONS 18 YEARS OF AGE AND OLDER, BY SELECTED CHARACTERISTICS: UNITED STATES, 1997** *(continued)*

| Selected Characteristic | All Persons 18 Years of Age and Older | Diabetes[1] | Ulcers[1] | Liver Disease[2] |
|---|---|---|---|---|
| Race, ethnicity, and age | Number in thousands[2] | | | |
| White non-Hispanic: | | | | |
| 18–44 years | 76,344 | 1,032 | 5,382 | 489 |
| 45–64 years | 43,072 | 2,634 | 4,977 | 548 |
| 65 years and older | 27,197 | 3,134 | 3,905 | 315 |
| Black non-Hispanic: | | | | |
| 18–44 years | 13,642 | 350 | 795 | 58 |
| 45–64 years | 5,503 | 836 | 720 | 74 |
| 65 years and older | 2,574 | 606 | 315 | 41 |
| Other non-Hispanic: | | | | |
| 18–44 years | 4,941 | 50 | 184 | 46 |
| 45–64 years | 2,143 | 199 | 219 | 18 |
| 65 years and older | 594 | 93 | 88 | 5 |
| Hispanic: | | | | |
| 18–44 years | 13,464 | 217 | 548 | 106 |
| 45–64 years | 4,159 | 513 | 346 | 57 |
| 65 years and older | 1,643 | 367 | 219 | 37 |
| Race, ethnicity, sex, and age | | | | |
| White non-Hispanic male: | | | | |
| 18–44 years | 38,086 | 492 | 2,564 | 310 |
| 45–64 years | 20,911 | 1,310 | 2,666 | 317 |
| 65 years and older | 11,514 | 1,335 | 1,933 | 126 |
| White non-Hispanic female: | | | | |
| 18–44 years | 38,259 | 540 | 2,819 | 179 |
| 45–64 years | 22,161 | 1,324 | 2,311 | 231 |
| 65 years and older | 15,683 | 1,799 | 1,972 | 189 |
| Black non-Hispanic male: | | | | |
| 18–44 years | 6,195 | 160 | 382 | 16 |
| 45–64 years | 2,435 | 357 | 373 | 62 |
| 65 years and older | 1,013 | 216 | 168 | 11 |
| Black non-Hispanic female: | | | | |
| 18–44 years | 7,447 | 190 | 413 | 42 |
| 45–64 years | 3,069 | 479 | 346 | 12 |
| 65 years and older | 1,561 | 391 | 147 | 31 |
| Hispanic male: | | | | |
| 18–44 years | 7,104 | 110 | 253 | 77 |
| 45–64 years | 2,017 | 262 | 141 | 23 |
| 65 years and older | 695 | 139 | 89 | 7 |
| Hispanic female: | | | | |
| 18–44 years | 6,360 | 107 | 296 | 29 |
| 45–64 years | 2,143 | 252 | 205 | 35 |
| 65 years and older | 949 | 228 | 130 | 29 |
| Poverty status and age | Number in thousands[2] | | | |
| Poor: | | | | |
| 18–44 years | 12,982 | 307 | 1,011 | 172 |
| 45–64 years | 4,050 | 652 | 758 | 140 |
| 65 years and older | 2,883 | 514 | 414 | 87 |
| Near poor: | | | | |
| 18–44 years | 17,370 | 318 | 1,301 | 132 |
| 45–64 years | 5,700 | 693 | 811 | 144 |
| 65 years and older | 6,898 | 1,025 | 1,183 | 118 |

| Selected Characteristic | All Persons 18 Years of Age and Older | Diabetes[1] | Ulcers[1] | Liver Disease[2] |
|---|---|---|---|---|
| Poverty status and age | Number in thousands[2] | | | |
| Not poor: | | | | |
| 18–44 years | 61,464 | 749 | 3,801 | 297 |
| 45–64 years | 34,531 | 1,983 | 3,848 | 332 |
| 65 years and older | 13,838 | 1,577 | 2,010 | 120 |

[1]In separate questions, respondents were asked whether they had ever been told by a doctor or other health professional that they had an ulcer (including a stomach, duodenal, or peptic ulcer) or diabetes (or sugar diabetes; female respondents were instructed to exclude pregnancy-related diabetes). Persons who said they had borderline diabetes were considered unknown with respect to diabetes. Persons may be represented in more than one column.

[2]Unknowns for the variable of interest are not included in the denominators when calculating percentages; nor are they shown in the frequencies. They are, however, included in the "All persons" column. Numbers may also be rounded.

[3]*Other non-Hispanic* includes non-Hispanic persons who identified their race as American Indian, Alaska Native, Asian, or Pacific Islander. These categories are too small to show separately. Persons of Hispanic origin may be of any race.

[4]Poverty status is based on family income and family size using U.S. Census Bureau's poverty thresholds. *Poor* persons are defined as below the poverty threshold. *Near poor* persons have income of 100 percent to less than 200 percent of the poverty threshold. *Not poor* persons have income 200 percent or greater than the poverty threshold.

## PERCENTAGES (WITH STANDARD ERRORS) OF SELECTED DISEASES AND CONDITIONS AMONG PERSONS 18 YEARS OF AGE AND OLDER, BY SELECTED CHARACTERISTICS: UNITED STATES, 1997

| Selected Characteristic | Diabetes[1] | Ulcers[1] | Liver Disease[2] |
|---|---|---|---|
| | Percentage[2] (Standard Error) | | |
| Total | 5.2 (0.14) | 9.1 (0.20) | 0.9 (0.06) |
| **Sex** | | | |
| Male | 4.9 (0.20) | 9.5 (0.28) | 1.0 (0.09) |
| Female | 5.5 (0.20) | 8.7 (0.23) | 0.8 (0.07) |
| **Age** | | | |
| 18–44 years | 1.5 (0.10) | 6.4 (0.21) | 0.7 (0.06) |
| 45–64 years | 7.8 (0.32) | 11.5 (0.38) | 1.3 (0.13) |
| 65–74 years | 14.7 (0.74) | 14.1 (0.68) | 1.6 (0.23) |
| 75 years and older | 12.0 (0.68) | 14.4 (0.76) | 0.8 (0.17) |
| **Race and ethnicity[3]** | | | |
| White non-Hispanic | 4.7 (0.15) | 9.8 (0.24) | 0.9 (0.07) |
| Black non-Hispanic | 8.4 (0.52) | 8.4 (0.48) | 0.8 (0.14) |
| Other non-Hispanic | 4.5 (0.64) | 6.4 (0.85) | *0.9 (0.29) |
| Hispanic | 5.8 (0.45) | 5.8 (0.38) | 1.0 (0.15) |
| **Poverty status[4]** | | | |
| Poor | 7.6 (0.46) | 11.0 (0.54) | 2.0 (0.23) |
| Near poor | 6.9 (0.37) | 11.0 (0.48) | 1.3 (0.17) |
| Not poor | 4.0 (0.17) | 8.8 (0.26) | 0.7 (0.07) |
| **Region** | | | |
| Northeast | 5.6 (0.30) | 7.1 (0.34) | 0.8 (0.13) |
| Midwest | 4.8 (0.27) | 9.2 (0.42) | 0.9 (0.10) |
| South | 5.8 (0.27) | 10.5 (0.38) | 1.0 (0.10) |
| West | 4.4 (0.29) | 8.5 (0.35) | 1.0 (0.13) |

*(continues)*

**PERCENTAGES (WITH STANDARD ERRORS) OF SELECTED DISEASES AND CONDITIONS AMONG PERSONS
18 YEARS OF AGE AND OLDER, BY SELECTED CHARACTERISTICS: UNITED STATES, 1997** *(continued)*

| Selected Characteristic | Diabetes[1] | Ulcers[1] | Liver Disease[2] |
|---|---|---|---|
| | Percentage[2] (Standard Error) | | |
| **Sex and age** | | | |
| Male: | | | |
| 18–44 years | 1.5 (0.15) | 6.1 (0.30) | 0.8 (0.10) |
| 45–64 years | 7.7 (0.47) | 12.7 (0.56) | 1.6 (0.21) |
| 65 years and older | 13.3 (0.82) | 16.8 (0.87) | 1.1 (0.22) |
| Female: | | | |
| 18–44 years | 1.6 (0.14) | 6.6 (0.28) | 0.5 (0.08) |
| 45–64 years | 7.8 (0.41) | 10.3 (0.46) | 1.0 (0.15) |
| 65 years and older | 13.7 (0.66) | 12.3 (0.58) | 1.4 (0.20) |
| **Race, ethnicity, and age** | | | |
| White non-Hispanic: | | | |
| 18–44 years | 1.4 (0.13) | 7.1 (0.27) | 0.6 (0.08) |
| 45–64 years | 6.2 (0.35) | 11.6 (0.44) | 1.3 (0.15) |
| 65 years and older | 11.9 (0.50) | 14.4 (0.59) | 1.2 (0.16) |
| Black non-Hispanic: | | | |
| 18–44 years | 2.6 (0.35) | 5.8 (0.51) | *0.4 (0.14) |
| 45–64 years | 15.5 (1.19) | 13.1 (1.12) | 1.3 (0.34) |
| 65 years and older | 24.2 (2.12) | 12.3 (1.32) | *1.6 (0.49) |
| Other non-Hispanic: | | | |
| 18–44 years | *1.0 (0.37) | 3.7 (0.74) | *0.9 (0.38) |
| 45–64 years | 9.4 (1.78) | 10.3 (2.12) | *0.8 (0.51) |
| 65 years and older | 16.5 (4.05) | 14.9 (4.04) | *0.9 (0.64) |
| Hispanic: | | | |
| 18–44 years | 1.6 (0.23) | 4.1 (0.39) | 0.8 (0.15) |
| 45–64 years | 12.7 (1.30) | 8.4 (0.96) | 1.4 (0.29) |
| 65 years and older | 22.9 (3.12) | 13.4 (1.91) | *2.3 (1.06) |
| **Race, ethnicity, sex, and age** | | | |
| White non-Hispanic male: | | | |
| 18–44 years | 1.3 (0.17) | 6.8 (0.37) | 0.8 (0.13) |
| 45–64 years | 6.4 (0.49) | 12.8 (0.68) | 1.5 (0.25) |
| 65 years and older | 12.0 (0.84) | 16.9 (0.97) | 1.1 (0.25) |
| White non-Hispanic female: | | | |
| 18–44 years | 1.4 (0.17) | 7.4 (0.36) | 0.5 (0.09) |
| 45–64 years | 6.1 (0.43) | 10.5 (0.53) | 1.1 (0.18) |
| 65 years and older | 11.8 (0.66) | 12.6 (0.64) | 1.2 (0.20) |
| Black non-Hispanic male: | | | |
| 18–44 years | 2.6 (0.60) | 6.2 (0.76) | *0.3 (0.12) |
| 45–64 years | 14.9 (1.91) | 15.4 (1.91) | 2.5 (0.71) |
| 65 years and older | 21.9 (3.69) | 16.8 (2.43) | *1.1 (0.57) |
| Black non-Hispanic female: | | | |
| 18–44 years | 2.6 (0.48) | 5.6 (0.60) | *0.6 (0.23) |
| 45–64 years | 15.9 (1.54) | 11.3 (1.26) | *0.4 (0.22) |
| 65 years and older | 25.7 (2.34) | 9.4 (1.37) | *2.0 (0.72) |
| Hispanic male: | | | |
| 18–44 years | 1.6 (0.38) | 3.6 (0.55) | 1.1 (0.26) |
| 45–64 years | 13.5 (2.27) | 7.1 (1.27) | *1.1 (0.40) |
| 65 years and older | 20.6 (3.34) | 12.9 (2.64) | *1.1 (0.85) |
| Hispanic female: | | | |
| 18–44 years | 1.7 (0.28) | 4.7 (0.49) | *0.5 (0.14) |
| 45–64 years | 11.9 (1.29) | 9.6 (1.39) | 1.6 (0.43) |
| 65 years and older | 24.5 (4.81) | 13.7 (2.67) | *3.1 (1.71) |

| Selected Characteristic | Diabetes[1] | Ulcers[1] | Liver Disease[2] |
|---|---|---|---|
| | Percentage[2] (Standard Error) | | |
| Poverty status and age | | | |
| Poor: | | | |
| 18–44 years | 2.4 (0.34) | 7.8 (0.57) | 1.3 (0.24) |
| 45–64 years | 16.3 (1.39) | 18.8 (1.37) | 3.5 (0.56) |
| 65 years and older | 18.3 (1.63) | 14.4 (1.52) | 3.0 (0.81) |
| Near poor: | | | |
| 18–44 years | 1.9 (0.28) | 7.5 (0.52) | 0.8 (0.17) |
| 45–64 years | 12.5 (1.18) | 14.3 (1.26) | 2.5 (0.60) |
| 65 years and older | 15.3 (1.02) | 17.2 (1.08) | 1.7 (0.32) |
| Not poor: | | | |
| 18–44 years | 1.2 (0.12) | 6.2 (0.29) | 0.5 (0.07) |
| 45–64 years | 5.8 (0.35) | 11.2 (0.49) | 1.0 (0.15) |
| 65 years and older | 11.7 (0.80) | 14.6 (0.81) | 0.9 (0.19) |

*Figure does not meet standard of reliability or precision.

[1]In separate questions, respondents were asked whether they had ever been told by a doctor or other health professional that they had an ulcer (including a stomach, duodenal, or peptic ulcer) or diabetes (or sugar diabetes; female respondents were instructed to exclude pregnancy-related diabetes). Persons who said they had borderline diabetes were considered unknown with respect to diabetes. Persons may be represented in more than one column.

[2]Unknowns for the variable of interest are not included in the denominators when calculating percentages.

[3]*Other non-Hispanic* includes non-Hispanic persons who identified their race as American, Indian, Alaska Native, Asian, or Pacific Islander. These categories are too small to show separately. Persons of Hispanic origin may be of any race.

[4]Poverty status is based on family income and family size using the U.S. Census Bureau's poverty thresholds. *Poor* persons are defined as below the poverty threshold. *Near poor* persons have income of 100 percent to less than 200 percent of the poverty threshold. *Not poor* persons have income 200 percent or greater than the poverty threshold.

# APPENDIX VIII
## WEB SITES THAT INCLUDE INFORMATION ON DIGESTIVE DISEASES

**American Academy of Allergy, Asthma and Immunology**
http://www.aaaai.org

**American Association for the Study of Liver Diseases**
http://www.aasld.org

**American Behçet's Disease Association**
http://www.behçets.com

**American Cancer Society**
http://www.cancer.org

**American College of Gastroenterology**
http://www.acgi.gi.org

**American Diabetes Association (ADA)**
http://www.diabetes.org/

**American Dietetic Association**
http://www.eatright.org

**American Gastroenterological Association (AGA)**
http://www.gastro.org

**American Hemochromatosis Society**
http://www.americanhs.org

**American Liver Foundation**
http://www.liverfoundation.org

**American Obesity Association**
http://www.obesity.org

**American Society for Gastrointestinal Endoscopy**
http://www.asge.org

**American Society for Parenteral and Enteral Nutrition (ASPEN)**
http://www.nutritioncare.org

**American Society of Abdominal Surgeons**
http://www.abdominalsurg.org

**American Society of Bariatric Physicians**
http://www.asbs.org

**American Society of Colon and Rectal Surgeons**
http://www.fascrs.org

**Association of Gastrointestinal Motility Disorders, Inc.**
http://www.digestivemotility.org

**Celiac Disease Foundation**
http://www.celiac.org

**Celiac Sprue Association**
http://www.csaceliacs.org

**Centers for Disease Control and Prevention (CDC)**
http://www.cdc.gov

**Colorectal Cancer Network**
http://www.colorectal-cancer.net

**Crohn's and Colitis Foundation of America**
http://www.ccfa.org

**The Cystic Fibrosis Foundation**
http://www.cff.org

**Digestive Disease National Coalition**
http://www.ddnc.org

**Food Allergy & Anaphylaxis Network**
http://www.foodallergy.org

**Food and Drug Administration**
http://www.fda.org

**Gastro-Intestinal Research Foundation**
http://www.girf.org

**Gluten Intolerance Group of North America**
http://www.gluten.net

**Hemochromatosis Foundation, Inc.**
http://www.hemochromatosis.org

**Hepatitis B Coalition/Immunization Action Coalition**
http://www.immunize.org

**Hepatitis B Foundation**
http://www.hepb.org

**Hepatitis Foundation International**
http://www.hepfi.org

**Hypoglycemia Support Foundation**
http://www.hypoglycemia.org

**International Foundation for Functional Gastrointestinal Disorders, Inc.**
http://www.iffgd.org

**Intestinal Disease Foundation**
http://www.intestinalfoundation.org

**Iron Overload Diseases Association**
http://www.ironoverload.org

**Juvenile Diabetes Research Foundation (JDF)**
http://www.jdf.org

**National Association of Anorexia Nervosa and Related Disorders**
http://www.anad.org

**National Association of Nutrition and Aging Service Programs**
http://www.nanasp.org

**National Clearinghouse for Alcohol and Drug Information**
http://www.health.org

**National Council on Alcoholism and Drug Dependence**
http://www.ncadd.org

**National Diabetes Information Clearinghouse**
http://www.niddk.nih.gov/health/diabetes.ndic.htm

**National Digestive Diseases Information Clearinghouse**
http://www.niddk.nih.gov

**National Eating Disorders Organization**
http://www./edap.org

**National Institute of Allergy and Infectious Diseases**
http://www.niaid.nih.gov

**National Institute of Diabetes and Digestive and Kidney Diseases**
http://www.niddk.nih.gov

**National Institute on Alcohol Abuse and Alcoholism**
http://www.niaaa.nih.gov

**National Organization for Rare Disorders**
http://www.rarediseases.org

**North American Society for Pediatric Gastroenterology, Hepatology and Nutrition**
http://www.naspghan.org

**Oley Foundation for Home Parenteral and Enteral Nutrition**
http://www.oley.org

**Pancreatic Cancer Action Network**
http://www.pancan.org

**Pediatric/Adolescent Gastroesophageal Reflux Association (PAGER)**
http://www.reflux.org

**Pediatric Crohn's & Colitis Association**
http://www.pcca.hypermart.net

**Scleroderma Foundation**
http://www.scleroderma.org

**Scleroderma Research Foundation**
http://www.srfcure.org

**Society for American Gastrointestinal Endoscopic Surgeons**
http://www.sages.org

**Society for Surgery of the Alimentary Tract**
http://www.ssat.com

**Transplant Recipient International Organization**
http://www.transweb.org

**United Network for Organ Sharing**
http://www.unos.org

**United States Department of Agriculture**
Food Safety and Inspection Service
http://www.fsis.usda.gov

**Wilson's Disease Association**
http://www.wilsonsdisease.org

# APPENDIX IX
## PERCENTAGES OF OVERWEIGHT ADULTS IN THE UNITED STATES BY BODY MASS INDEX

**PERCENTAGE OF ADULTS 18 YEARS OF AGE AND OLDER WHO WERE OVERWEIGHT, BY SELECTED CHARACTERISTICS: UNITED STATES, AVERAGE ANNUAL, 1997–1998**

| Selected Characteristic | Overweight (BMI of 25 or more)[1] | | |
| --- | --- | --- | --- |
| | Both Sexes | Men | Women |
| | Percentage of adults (standard error) | | |
| Ages 18 years and older (age-adjusted)[2,3] | 54.7 (0.25) | 62.7 (0.37) | 46.9 (0.33) |
| Ages 18 years and older (crude)[2] | 54.6 (0.26) | 62.9 (0.38) | 46.8 (0.33) |
| **Age** | | | |
| 18–24 years | 37.5 (0.72) | 42.5 (1.06) | 32.3 (0.95) |
| 25–44 years | 53.7 (0.36) | 64.3 (0.48) | 43.2 (0.47) |
| 45–64 years | 63.5 (0.43) | 71.5 (0.61) | 55.7 (0.61) |
| 65–74 years | 61.1 (0.67) | 67.0 (0.93) | 56.2 (0.91) |
| 75 years and older | 47.2 (0.75) | 50.0 (1.31) | 45.3 (0.88) |
| **Race-ethnicity[3]** | | | |
| Hispanic | 61.6 (0.70) | 66.2 (0.95) | 56.6 (0.92) |
| White non-Hispanic | 53.0 (0.29) | 62.7 (0.41) | 43.4 (0.39) |
| Black non-Hispanic | 65.5 (0.59) | 65.7 (1.00) | 65.2 (0.70) |
| Asian/Pacific Islander non-Hispanic | 31.6 (1.67) | 36.7 (2.50) | 27.1 (1.91) |
| **Education[3]** | | | |
| Less than high school graduate | 60.4 (0.52) | 62.0 (0.75) | 58.7 (0.75) |
| GED diploma[4] | 60.3 (1.34) | 64.3 (1.92) | 56.0 (1.93) |
| High school graduate | 56.8 (0.44) | 64.7 (0.65) | 49.7 (0.55) |
| Some college—no degree | 55.3 (0.54) | 65.6 (0.77) | 45.6 (0.69) |
| Associate of arts degree | 55.3 (0.87) | 66.2 (1.24) | 46.3 (1.12) |
| Bachelor of arts, science degree | 47.5 (0.60) | 59.0 (0.89) | 35.7 (0.85) |
| Master's, doctorate, medical degree | 42.4 (0.99) | 53.7 (1.73) | 29.2 (0.96) |
| **Poverty status[3,5]** | | | |
| Below poverty level | 56.9 (0.66) | 57.0 (1.10) | 56.6 (0.83) |
| 1.00–1.99 times poverty level | 58.7 (0.60) | 62.4 (0.84) | 55.4 (0.78) |
| 2.00–3.99 times poverty level | 56.7 (0.43) | 63.5 (0.65) | 49.7 (0.58) |
| 4.00 times poverty level or more | 51.7 (0.48) | 63.6 (0.69) | 38.1 (0.63) |
| **Marital status[3]** | | | |
| Never married | 51.4 (0.65) | 54.4 (0.99) | 48.2 (0.93) |
| Married | 56.0 (0.36) | 65.6 (0.54) | 46.4 (0.48) |
| Cohabiting | 53.4 (1.37) | 59.8 (1.75) | 46.7 (2.74) |
| Divorced or separated | 54.0 (0.72) | 58.7 (1.20) | 50.8 (0.90) |
| Widowed | 51.0 (1.85) | 61.1 (3.30) | 48.7 (2.20) |

*(continues)*

**PERCENTAGE OF ADULTS 18 YEARS OF AGE AND OLDER WHO WERE OVERWEIGHT,
BY SELECTED CHARACTERISTICS: UNITED STATES, AVERAGE ANNUAL, 1997–1998 *(continued)***

| Selected Characteristic | Overweight (BMI of 25 or more)[1] | | |
|---|---|---|---|
| | Both Sexes | Men | Women |
| | Percentage of adults (standard error) | | |
| Geographic region[3] | | | |
| Northeast | 54.0 (0.57) | 63.1 (0.80) | 45.5 (0.66) |
| Midwest | 56.4 (0.43) | 64.6 (0.65) | 48.3 (0.63) |
| South | 55.4 (0.44) | 62.7 (0.66) | 48.4 (0.58) |
| West | 51.6 (0.60) | 59.7 (0.87) | 43.4 (0.69) |
| Place of residence[3] | | | |
| MSA, central city[6] | 53.7 (0.45) | 59.6 (0.66) | 48.1 (0.61) |
| MSA, not central city[6] | 54.2 (0.37) | 63.6 (0.47) | 45.0 (0.51) |
| Not MSA[6] | 57.4 (0.57) | 64.9 (0.85) | 49.9 (0.68) |

[1]Body mass index (BMI) is calculated as kilograms per square meters (k/m[2]) using self-reported height and weight. Overweight is defined as a BMI of 25 or more, which includes obese.
[2]Persons of other races and unknown race and ethnicity, unknown education, unknown poverty status, and unknown marital status are included in the total.
[3]Age adjusted to the 2000 projected U.S. population using age groups 18–24 years, 25–44 years, 45–64 years, 65–74 years, and 75 years and older.
[4] GED is General Educational Development high school equivalency diploma.
[5]Poverty status is based on family income and family size using the U.S. Census Bureau poverty thresholds for 1996 and 1997.
[6]MSA is metropolitan statistical area (see Technical notes).
Note: Denominator for each percentage excludes persons with unknown body mass index.

**PERCENTAGE DISTRIBUTION OF BODY WEIGHT STATUS FOR ADULTS 18 YEARS OF AGE
AND OLDER, BY SELECTED CHARACTERISTICS: UNITED STATES, AVERAGE ANNUAL, 1997–1998**

| Selected Characteristic | Total | Body Weight Status[1] | | | |
|---|---|---|---|---|---|
| | | Not Overweight | | Overweight | |
| | | Underweight | Healthy Weight | Overweight (but not obese) | Obese |
| Both sexes | | Percentage distribution (standard error) | | | |
| Ages 18 years and older (age-adjusted)[2,3] | 100.0 | 2.3 (0.08) | 43.0 (0.25) | 35.2 (0.22) | 19.5 (0.19) |
| Ages 18 years and older (crude)[2] | 100.0 | 2.3 (0.08) | 43.1 (0.26) | 35.1 (0.23) | 19.5 (0.19) |
| Age | | | | | |
| 18–24 years | 100.0 | 4.7 (0.35) | 57.8 (0.75) | 24.7 (0.60) | 12.8 (0.50) |
| 25–44 years | 100.0 | 2.0 (0.10) | 44.2 (0.35) | 34.4 (0.34) | 19.4 (0.27) |
| 45–64 years | 100.0 | 1.2 (0.09) | 35.3 (0.43) | 39.2 (0.41) | 24.3 (0.39) |
| 65–74 years | 100.0 | 1.6 (0.16) | 37.3 (0.65) | 41.1 (0.73) | 20.0 (0.56) |
| 75 years and older | 100.0 | 5.0 (0.35) | 47.8 (0.79) | 34.4 (0.69) | 12.8 (0.46) |
| Race-ethnicity[3] | | | | | |
| Hispanic | 100.0 | 1.4 (0.15) | 37.0 (0.68) | 39.0 (0.61) | 22.6 (0.52) |
| White non-Hispanic | 100.0 | 2.4 (0.10) | 44.6 (0.29) | 34.8 (0.25) | 18.2 (0.23) |
| Black non-Hispanic | 100.0 | 1.4 (0.13) | 33.1 (0.61) | 36.6 (0.59) | 29.0 (0.56) |
| Asian/Pacific Islander non-Hispanic | 100.0 | 6.2 (0.76) | 62.3 (1.79) | 25.2 (1.44) | 6.3 (0.83) |

| Selected Characteristic | Total | Body Weight Status[1] | | | |
| | | Not Overweight | | Overweight | |
| | | Underweight | Healthy Weight | Overweight (but not obese) | Obese |
|---|---|---|---|---|---|
| Education[3] | Percentage distribution (standard error) | | | | |
| Less than high school graduate | 100.0 | 2.5 (0.19) | 37.1 (0.54) | 35.7 (0.56) | 24.7 (0.50) |
| GED diploma[4] | 100.0 | 2.5 (0.63) | 37.1 (1.36) | 35.3 (1.37) | 25.0 (1.15) |
| High school graduate | 100.0 | 2.4 (0.14) | 40.9 (0.44) | 35.9 (0.43) | 20.9 (0.35) |
| Some college—no degree | 100.0 | 2.2 (0.14) | 42.5 (0.54) | 35.6 (0.51) | 19.7 (0.42) |
| Associate of arts degree | 100.0 | 1.9 (0.22) | 42.8 (0.88) | 35.8 (0.78) | 19.5 (0.69) |
| Bachelor of arts, science degree | 100.0 | 2.5 (0.23) | 50.0 (0.60) | 33.9 (0.57) | 13.6 (0.41) |
| Master's, doctorate, medical degree | 100.0 | 2.5 (0.53) | 55.2 (1.08) | 31.0 (0.95) | 11.3 (0.48) |
| Poverty status[3,5] | | | | | |
| Below poverty level | 100.0 | 3.2 (0.23) | 39.9 (0.66) | 30.9 (0.67) | 26.0 (0.59) |
| 1.00–1.99 times poverty level | 100.0 | 2.2 (0.18) | 39.0 (0.59) | 34.5 (0.58) | 24.2 (0.51) |
| 2.00–3.99 times poverty level | 100.0 | 2.3 (0.14) | 41.0 (0.44) | 36.1 (0.41) | 20.6 (0.37) |
| 4.00 times poverty level or more | 100.0 | 2.0 (0.16) | 46.3 (0.49) | 35.9 (0.45) | 15.8 (0.34) |
| Marital status[3] | | | | | |
| Never married | 100.0 | 2.8 (0.22) | 45.9 (0.67) | 31.2 (0.61) | 20.2 (0.55) |
| Married | 100.0 | 2.1 (0.12) | 41.9 (0.37) | 36.7 (0.33) | 19.3 (0.27) |
| Cohabiting | 100.0 | 1.9 (0.31) | 44.7 (1.37) | 36.8 (1.35) | 16.6 (0.95) |
| Divorced or separated | 100.0 | 2.5 (0.26) | 43.4 (0.73) | 33.4 (0.68) | 20.6 (0.54) |
| Widowed | 100.0 | *3.4 (1.34) | 45.6 (2.12) | 29.0 (1.68) | 22.0 (1.46) |
| Geographic region[3] | | | | | |
| Northeast | 100.0 | 2.1 (0.17) | 43.9 (0.58) | 35.1 (0.42) | 18.9 (0.49) |
| Midwest | 100.0 | 2.2 (0.14) | 41.4 (0.43) | 35.7 (0.42) | 20.8 (0.39) |
| South | 100.0 | 2.6 (0.14) | 42.0 (0.44) | 35.1 (0.40) | 20.4 (0.34) |
| West | 100.0 | 2.4 (0.18) | 46.1 (0.62) | 34.6 (0.47) | 17.0 (0.33) |
| Place of residence[3] | | | | | |
| MSA, central city[6] | 100.0 | 2.6 (0.12) | 43.8 (0.46) | 34.1 (0.37) | 19.5 (0.34) |
| MSA, not central city[6] | 100.0 | 2.2 (0.11) | 43.6 (0.36) | 35.6 (0.29) | 18.6 (0.29) |
| Not MSA[6] | 100.0 | 2.2 (0.16) | 40.4 (0.55) | 35.7 (0.51) | 21.7 (0.41) |
| Men | | | | | |
| Ages 18 years and older (age-adjusted)[2,3] | 100.0 | 0.9 (0.07) | 36.3 (0.37) | 43.4 (0.35) | 19.3 (0.29) |
| Ages 18 years and older (crude)[2] | 100.0 | 0.9 (0.07) | 36.2 (0.37) | 43.4 (0.35) | 19.4 (0.29) |
| Age | | | | | |
| 18–24 years | 100.0 | 2.2 (0.33) | 55.2 (1.09) | 29.8 (0.91) | 12.7 (0.74) |
| 25–44 years | 100.0 | 0.6 (0.07) | 35.1 (0.48) | 44.3 (0.49) | 20.0 (0.40) |
| 45–64 years | 100.0 | 0.6 (0.10) | 27.9 (0.61) | 47.7 (0.65) | 23.8 (0.56) |
| 65–74 years | 100.0 | 0.7 (0.16) | 32.3 (0.92) | 48.0 (1.02) | 18.9 (0.84) |
| 75 years and older | 100.0 | 2.3 (0.39) | 47.7 (1.30) | 40.0 (1.22) | 10.0 (0.70) |
| Race-ethnicity[3] | | | | | |
| Hispanic | 100.0 | 1.0 (0.23) | 32.7 (0.96) | 44.4 (0.88) | 21.8 (0.79) |
| White non-Hispanic | 100.0 | 0.9 (0.08) | 36.4 (0.41) | 44.0 (0.40) | 18.7 (0.34) |
| Black non-Hispanic | 100.0 | 0.7 (0.14) | 33.6 (1.00) | 41.7 (0.99) | 24.0 (0.88) |
| Asian/Pacific Islander non-Hispanic | 100.0 | *2.3 (0.78) | 61.0 (2.58) | 29.7 (2.02) | 7.1 (1.22) |

*(continues)*

**PERCENTAGE DISTRIBUTION OF BODY WEIGHT STATUS FOR ADULTS 18 YEARS OF AGE AND OLDER, BY SELECTED CHARACTERISTICS: UNITED STATES, AVERAGE ANNUAL, 1997–1998** *(continued)*

| | | Body Weight Status[1] | | | |
| | | Not Overweight | | Overweight | |
| Selected Characteristic | Total | Underweight | Healthy Weight | Overweight (but not obese) | Obese |
| --- | --- | --- | --- | --- | --- |
| Education[3] | | Percentage distribution (standard error) | | | |
| Less than high school graduate | 100.0 | 1.4 (0.17) | 36.6 (0.75) | 40.2 (0.79) | 21.8 (0.67) |
| GED diploma[4] | 100.0 | *2.0 (0.80) | 33.8 (1.89) | 39.9 (2.05) | 24.4 (1.71) |
| High school graduate | 100.0 | 1.1 (0.15) | 34.2 (0.64) | 43.9 (0.70) | 20.9 (0.55) |
| Some college—no degree | 100.0 | 0.6 (0.11) | 33.8 (0.76) | 45.0 (0.77) | 20.6 (0.65) |
| Associate of arts degree | 100.0 | *0.5 (0.16) | 33.3 (1.24) | 46.0 (1.25) | 20.1 (0.97) |
| Bachelor of arts, science degree | 100.0 | 1.0 (0.24) | 39.9 (0.90) | 44.3 (0.94) | 14.8 (0.68) |
| Master's, doctorate, medical degree | 100.0 | *0.4 (0.15) | 45.9 (1.74) | 41.7 (1.75) | 12.0 (0.69) |
| Poverty status[3,5] | | | | | |
| Below poverty level | 100.0 | 1.9 (0.30) | 41.1 (1.11) | 35.3 (1.04) | 21.7 (1.04) |
| 1.00–1.99 times poverty level | 100.0 | 1.2 (0.20) | 36.4 (0.83) | 39.6 (0.90) | 22.8 (0.75) |
| 2.00–3.99 times poverty level | 100.0 | 1.0 (0.15) | 35.4 (0.65) | 43.3 (0.66) | 20.2 (0.51) |
| 4.00 times poverty level or more | 100.0 | 0.5 (0.11) | 35.9 (0.70) | 45.9 (0.63) | 17.7 (0.48) |
| Marital status[3] | | | | | |
| Never married | 100.0 | 1.1 (0.19) | 44.5 (0.99) | 36.7 (0.91) | 17.6 (0.77) |
| Married | 100.0 | 0.9 (0.13) | 33.5 (0.54) | 45.3 (0.55) | 20.4 (0.43) |
| Cohabiting | 100.0 | *1.0 (0.38) | 39.2 (1.76) | 42.7 (1.82) | 17.1 (1.34) |
| Divorced or separated | 100.0 | 0.9 (0.22) | 40.4 (1.20) | 41.9 (1.21) | 16.8 (0.75) |
| Widowed | 100.0 | *0.8 (0.33) | 38.1 (3.30) | 41.6 (3.93) | 19.5 (3.86) |
| Geographic region[3] | | | | | |
| Northeast | 100.0 | 0.8 (0.13) | 36.1 (0.80) | 44.0 (0.75) | 19.1 (0.74) |
| Midwest | 100.0 | 0.8 (0.12) | 34.6 (0.65) | 44.7 (0.73) | 19.9 (0.61) |
| South | 100.0 | 1.2 (0.14) | 36.1 (0.66) | 42.7 (0.58) | 20.1 (0.47) |
| West | 100.0 | 0.9 (0.15) | 39.4 (0.87) | 42.5 (0.75) | 17.2 (0.53) |
| Place of residence[3] | | | | | |
| MSA, central city[6] | 100.0 | 1.0 (0.12) | 39.4 (0.67) | 41.3 (0.63) | 18.3 (0.48) |
| MSA, not central city[6] | 100.0 | 0.9 (0.10) | 35.5 (0.48) | 44.5 (0.43) | 19.1 (0.43) |
| Not MSA[6] | 100.0 | 1.0 (0.16) | 34.1 (0.83) | 43.8 (0.80) | 21.1 (0.56) |
| Women | | | | | |
| Ages 18 years and older (age-adjusted)[2,3] | 100.0 | 3.6 (0.13) | 49.5 (0.33) | 27.2 (0.27) | 19.7 (0.26) |
| Ages 18 years and older (crude)[2] | 100.0 | 3.7 (0.13) | 49.5 (0.33) | 27.2 (0.28) | 19.6 (0.25) |
| Age | | | | | |
| 18–24 years | 100.0 | 7.2 (0.60) | 60.4 (1.01) | 19.5 (0.78) | 12.9 (0.63) |
| 25–44 years | 100.0 | 3.5 (0.18) | 53.3 (0.45) | 24.5 (0.40) | 18.8 (0.36) |
| 45–64 years | 100.0 | 1.8 (0.16) | 42.5 (0.62) | 30.9 (0.53) | 24.7 (0.54) |
| 65–74 years | 100.0 | 2.4 (0.27) | 41.4 (0.91) | 35.3 (0.94) | 20.9 (0.72) |
| 75 years and older | 100.0 | 6.7 (0.50) | 47.9 (0.92) | 30.7 (0.84) | 14.7 (0.63) |
| Race-ethnicity[3] | | | | | |
| Hispanic | 100.0 | 1.9 (0.18) | 41.5 (0.89) | 33.4 (0.86) | 23.3 (0.69) |
| White non-Hispanic | 100.0 | 3.8 (0.16) | 52.8 (0.40) | 25.8 (0.31) | 17.6 (0.30) |
| Black non-Hispanic | 100.0 | 2.0 (0.22) | 32.8 (0.70) | 32.3 (0.76) | 32.9 (0.71) |
| Asian/Pacific Islander non-Hispanic | 100.0 | 9.9 (1.20) | 63.0 (1.89) | 21.2 (1.61) | 5.8 (1.19) |

| Selected Characteristic | Total | Body Weight Status[1] | | | |
| | | Not Overweight | | Overweight | |
| | | Underweight | Healthy Weight | Overweight (but not obese) | Obese |
|---|---|---|---|---|---|
| Education[3] | Percentage distribution (standard error) | | | | |
| Less than high school graduate | 100.0 | 3.6 (0.32) | 37.6 (0.78) | 31.3 (0.71) | 27.4 (0.70) |
| GED diploma[4] | 100.0 | 3.0 (0.78) | 41.0 (1.96) | 30.0 (1.85) | 26.1 (1.68) |
| High school graduate | 100.0 | 3.5 (0.23) | 46.8 (0.56) | 28.9 (0.53) | 20.8 (0.46) |
| Some college—no degree | 100.0 | 3.7 (0.26) | 50.7 (0.72) | 26.7 (0.60) | 18.9 (0.55) |
| Associate of arts degree | 100.0 | 3.0 (0.39) | 50.6 (1.12) | 27.4 (0.93) | 19.0 (0.83) |
| Bachelor of arts, science degree | 100.0 | 3.9 (0.37) | 60.4 (0.86) | 23.2 (0.73) | 12.5 (0.52) |
| Master's, doctorate, medical degree | 100.0 | 4.4 (0.88) | 66.5 (1.24) | 18.6 (0.88) | 10.5 (0.67) |
| Poverty status[3,5] | | | | | |
| Below poverty level | 100.0 | 4.1 (0.33) | 39.3 (0.84) | 27.9 (0.80) | 28.7 (0.76) |
| 1.00–1.99 times poverty level | 100.0 | 3.2 (0.28) | 41.4 (0.76) | 30.0 (0.76) | 25.4 (0.68) |
| 2.00–3.99 times poverty level | 100.0 | 3.6 (0.24) | 46.7 (0.59) | 28.8 (0.57) | 20.9 (0.49) |
| 4.00 times poverty level or more | 100.0 | 3.7 (0.31) | 58.2 (0.67) | 24.4 (0.56) | 13.7 (0.47) |
| Marital status[3] | | | | | |
| Never married | 100.0 | 4.4 (0.37) | 47.4 (0.94) | 25.0 (0.84) | 23.1 (0.79) |
| Married | 100.0 | 3.4 (0.20) | 50.3 (0.48) | 28.0 (0.40) | 18.4 (0.36) |
| Cohabiting | 100.0 | 2.6 (0.43) | 50.7 (2.73) | 30.3 (2.67) | 16.4 (1.35) |
| Divorced or separated | 100.0 | 3.6 (0.39) | 45.6 (0.92) | 27.6 (0.80) | 23.2 (0.72) |
| Widowed | 100.0 | *5.6 (2.64) | 45.7 (2.99) | 25.9 (1.84) | 22.8 (1.61) |
| Geographic region[3] | | | | | |
| Northeast | 100.0 | 3.3 (0.31) | 51.2 (0.68) | 26.9 (0.60) | 18.6 (0.58) |
| Midwest | 100.0 | 3.4 (0.25) | 48.3 (0.62) | 26.8 (0.55) | 21.5 (0.51) |
| South | 100.0 | 3.9 (0.22) | 47.8 (0.58) | 27.8 (0.48) | 20.5 (0.45) |
| West | 100.0 | 3.8 (0.31) | 52.7 (0.75) | 26.8 (0.55) | 16.6 (0.46) |
| Place of residence[3] | | | | | |
| MSA, central city[6] | 100.0 | 4.0 (0.21) | 48.0 (0.63) | 27.5 (0.53) | 20.6 (0.44) |
| MSA, not central city[6] | 100.0 | 3.5 (0.19) | 51.5 (0.49) | 26.9 (0.40) | 18.1 (0.38) |
| Not MSA[6] | 100.0 | 3.4 (0.29) | 46.7 (0.66) | 27.7 (0.54) | 22.2 (0.55) |

*Figure does not meet standards of reliability or precision (see Technical notes).

[1]Body weight status was based on body mass index (BMI) using self-reported height and weight. The formula for BMI is kilograms per square meters ($kg/m^2$). Underweight is defined as a BMI of less than 18.5; healthy weight is defined as a BMI of at least 18.5 and less than 25; overweight, and not obese, is defined as a BMI of at least 25 and less than 30; and obese is defined as a BMI of 30 or more.

[2]Persons of other races and unknown race and ethnicity, unknown education, unknown poverty status, and unknown marital status are included in the total.

[3]Age adjusted to the 2000 projected U.S. population using age groups 18–24 years, 25–44 years, 45–64 years, 65–74 years, and 75 years and older.

[4]GED is General Educational Development high school equivalency diploma.

[5]Poverty status is based on family income and family size using the U.S. Census Bureau poverty thresholds for 1996 and 1997.

[6]MSA is metropolitan statistical area (see Technical notes).

Note: Denominator for each percentage distribution excludes persons with unknown body mass index.

# APPENDIX X
## BODY MASS INDEX (BMI) CHARTS FOR CHILDREN

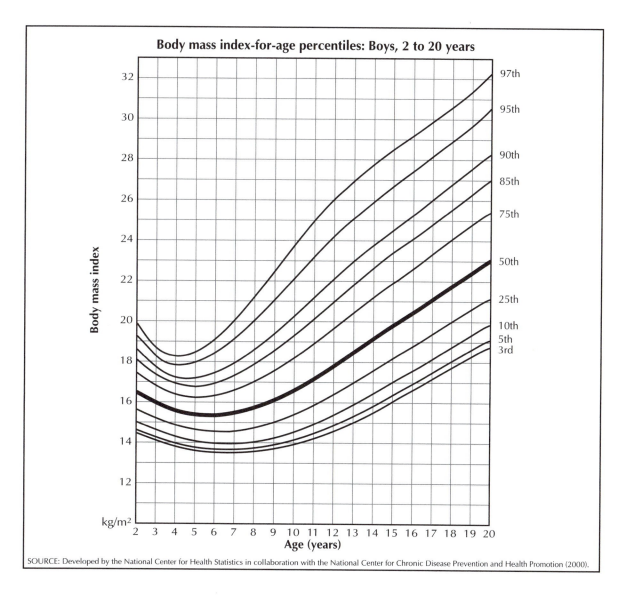

**Body mass index-for-age percentiles: Boys, 2 to 20 years**

SOURCE: Developed by the National Center for Health Statistics in collaboration with the National Center for Chronic Disease Prevention and Health Promotion (2000).

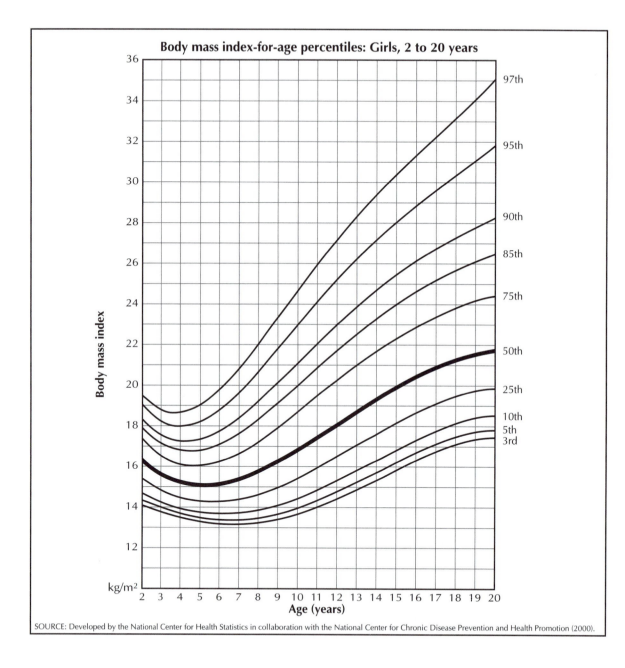

**Body mass index-for-age percentiles: Girls, 2 to 20 years**

SOURCE: Developed by the National Center for Health Statistics in collaboration with the National Center for Chronic Disease Prevention and Health Promotion (2000).

## CALCULATED BODY MASS INDEX    29 in.–37 in. AND 18 LB–26 LB

| Height | | Weight | | | | | | | | | | | | | | | | |
|---|---|---|---|---|---|---|---|---|---|---|---|---|---|---|---|---|---|---|
| cm | in | kg | 8.2 | 8.4 | 8.6 | 8.8 | 9.1 | 9.3 | 9.5 | 9.8 | 10.0 | 10.2 | 10.4 | 10.7 | 10.9 | 11.1 | 11.3 | 11.6 | 11.8 |
| | | lb | 18 | 18.5 | 19 | 19.5 | 20 | 20.5 | 21 | 21.5 | 22 | 22.5 | 23 | 23.5 | 24 | 24.5 | 25 | 25.5 | 26 |
| 73.7 | 29 | | 15.0 | 15.5 | 15.9 | 16.3 | 16.7 | 17.1 | 17.6 | 18.0 | 18.4 | 18.8 | 19.2 | 19.6 | 20.1 | 20.5 | 20.9 | 21.3 | 21.7 |
| 74.9 | 29.5 | | 14.5 | 14.9 | 15.3 | 15.8 | 16.2 | 16.6 | 17.0 | 17.4 | 17.8 | 18.2 | 18.6 | 19.0 | 19.4 | 19.8 | 20.2 | 20.6 | 21.0 |
| 76.2 | 30 | | 14.1 | 14.5 | 14.8 | 15.2 | 15.6 | 16.0 | 16.4 | 16.8 | 17.2 | 17.6 | 18.0 | 18.4 | 18.7 | 19.1 | 19.5 | 19.9 | 20.3 |
| 77.5 | 30.5 | | 13.6 | 14.0 | 14.4 | 14.7 | 15.1 | 15.5 | 15.9 | 16.2 | 16.6 | 17.0 | 17.4 | 17.8 | 18.1 | 18.5 | 18.9 | 19.3 | 19.7 |
| 78.7 | 31 | | 13.2 | 13.5 | 13.9 | 14.3 | 14.6 | 15.0 | 15.4 | 15.7 | 16.1 | 16.5 | 16.8 | 17.2 | 17.6 | 17.9 | 18.3 | 18.7 | 19.0 |
| 80.0 | 31.5 | | | 13.1 | 13.5 | 13.8 | 14.2 | 14.5 | 14.9 | 15.2 | 15.6 | 15.9 | 16.3 | 16.7 | 17.0 | 17.4 | 17.7 | 18.1 | 18.4 |
| 81.3 | 32 | | | | 13.0 | 13.4 | 13.7 | 14.1 | 14.4 | 14.8 | 15.1 | 15.4 | 15.8 | 16.1 | 16.5 | 16.8 | 17.2 | 17.5 | 17.9 |
| 82.6 | 32.5 | | | | | | 13.3 | 13.6 | 14.0 | 14.3 | 14.6 | 15.0 | 15.3 | 15.6 | 16.0 | 16.3 | 16.6 | 17.0 | 17.3 |
| 83.8 | 33 | | | | | | | 13.2 | 13.6 | 13.9 | 14.2 | 14.5 | 14.8 | 15.2 | 15.5 | 15.8 | 16.1 | 16.5 | 16.8 |
| 85.1 | 33.5 | | | | | | | | 13.2 | 13.5 | 13.8 | 14.1 | 14.4 | 14.7 | 15.0 | 15.3 | 15.7 | 16.0 | 16.3 |
| 86.4 | 34 | | | | | | | | | 13.1 | 13.4 | 13.7 | 14.0 | 14.3 | 14.6 | 14.9 | 15.2 | 15.5 | 15.8 |
| 87.6 | 34.5 | | | | | | | | | | | 13.3 | 13.6 | 13.9 | 14.2 | 14.5 | 14.8 | 15.1 | 15.4 |
| 88.9 | 35 | | | | | | | | | | | | 13.2 | 13.5 | 13.8 | 14.1 | 14.3 | 14.6 | 14.9 |
| 90.2 | 35.5 | | | | | | | | | | | | | 13.1 | 13.4 | 13.7 | 13.9 | 14.2 | 14.5 |
| 91.4 | 36 | | | | | | | | | | | | | | 13.0 | 13.3 | 13.6 | 13.8 | 14.1 |
| 92.7 | 36.5 | | | | | | | | | | | | | | | | 13.2 | 13.5 | 13.7 |
| 94.0 | 37 | | | | | | | | | | | | | | | | | | 13.4 |

*Whenever a child's specific height or weight measurement is not listed, round to the closest number in the table.*

CALCULATED BODY MASS INDEX    29 in.–43 in. AND 26.5 LB–34.5 LB

| Height | | | Weight | | | | | | | | | | | | | | | | | |
|---|---|---|---|---|---|---|---|---|---|---|---|---|---|---|---|---|---|---|---|---|
| cm | in | kg | 12.0 | 12.2 | 12.5 | 12.7 | 12.9 | 13.2 | 13.4 | 13.6 | 13.8 | 14.1 | 14.3 | 14.5 | 14.7 | 15.0 | 15.2 | 15.4 | 15.6 |
| | | lb | 26.5 | 27 | 27.5 | 28 | 28.5 | 29 | 29.5 | 30 | 30.5 | 31 | 31.5 | 32 | 32.5 | 33 | 33.5 | 34 | 34.5 |
| 73.7 | 29 | | 22.2 | 22.6 | 23.0 | 23.4 | 23.8 | 24.2 | 24.7 | 25.1 | 25.5 | 25.9 | 26.3 | 26.8 | 27.2 | 27.6 | 28.0 | 28.4 | 28.8 |
| 74.9 | 29.5 | | 21.4 | 21.8 | 22.2 | 22.6 | 23.0 | 23.4 | 23.8 | 24.2 | 24.6 | 25.0 | 25.4 | 25.9 | 26.3 | 26.7 | 27.1 | 27.5 | 27.9 |
| 76.2 | 30 | | 20.7 | 21.1 | 21.5 | 21.9 | 22.3 | 22.7 | 23.0 | 23.4 | 23.8 | 24.2 | 24.6 | 25.0 | 25.4 | 25.8 | 26.2 | 26.6 | 27.0 |
| 77.5 | 30.5 | | 20.0 | 20.4 | 20.8 | 21.2 | 21.5 | 21.9 | 22.3 | 22.7 | 23.1 | 23.4 | 23.8 | 24.2 | 24.6 | 24.9 | 25.3 | 25.7 | 26.1 |
| 78.7 | 31 | | 19.4 | 19.8 | 20.1 | 20.5 | 20.9 | 21.2 | 21.6 | 21.9 | 22.3 | 22.7 | 23.0 | 23.4 | 23.8 | 24.1 | 24.5 | 24.9 | 25.2 |
| 80.0 | 31.5 | | 18.8 | 19.1 | 19.5 | 19.8 | 20.2 | 20.5 | 20.9 | 21.3 | 21.6 | 22.0 | 22.3 | 22.7 | 23.0 | 23.4 | 23.7 | 24.1 | 24.4 |
| 81.3 | 32 | | 18.2 | 18.5 | 18.9 | 19.2 | 19.6 | 19.9 | 20.3 | 20.6 | 20.9 | 21.3 | 21.6 | 22.0 | 22.3 | 22.7 | 23.0 | 23.3 | 23.7 |
| 82.6 | 32.5 | | 17.6 | 18.0 | 18.3 | 18.6 | 19.0 | 19.3 | 19.6 | 20.0 | 20.3 | 20.6 | 21.0 | 21.3 | 21.6 | 22.0 | 22.3 | 22.6 | 23.0 |
| 83.8 | 33 | | 17.1 | 17.4 | 17.8 | 18.1 | 18.4 | 18.7 | 19.0 | 19.4 | 19.7 | 20.0 | 20.3 | 20.7 | 21.0 | 21.3 | 21.6 | 22.0 | 22.3 |
| 85.1 | 33.5 | | 16.6 | 16.9 | 17.2 | 17.5 | 17.9 | 18.2 | 18.5 | 18.8 | 19.1 | 19.4 | 19.7 | 20.0 | 20.4 | 20.7 | 21.0 | 21.3 | 21.6 |
| 86.4 | 34 | | 16.1 | 16.4 | 16.7 | 17.0 | 17.3 | 17.6 | 17.9 | 18.2 | 18.5 | 18.9 | 19.2 | 19.5 | 19.8 | 20.1 | 20.4 | 20.7 | 21.0 |
| 87.6 | 34.5 | | 15.7 | 15.9 | 16.2 | 16.5 | 16.8 | 17.1 | 17.4 | 17.7 | 18.0 | 18.3 | 18.6 | 18.9 | 19.2 | 19.5 | 19.8 | 20.1 | 20.4 |
| 88.9 | 35 | | 15.2 | 15.5 | 15.8 | 16.1 | 16.4 | 16.6 | 16.9 | 17.2 | 17.5 | 17.8 | 18.1 | 18.4 | 18.7 | 18.9 | 19.2 | 19.5 | 19.8 |
| 90.2 | 35.5 | | 14.8 | 15.1 | 15.3 | 15.6 | 15.9 | 16.2 | 16.5 | 16.7 | 17.0 | 17.3 | 17.6 | 17.9 | 18.1 | 18.4 | 18.7 | 19.0 | 19.2 |
| 91.4 | 36 | | 14.4 | 14.6 | 14.9 | 15.2 | 15.5 | 15.7 | 16.0 | 16.3 | 16.5 | 16.8 | 17.1 | 17.4 | 17.6 | 17.9 | 18.2 | 18.4 | 18.7 |
| 92.7 | 36.5 | | 14.0 | 14.2 | 14.5 | 14.8 | 15.0 | 15.3 | 15.6 | 15.8 | 16.1 | 16.4 | 16.6 | 16.9 | 17.2 | 17.4 | 17.7 | 17.9 | 18.2 |
| 94.0 | 37 | | 13.6 | 13.9 | 14.1 | 14.4 | 14.6 | 14.9 | 15.2 | 15.4 | 15.7 | 15.9 | 16.2 | 16.4 | 16.7 | 16.9 | 17.2 | 17.5 | 17.7 |
| 95.3 | 37.5 | | 13.2 | 13.5 | 13.7 | 14.0 | 14.2 | 14.5 | 14.7 | 15.0 | 15.2 | 15.5 | 15.7 | 16.0 | 16.2 | 16.5 | 16.7 | 17.0 | 17.2 |
| 96.5 | 38 | | | 13.1 | 13.4 | 13.6 | 13.9 | 14.1 | 14.4 | 14.6 | 14.9 | 15.1 | 15.3 | 15.6 | 15.8 | 16.1 | 16.3 | 16.6 | 16.8 |
| 97.8 | 38.5 | | | | 13.0 | 13.3 | 13.5 | 13.8 | 14.0 | 14.2 | 14.5 | 14.7 | 14.9 | 15.2 | 15.4 | 15.7 | 15.9 | 16.1 | 16.4 |
| 99.1 | 39 | | | | | | 13.2 | 13.4 | 13.6 | 13.9 | 14.1 | 14.3 | 14.6 | 14.8 | 15.0 | 15.3 | 15.5 | 15.7 | 15.9 |
| 100.3 | 39.5 | | | | | | | 13.1 | 13.3 | 13.5 | 13.7 | 14.0 | 14.2 | 14.4 | 14.6 | 14.9 | 15.1 | 15.3 | 15.5 |
| 101.6 | 40 | | | | | | | | | 13.2 | 13.4 | 13.6 | 13.8 | 14.1 | 14.3 | 14.5 | 14.7 | 14.9 | 15.2 |
| 102.9 | 40.5 | | | | | | | | | | | 13.3 | 13.5 | 13.7 | 13.9 | 14.1 | 14.4 | 14.6 | 14.8 |
| 104.1 | 41 | | | | | | | | | | | | 13.2 | 13.4 | 13.6 | 13.8 | 14.0 | 14.2 | 14.4 |
| 105.4 | 41.5 | | | | | | | | | | | | | 13.1 | 13.3 | 13.5 | 13.7 | 13.9 | 14.1 |
| 106.7 | 42 | | | | | | | | | | | | | | | 13.2 | 13.4 | 13.6 | 13.8 |
| 108.0 | 42.5 | | | | | | | | | | | | | | | | 13.0 | 13.2 | 13.4 |
| 109.2 | 43 | | | | | | | | | | | | | | | | | | 13.1 |

*Whenever a child's specific height or weight measurement is not listed, round to the closest number in the table.*

## CALCULATED BODY MASS INDEX    29 in.–43 in. AND 35 LB–43 LB

| | | Weight | | | | | | | | | | | | | | | | |
|---|---|---|---|---|---|---|---|---|---|---|---|---|---|---|---|---|---|---|
| Height | | kg | 15.9 | 16.1 | 16.3 | 16.6 | 16.8 | 17.0 | 17.2 | 17.5 | 17.7 | 17.9 | 18.1 | 18.4 | 18.6 | 18.8 | 19.1 | 19.3 | 19.5 |
| cm | in | lb | 35 | 35.5 | 36 | 36.5 | 37 | 37.5 | 38 | 38.5 | 39 | 39.5 | 40 | 40.5 | 41 | 41.5 | 42 | 42.5 | 43 |
| 73.7 | 29 | | 29.3 | 29.7 | 30.1 | 30.5 | 30.9 | 31.3 | 31.8 | 32.2 | 32.6 | 33.0 | 33.4 | 33.9 | 34.3 | 34.7 | | | |
| 74.9 | 29.5 | | 28.3 | 28.7 | 29.1 | 29.5 | 29.9 | 30.3 | 30.7 | 31.1 | 31.5 | 31.9 | 32.3 | 32.7 | 33.1 | 33.5 | 33.9 | 34.3 | 34.7 |
| 76.2 | 30 | | 27.3 | 27.7 | 28.1 | 28.5 | 28.9 | 29.3 | 29.7 | 30.1 | 30.5 | 30.9 | 31.2 | 31.6 | 32.0 | 32.4 | 32.8 | 33.2 | 33.6 |
| 77.5 | 30.5 | | 26.5 | 26.8 | 27.2 | 27.6 | 28.0 | 28.3 | 28.7 | 29.1 | 29.5 | 29.9 | 30.2 | 30.6 | 31.0 | 31.4 | 31.7 | 32.1 | 32.5 |
| 78.7 | 31 | | 25.6 | 26.0 | 26.3 | 26.7 | 27.1 | 27.4 | 27.8 | 28.2 | 28.5 | 28.9 | 29.3 | 29.6 | 30.0 | 30.4 | 30.7 | 31.1 | 31.5 |
| 80.0 | 31.5 | | 24.8 | 25.2 | 25.5 | 25.9 | 26.2 | 26.6 | 26.9 | 27.3 | 27.6 | 28.0 | 28.3 | 28.7 | 29.1 | 29.4 | 29.8 | 30.1 | 30.5 |
| 81.3 | 32 | | 24.0 | 24.4 | 24.7 | 25.1 | 25.4 | 25.7 | 26.1 | 26.4 | 26.8 | 27.1 | 27.5 | 27.8 | 28.2 | 28.5 | 28.8 | 29.2 | 29.5 |
| 82.6 | 32.5 | | 23.3 | 23.6 | 24.0 | 24.3 | 24.6 | 25.0 | 25.3 | 25.6 | 26.0 | 26.3 | 26.6 | 27.0 | 27.3 | 27.6 | 28.0 | 28.3 | 28.6 |
| 83.8 | 33 | | 22.6 | 22.9 | 23.2 | 23.6 | 23.9 | 24.2 | 24.5 | 24.9 | 25.2 | 25.5 | 25.8 | 26.1 | 26.5 | 26.8 | 27.1 | 27.4 | 27.8 |
| 85.1 | 33.5 | | 21.9 | 22.2 | 22.6 | 22.9 | 23.2 | 23.5 | 23.8 | 24.1 | 24.4 | 24.7 | 25.1 | 25.4 | 25.7 | 26.0 | 26.3 | 26.6 | 26.9 |
| 86.4 | 34 | | 21.3 | 21.6 | 21.9 | 22.2 | 22.5 | 22.8 | 23.1 | 23.4 | 23.7 | 24.0 | 24.3 | 24.6 | 24.9 | 25.2 | 25.5 | 25.8 | 26.2 |
| 87.6 | 34.5 | | 20.7 | 21.0 | 21.3 | 21.6 | 21.9 | 22.2 | 22.4 | 22.7 | 23.0 | 23.3 | 23.6 | 23.9 | 24.2 | 24.5 | 24.8 | 25.1 | 25.4 |
| 88.9 | 35 | | 20.1 | 20.4 | 20.7 | 20.9 | 21.2 | 21.5 | 21.8 | 22.1 | 22.4 | 22.7 | 23.0 | 23.2 | 23.5 | 23.8 | 24.1 | 24.4 | 24.7 |
| 90.2 | 35.5 | | 19.5 | 19.8 | 20.1 | 20.4 | 20.6 | 20.9 | 21.2 | 21.5 | 21.8 | 22.0 | 22.3 | 22.6 | 22.9 | 23.2 | 23.4 | 23.7 | 24.0 |
| 91.4 | 36 | | 19.0 | 19.3 | 19.5 | 19.8 | 20.1 | 20.3 | 20.6 | 20.9 | 21.2 | 21.4 | 21.7 | 22.0 | 22.2 | 22.5 | 22.8 | 23.1 | 23.3 |
| 92.7 | 36.5 | | 18.5 | 18.7 | 19.0 | 19.3 | 19.5 | 19.8 | 20.1 | 20.3 | 20.6 | 20.8 | 21.1 | 21.4 | 21.6 | 21.9 | 22.2 | 22.4 | 22.7 |
| 94.0 | 37 | | 18.0 | 18.2 | 18.5 | 18.7 | 19.0 | 19.3 | 19.5 | 19.8 | 20.0 | 20.3 | 20.5 | 20.8 | 21.1 | 21.3 | 21.6 | 21.8 | 22.1 |
| 95.3 | 37.5 | | 17.5 | 17.7 | 18.0 | 18.2 | 18.5 | 18.7 | 19.0 | 19.2 | 19.5 | 19.7 | 20.0 | 20.2 | 20.5 | 20.7 | 21.0 | 21.2 | 21.5 |
| 96.5 | 38 | | 17.0 | 17.3 | 17.5 | 17.8 | 18.0 | 18.3 | 18.5 | 18.7 | 19.0 | 19.2 | 19.5 | 19.7 | 20.0 | 20.2 | 20.4 | 20.7 | 20.9 |
| 97.8 | 38.5 | | 16.6 | 16.8 | 17.1 | 17.3 | 17.6 | 17.8 | 18.0 | 18.3 | 18.5 | 18.7 | 19.0 | 19.2 | 19.4 | 19.7 | 19.9 | 20.2 | 20.4 |
| 99.1 | 39 | | 16.2 | 16.4 | 16.6 | 16.9 | 17.1 | 17.3 | 17.6 | 17.8 | 18.0 | 18.3 | 18.5 | 18.7 | 19.0 | 19.2 | 19.4 | 19.6 | 19.9 |
| 100.3 | 39.5 | | 15.8 | 16.0 | 16.2 | 16.4 | 16.7 | 16.9 | 17.1 | 17.3 | 17.6 | 17.8 | 18.0 | 18.2 | 18.5 | 18.7 | 18.9 | 19.2 | 19.4 |
| 101.6 | 40 | | 15.4 | 15.6 | 15.8 | 16.0 | 16.3 | 16.5 | 16.7 | 16.9 | 17.1 | 17.4 | 17.6 | 17.8 | 18.0 | 18.2 | 18.5 | 18.7 | 18.9 |
| 102.9 | 40.5 | | 15.0 | 15.2 | 15.4 | 15.6 | 15.9 | 16.1 | 16.3 | 16.5 | 16.7 | 16.9 | 17.1 | 17.4 | 17.6 | 17.8 | 18.0 | 18.2 | 18.4 |
| 104.1 | 41 | | 14.6 | 14.8 | 15.1 | 15.3 | 15.5 | 15.7 | 15.9 | 16.1 | 16.3 | 16.5 | 16.7 | 16.9 | 17.1 | 17.4 | 17.6 | 17.8 | 18.0 |
| 105.4 | 41.5 | | 14.3 | 14.5 | 14.7 | 14.9 | 15.1 | 15.3 | 15.5 | 15.7 | 15.9 | 16.1 | 16.3 | 16.5 | 16.7 | 16.9 | 17.1 | 17.3 | 17.6 |
| 106.7 | 42 | | 13.9 | 14.1 | 14.3 | 14.5 | 14.7 | 14.9 | 15.1 | 15.3 | 15.5 | 15.7 | 15.9 | 16.1 | 16.3 | 16.5 | 16.7 | 16.9 | 17.1 |
| 108.0 | 42.5 | | 13.6 | 13.8 | 14.0 | 14.2 | 14.4 | 14.6 | 14.8 | 15.0 | 15.2 | 15.4 | 15.6 | 15.8 | 16.0 | 16.2 | 16.3 | 16.5 | 16.7 |
| 109.2 | 43 | | 13.3 | 13.5 | 13.7 | 13.9 | 14.1 | 14.3 | 14.4 | 14.6 | 14.8 | 15.0 | 15.2 | 15.4 | 15.6 | 15.8 | 16.0 | 16.2 | 16.4 |

*Whenever a child's specific height or weight measurement is not listed, round to the closest number in the table.*

## CALCULATED BODY MASS INDEX   43.5 in.–48 in. AND 35 LB–43 LB

| Height cm | Height in | Weight kg 15.9 | 16.1 | 16.3 | 16.6 | 16.8 | 17.0 | 17.2 | 17.5 | 17.7 | 17.9 | 18.1 | 18.4 | 18.6 | 18.8 | 19.1 | 19.3 | 19.5 |
|---|---|---|---|---|---|---|---|---|---|---|---|---|---|---|---|---|---|---|
| | | lb 35 | 35.5 | 36 | 36.5 | 37 | 37.5 | 38 | 38.5 | 39 | 39.5 | 40 | 40.5 | 41 | 41.5 | 42 | 42.5 | 43 |
| 110.5 | 43.5 | 13.0 | 13.2 | 13.4 | 13.6 | 13.7 | 13.9 | 14.1 | 14.3 | 14.5 | 14.7 | 14.9 | 15.0 | 15.2 | 15.4 | 15.6 | 15.8 | 16.0 |
| 111.8 | 44 | | 13.1 | 13.1 | 13.3 | 13.4 | 13.6 | 13.8 | 14.0 | 14.2 | 14.3 | 14.5 | 14.7 | 14.9 | 15.1 | 15.3 | 15.4 | 15.6 |
| 113.0 | 44.5 | | | | | 13.1 | 13.3 | 13.5 | 13.7 | 13.8 | 14.0 | 14.2 | 14.4 | 14.6 | 14.7 | 14.9 | 15.1 | 15.3 |
| 114.3 | 45 | | | | | | 13.0 | 13.2 | 13.4 | 13.5 | 13.7 | 13.9 | 14.1 | 14.2 | 14.4 | 14.6 | 14.8 | 14.9 |
| 115.6 | 45.5 | | | | | | | | 13.1 | 13.2 | 13.4 | 13.6 | 13.8 | 13.9 | 14.1 | 14.3 | 14.4 | 14.6 |
| 116.8 | 46 | | | | | | | | | | 13.1 | 13.3 | 13.5 | 13.6 | 13.8 | 14.0 | 14.1 | 14.3 |
| 118.1 | 46.5 | | | | | | | | | | | 13.0 | 13.2 | 13.3 | 13.5 | 13.7 | 13.8 | 14.0 |
| 119.4 | 47 | | | | | | | | | | | | | 13.0 | 13.2 | 13.4 | 13.5 | 13.7 |
| 120.7 | 47.5 | | | | | | | | | | | | | | | 13.1 | 13.2 | 13.4 |
| 121.9 | 48 | | | | | | | | | | | | | | | | | 13.1 |

*Whenever a child's specific height or weight measurement is not listed, round to the closest number in the table.*

## CALCULATED BODY MASS INDEX    30 in.–44 in. AND 43.5 LB–51.5 LB

| Height | | Weight | | | | | | | | | | | | | | | | |
|---|---|---|---|---|---|---|---|---|---|---|---|---|---|---|---|---|---|---|
| cm | in | kg 19.7 | 20.0 | 20.2 | 20.4 | 20.6 | 20.9 | 21.1 | 21.3 | 21.5 | 21.8 | 22.0 | 22.2 | 22.5 | 22.7 | 22.9 | 23.1 | 23.4 |
| | | lb 43.5 | 44 | 44.5 | 45 | 45.5 | 46 | 46.5 | 47 | 47.5 | 48 | 48.5 | 49 | 49.5 | 50 | 50.5 | 51 | 51.5 |
| 76.2 | 30 | 34.0 | 34.4 | 34.8 | | | | | | | | | | | | | | |
| 77.5 | 30.5 | 32.9 | 33.3 | 33.6 | 34.0 | 34.4 | 34.8 | | | | | | | | | | | |
| 78.7 | 31 | 31.8 | 32.2 | 32.6 | 32.9 | 33.3 | 33.7 | 34.0 | 34.4 | 34.8 | | | | | | | | |
| 80.0 | 31.5 | 30.8 | 31.2 | 31.5 | 31.9 | 32.2 | 32.6 | 32.9 | 33.3 | 33.7 | 34.0 | 34.4 | 34.7 | | | | | |
| 81.3 | 32 | 29.9 | 30.2 | 30.6 | 30.9 | 31.2 | 31.6 | 31.9 | 32.3 | 32.6 | 33.0 | 33.3 | 33.6 | 34.0 | 34.3 | 34.7 | | |
| 82.6 | 32.5 | 29.0 | 29.3 | 29.6 | 30.0 | 30.3 | 30.6 | 31.0 | 31.3 | 31.6 | 32.0 | 32.3 | 32.6 | 32.9 | 33.3 | 33.6 | 33.9 | 34.3 |
| 83.8 | 33 | 28.1 | 28.4 | 28.7 | 29.1 | 29.4 | 29.7 | 30.0 | 30.3 | 30.7 | 31.0 | 31.3 | 31.6 | 32.0 | 32.3 | 32.6 | 32.9 | 33.2 |
| 85.1 | 33.5 | 27.3 | 27.6 | 27.9 | 28.2 | 28.5 | 28.8 | 29.1 | 29.4 | 29.8 | 30.1 | 30.4 | 30.7 | 31.0 | 31.3 | 31.6 | 32.0 | 32.3 |
| 86.4 | 34 | 26.5 | 26.8 | 27.1 | 27.4 | 27.7 | 28.0 | 28.3 | 28.6 | 28.9 | 29.2 | 29.5 | 29.8 | 30.1 | 30.4 | 30.7 | 31.0 | 31.3 |
| 87.6 | 34.5 | 25.7 | 26.0 | 26.3 | 26.6 | 26.9 | 27.2 | 27.5 | 27.8 | 28.1 | 28.4 | 28.6 | 28.9 | 29.2 | 29.5 | 29.8 | 30.1 | 30.4 |
| 88.9 | 35 | 25.0 | 25.3 | 25.5 | 25.8 | 26.1 | 26.4 | 26.7 | 27.0 | 27.3 | 27.5 | 27.8 | 28.1 | 28.4 | 28.7 | 29.0 | 29.3 | 29.6 |
| 90.2 | 35.5 | 24.3 | 24.5 | 24.8 | 25.1 | 25.4 | 25.7 | 25.9 | 26.2 | 26.5 | 26.8 | 27.1 | 27.3 | 27.6 | 27.9 | 28.2 | 28.5 | 28.7 |
| 91.4 | 36 | 23.6 | 23.9 | 24.1 | 24.4 | 24.7 | 25.0 | 25.2 | 25.5 | 25.8 | 26.0 | 26.3 | 26.6 | 26.9 | 27.1 | 27.4 | 27.7 | 27.9 |
| 92.7 | 36.5 | 23.0 | 23.2 | 23.5 | 23.7 | 24.0 | 24.3 | 24.5 | 24.8 | 25.1 | 25.3 | 25.6 | 25.9 | 26.1 | 26.4 | 26.7 | 26.9 | 27.2 |
| 94.0 | 37 | 22.3 | 22.6 | 22.9 | 23.1 | 23.4 | 23.6 | 23.9 | 24.1 | 24.4 | 24.7 | 24.9 | 25.2 | 25.4 | 25.7 | 25.9 | 26.2 | 26.4 |
| 95.3 | 37.5 | 21.7 | 22.0 | 22.2 | 22.5 | 22.7 | 23.0 | 23.2 | 23.5 | 23.7 | 24.0 | 24.2 | 24.5 | 24.7 | 25.0 | 25.2 | 25.5 | 25.7 |
| 96.5 | 38 | 21.2 | 21.4 | 21.7 | 21.9 | 22.2 | 22.4 | 22.6 | 22.9 | 23.1 | 23.4 | 23.6 | 23.9 | 24.1 | 24.3 | 24.6 | 24.8 | 25.1 |
| 97.8 | 38.5 | 20.6 | 20.9 | 21.1 | 21.3 | 21.6 | 21.8 | 22.1 | 22.3 | 22.5 | 22.8 | 23.0 | 23.2 | 23.5 | 23.7 | 24.0 | 24.2 | 24.4 |
| 99.1 | 39 | 20.1 | 20.3 | 20.6 | 20.8 | 21.0 | 21.3 | 21.5 | 21.7 | 22.0 | 22.2 | 22.4 | 22.6 | 22.9 | 23.1 | 23.3 | 23.6 | 23.8 |
| 100.3 | 39.5 | 19.6 | 19.8 | 20.1 | 20.3 | 20.5 | 20.7 | 21.0 | 21.2 | 21.4 | 21.6 | 21.9 | 22.1 | 22.3 | 22.5 | 22.8 | 23.0 | 23.2 |
| 101.6 | 40 | 19.1 | 19.3 | 19.6 | 19.8 | 20.0 | 20.2 | 20.4 | 20.7 | 20.9 | 21.1 | 21.3 | 21.5 | 21.8 | 22.0 | 22.2 | 22.4 | 22.6 |
| 102.9 | 40.5 | 18.6 | 18.9 | 19.1 | 19.3 | 19.5 | 19.7 | 19.9 | 20.1 | 20.4 | 20.6 | 20.8 | 21.0 | 21.2 | 21.4 | 21.6 | 21.9 | 22.1 |
| 104.1 | 41 | 18.2 | 18.4 | 18.6 | 18.8 | 19.0 | 19.2 | 19.4 | 19.7 | 19.9 | 20.1 | 20.3 | 20.5 | 20.7 | 20.9 | 21.1 | 21.3 | 21.5 |
| 105.4 | 41.5 | 17.8 | 18.0 | 18.2 | 18.4 | 18.6 | 18.8 | 19.0 | 19.2 | 19.4 | 19.6 | 19.8 | 20.0 | 20.2 | 20.4 | 20.6 | 20.8 | 21.0 |
| 106.7 | 42 | 17.3 | 17.5 | 17.7 | 17.9 | 18.1 | 18.3 | 18.5 | 18.7 | 18.9 | 19.1 | 19.3 | 19.5 | 19.7 | 19.9 | 20.1 | 20.3 | 20.5 |
| 108.0 | 42.5 | 16.9 | 17.1 | 17.3 | 17.5 | 17.7 | 17.9 | 18.1 | 18.3 | 18.5 | 18.7 | 18.9 | 19.1 | 19.3 | 19.5 | 19.7 | 19.9 | 20.0 |
| 109.2 | 43 | 16.5 | 16.7 | 16.9 | 17.1 | 17.3 | 17.5 | 17.7 | 17.9 | 18.1 | 18.3 | 18.4 | 18.6 | 18.8 | 19.0 | 19.2 | 19.4 | 19.6 |
| 110.5 | 43.5 | 16.2 | 16.3 | 16.5 | 16.7 | 16.9 | 17.1 | 17.3 | 17.5 | 17.6 | 17.8 | 18.0 | 18.2 | 18.4 | 18.6 | 18.8 | 18.9 | 19.1 |
| 111.8 | 44 | 15.8 | 16.0 | 16.2 | 16.3 | 16.5 | 16.7 | 16.9 | 17.1 | 17.2 | 17.4 | 17.6 | 17.8 | 18.0 | 18.2 | 18.3 | 18.5 | 18.7 |

*Whenever a child's specific height or weight measurement is not listed, round to the closest number in the table.*

## CALCULATED BODY MASS INDEX   44.5 in.–51 in. AND 43.5 LB–51.5 LB

| Height | | Weight (kg) | | | | | | | | | | | | | | | | |
|---|---|---|---|---|---|---|---|---|---|---|---|---|---|---|---|---|---|---|
| cm | in | 19.7 | 20.0 | 20.2 | 20.4 | 20.6 | 20.9 | 21.1 | 21.3 | 21.5 | 21.8 | 22.0 | 22.2 | 22.5 | 22.7 | 22.9 | 23.1 | 23.4 |
| | | **lb** | | | | | | | | | | | | | | | | |
| | | 43.5 | 44 | 44.5 | 45 | 45.5 | 46 | 46.5 | 47 | 47.5 | 48 | 48.5 | 49 | 49.5 | 50 | 50.5 | 51 | 51.5 |
| 110.5 | 43.5 | 13.0 | 13.2 | 13.4 | 13.6 | 13.7 | 13.9 | 14.1 | 14.3 | 14.5 | 14.7 | 14.9 | 15.0 | 15.2 | 15.4 | 15.6 | 15.8 | 16.0 |
| 113.0 | 44.5 | 15.4 | 15.6 | 15.8 | 16.0 | 16.2 | 16.3 | 16.5 | 16.7 | 16.9 | 17.0 | 17.2 | 17.4 | 17.6 | 17.8 | 17.9 | 18.1 | 18.3 |
| 114.3 | 45 | 15.1 | 15.3 | 15.5 | 15.6 | 15.8 | 16.0 | 16.1 | 16.3 | 16.5 | 16.7 | 16.8 | 17.0 | 17.2 | 17.4 | 17.5 | 17.7 | 17.9 |
| 115.6 | 45.5 | 14.8 | 14.9 | 15.1 | 15.3 | 15.5 | 15.6 | 15.8 | 16.0 | 16.1 | 16.3 | 16.5 | 16.6 | 16.8 | 17.0 | 17.2 | 17.3 | 17.5 |
| 116.8 | 46 | 14.5 | 14.6 | 14.8 | 15.0 | 15.1 | 15.3 | 15.5 | 15.6 | 15.8 | 15.9 | 16.1 | 16.3 | 16.4 | 16.6 | 16.8 | 16.9 | 17.1 |
| 118.1 | 46.5 | 14.1 | 14.3 | 14.5 | 14.6 | 14.8 | 15.0 | 15.1 | 15.3 | 15.4 | 15.6 | 15.8 | 15.9 | 16.1 | 16.3 | 16.4 | 16.6 | 16.7 |
| 119.4 | 47 | 13.8 | 14.0 | 14.2 | 14.3 | 14.5 | 14.6 | 14.8 | 15.0 | 15.1 | 15.3 | 15.4 | 15.6 | 15.8 | 15.9 | 16.1 | 16.2 | 16.4 |
| 120.7 | 47.5 | 13.6 | 13.7 | 13.9 | 14.0 | 14.2 | 14.3 | 14.5 | 14.6 | 14.8 | 15.0 | 15.1 | 15.3 | 15.4 | 15.6 | 15.7 | 15.9 | 16.0 |
| 121.9 | 48 | 13.3 | 13.4 | 13.6 | 13.7 | 13.9 | 14.0 | 14.2 | 14.3 | 14.5 | 14.6 | 14.8 | 15.0 | 15.1 | 15.3 | 15.4 | 15.6 | 15.7 |
| 124.5 | 49 | | | 13.0 | 13.2 | 13.3 | 13.5 | 13.6 | 13.8 | 13.9 | 14.1 | 14.2 | 14.3 | 14.5 | 14.6 | 14.8 | 14.9 | 15.1 |
| 127.0 | 50 | | | | | | | 13.1 | 13.2 | 13.4 | 13.5 | 13.6 | 13.8 | 13.9 | 14.1 | 14.2 | 14.3 | 14.5 |
| 129.5 | 51 | | | | | | | | | | | 13.1 | 13.2 | 13.4 | 13.5 | 13.7 | 13.8 | 13.9 |
| 132.1 | 52 | | | | | | | | | | | | | | 13.0 | 13.1 | 13.3 | 13.4 |

*Whenever a child's specific height or weight measurement is not listed, round to the closest number in the table.*

## CALCULATED BODY MASS INDEX   47 in.–56 in. AND 52 LB–60 LB

| Height (cm) | Height (in) | kg 23.6 / lb 52 | 23.8 / 52.5 | 24.0 / 53 | 24.3 / 53.5 | 24.5 / 54 | 24.7 / 54.5 | 24.9 / 55 | 25.2 / 55.5 | 25.4 / 56 | 25.6 / 56.5 | 25.9 / 57 | 26.1 / 57.5 | 26.3 / 58 | 26.5 / 58.5 | 26.8 / 59 | 27.0 / 59.5 | 27.2 / 60 |
|---|---|---|---|---|---|---|---|---|---|---|---|---|---|---|---|---|---|---|
| 119.4 | 47 | 16.6 | 16.7 | 16.9 | 17.0 | 17.2 | 17.3 | 17.5 | 17.7 | 17.8 | 18.0 | 18.1 | 18.3 | 18.5 | 18.6 | 18.8 | 18.9 | 19.1 |
| 120.7 | 47.5 | 16.2 | 16.4 | 16.5 | 16.7 | 16.8 | 17.0 | 17.1 | 17.3 | 17.5 | 17.6 | 17.8 | 17.9 | 18.1 | 18.2 | 18.4 | 18.5 | 18.7 |
| 121.9 | 48 | 15.9 | 16.0 | 16.2 | 16.3 | 16.5 | 16.6 | 16.8 | 16.9 | 17.1 | 17.2 | 17.4 | 17.5 | 17.7 | 17.9 | 18.0 | 18.2 | 18.3 |
| 124.5 | 49 | 15.2 | 15.4 | 15.5 | 15.7 | 15.8 | 16.0 | 16.1 | 16.3 | 16.4 | 16.5 | 16.7 | 16.8 | 17.0 | 17.1 | 17.3 | 17.4 | 17.6 |
| 127.0 | 50 | 14.6 | 14.8 | 14.9 | 15.0 | 15.2 | 15.3 | 15.5 | 15.6 | 15.7 | 15.9 | 16.0 | 16.2 | 16.3 | 16.5 | 16.6 | 16.7 | 16.9 |
| 129.5 | 51 | 14.1 | 14.2 | 14.3 | 14.5 | 14.6 | 14.7 | 14.9 | 15.0 | 15.1 | 15.3 | 15.4 | 15.5 | 15.7 | 15.8 | 15.9 | 16.1 | 16.2 |
| 132.1 | 52 | 13.5 | 13.7 | 13.8 | 13.9 | 14.0 | 14.2 | 14.3 | 14.4 | 14.6 | 14.7 | 14.8 | 15.0 | 15.1 | 15.2 | 15.3 | 15.5 | 15.6 |
| 134.6 | 53 | 13.0 | 13.1 | 13.3 | 13.4 | 13.5 | 13.6 | 13.8 | 13.9 | 14.0 | 14.1 | 14.3 | 14.4 | 14.5 | 14.6 | 14.8 | 14.9 | 15.0 |
| 137.2 | 54 | | | | | 13.0 | 13.1 | 13.3 | 13.4 | 13.5 | 13.6 | 13.7 | 13.9 | 14.0 | 14.1 | 14.2 | 14.3 | 14.5 |
| 139.7 | 55 | | | | | | | | | 13.0 | 13.1 | 13.2 | 13.4 | 13.5 | 13.6 | 13.7 | 13.8 | 13.9 |
| 142.2 | 56 | | | | | | | | | | | | | 13.0 | 13.1 | 13.2 | 13.3 | 13.5 |

*Whenever a child's specific height or weight measurement is not listed, round to the closest number in the table.*

CALCULATED BODY MASS INDEX    35.5 in.–51 in. AND 61 LB–77 LB

Weight

| Height cm | in | kg → 27.7 / lb 61 | 28.1 / 62 | 28.6 / 63 | 29.0 / 64 | 29.5 / 65 | 29.9 / 66 | 30.4 / 67 | 30.8 / 68 | 31.3 / 69 | 31.8 / 70 | 32.2 / 71 | 32.7 / 72 | 33.1 / 73 | 33.6 / 74 | 34.0 / 75 | 34.5 / 76 | 34.9 / 77 |
|---|---|---|---|---|---|---|---|---|---|---|---|---|---|---|---|---|---|---|
| 90.2 | 35.5 | 34.0 | 34.6 | | | | | | | | | | | | | | | |
| 91.4 | 36 | 33.1 | 33.6 | 34.2 | 34.7 | | | | | | | | | | | | | |
| 92.7 | 36.5 | 32.2 | 32.7 | 33.2 | 33.8 | 34.3 | 34.8 | | | | | | | | | | | |
| 94.0 | 37 | 31.3 | 31.8 | 32.4 | 32.9 | 33.4 | 33.9 | 34.4 | 34.9 | | | | | | | | | |
| 95.3 | 37.5 | 30.5 | 31.0 | 31.5 | 32.0 | 32.5 | 33.0 | 33.5 | 34.0 | 34.5 | 35.0 | | | | | | | |
| 96.5 | 38 | 29.7 | 30.2 | 30.7 | 31.2 | 31.6 | 32.1 | 32.6 | 33.1 | 33.6 | 34.1 | 34.6 | | | | | | |
| 97.8 | 38.5 | 28.9 | 29.4 | 29.9 | 30.4 | 30.8 | 31.3 | 31.8 | 32.3 | 32.7 | 33.2 | 33.7 | 34.2 | 34.6 | | | | |
| 99.1 | 39 | 28.2 | 28.7 | 29.1 | 29.6 | 30.0 | 30.5 | 31.0 | 31.4 | 31.9 | 32.4 | 32.8 | 33.3 | 33.7 | 34.2 | 34.7 | | |
| 100.3 | 39.5 | 27.5 | 27.9 | 28.4 | 28.8 | 29.3 | 29.7 | 30.2 | 30.6 | 31.1 | 31.5 | 32.0 | 32.4 | 32.9 | 33.3 | 33.8 | 34.2 | 34.7 |
| 101.6 | 40 | 26.8 | 27.2 | 27.7 | 28.1 | 28.6 | 29.0 | 29.4 | 29.9 | 30.3 | 30.8 | 31.2 | 31.6 | 32.1 | 32.5 | 33.0 | 33.4 | 33.8 |
| 102.9 | 40.5 | 26.1 | 26.6 | 27.0 | 27.4 | 27.9 | 28.3 | 28.7 | 29.1 | 29.6 | 30.0 | 30.4 | 30.9 | 31.3 | 31.7 | 32.1 | 32.6 | 33.0 |
| 104.1 | 41 | 25.5 | 25.9 | 26.3 | 26.8 | 27.2 | 27.6 | 28.0 | 28.4 | 28.9 | 29.3 | 29.7 | 30.1 | 30.5 | 31.0 | 31.4 | 31.8 | 32.2 |
| 105.4 | 41.5 | 24.9 | 25.3 | 25.7 | 26.1 | 26.5 | 26.9 | 27.4 | 27.8 | 28.2 | 28.6 | 29.0 | 29.4 | 29.8 | 30.2 | 30.6 | 31.0 | 31.4 |
| 106.7 | 42 | 24.3 | 24.7 | 25.1 | 25.5 | 25.9 | 26.3 | 26.7 | 27.1 | 27.5 | 27.9 | 28.3 | 28.7 | 29.1 | 29.5 | 29.9 | 30.3 | 30.7 |
| 108.0 | 42.5 | 23.7 | 24.1 | 24.5 | 24.9 | 25.3 | 25.7 | 26.1 | 26.5 | 26.9 | 27.2 | 27.6 | 28.0 | 28.4 | 28.8 | 29.2 | 29.6 | 30.0 |
| 109.2 | 43 | 23.2 | 23.6 | 24.0 | 24.3 | 24.7 | 25.1 | 25.5 | 25.9 | 26.2 | 26.6 | 27.0 | 27.4 | 27.8 | 28.1 | 28.5 | 28.9 | 29.3 |
| 110.5 | 43.5 | 22.7 | 23.0 | 23.4 | 23.8 | 24.2 | 24.5 | 24.9 | 25.3 | 25.6 | 26.0 | 26.4 | 26.8 | 27.1 | 27.5 | 27.9 | 28.2 | 28.6 |
| 111.8 | 44 | 22.2 | 22.5 | 22.9 | 23.2 | 23.6 | 24.0 | 24.3 | 24.7 | 25.1 | 25.4 | 25.8 | 26.1 | 26.5 | 26.9 | 27.2 | 27.6 | 28.0 |
| 113.0 | 44.5 | 21.7 | 22.0 | 22.4 | 22.7 | 23.1 | 23.4 | 23.8 | 24.1 | 24.5 | 24.9 | 25.2 | 25.6 | 25.9 | 26.3 | 26.6 | 27.0 | 27.3 |
| 114.3 | 45 | 21.2 | 21.5 | 21.9 | 22.2 | 22.6 | 22.9 | 23.3 | 23.6 | 24.0 | 24.3 | 24.7 | 25.0 | 25.3 | 25.7 | 26.0 | 26.4 | 26.7 |
| 115.6 | 45.5 | 20.7 | 21.1 | 21.4 | 21.7 | 22.1 | 22.4 | 22.8 | 23.1 | 23.4 | 23.8 | 24.1 | 24.5 | 24.8 | 25.1 | 25.5 | 25.8 | 26.1 |
| 116.8 | 46 | 20.3 | 20.6 | 20.9 | 21.3 | 21.6 | 21.9 | 22.3 | 22.6 | 22.9 | 23.3 | 23.6 | 23.9 | 24.3 | 24.6 | 24.9 | 25.3 | 25.6 |
| 118.1 | 46.5 | 19.8 | 20.2 | 20.5 | 20.8 | 21.1 | 21.5 | 21.8 | 22.1 | 22.4 | 22.8 | 23.1 | 23.4 | 23.7 | 24.1 | 24.4 | 24.7 | 25.0 |
| 119.4 | 47 | 19.4 | 19.7 | 20.1 | 20.4 | 20.7 | 21.0 | 21.3 | 21.6 | 22.0 | 22.3 | 22.6 | 22.9 | 23.2 | 23.6 | 23.9 | 24.2 | 24.5 |
| 120.7 | 47.5 | 19.0 | 19.3 | 19.6 | 19.9 | 20.3 | 20.6 | 20.9 | 21.2 | 21.5 | 21.8 | 22.1 | 22.4 | 22.7 | 23.1 | 23.4 | 23.7 | 24.0 |
| 121.9 | 48 | 18.6 | 18.9 | 19.2 | 19.5 | 19.8 | 20.1 | 20.4 | 20.8 | 21.1 | 21.4 | 21.7 | 22.0 | 22.3 | 22.6 | 22.9 | 23.2 | 23.5 |
| 124.5 | 49 | 17.9 | 18.2 | 18.4 | 18.7 | 19.0 | 19.3 | 19.6 | 19.9 | 20.2 | 20.5 | 20.8 | 21.1 | 21.4 | 21.7 | 22.0 | 22.3 | 22.5 |
| 127.0 | 50 | 17.2 | 17.4 | 17.7 | 18.0 | 18.3 | 18.6 | 18.8 | 19.1 | 19.4 | 19.7 | 20.0 | 20.2 | 20.5 | 20.8 | 21.1 | 21.4 | 21.7 |
| 129.5 | 51 | 16.5 | 16.8 | 17.0 | 17.3 | 17.6 | 17.8 | 18.1 | 18.4 | 18.7 | 18.9 | 19.2 | 19.5 | 19.7 | 20.0 | 20.3 | 20.5 | 20.8 |

*Whenever a child's specific height or weight measurement is not listed, round to the closest number in the table.*

## CALCULATED BODY MASS INDEX   52 in.–64 in. AND 61 LB–77 LB

| Height | | Weight | | | | | | | | | | | | | | | | |
|---|---|---|---|---|---|---|---|---|---|---|---|---|---|---|---|---|---|---|
| | | kg | 27.7 | 28.1 | 28.6 | 29.0 | 29.5 | 29.9 | 30.4 | 30.8 | 31.3 | 31.8 | 32.2 | 32.7 | 33.1 | 33.6 | 34.0 | 34.5 | 34.9 |
| cm | in | lb | 61 | 62 | 63 | 64 | 65 | 66 | 67 | 68 | 69 | 70 | 71 | 72 | 73 | 74 | 75 | 76 | 77 |
| 132.1 | 52 | | 15.9 | 16.1 | 16.4 | 16.6 | 16.9 | 17.2 | 17.4 | 17.7 | 17.9 | 18.2 | 18.5 | 18.7 | 19.0 | 19.2 | 19.5 | 19.8 | 20.0 |
| 134.6 | 53 | | 15.3 | 15.5 | 15.8 | 16.0 | 16.3 | 16.5 | 16.8 | 17.0 | 17.3 | 17.5 | 17.8 | 18.0 | 18.3 | 18.5 | 18.8 | 19.0 | 19.3 |
| 137.2 | 54 | | 14.7 | 14.9 | 15.2 | 15.4 | 15.7 | 15.9 | 16.2 | 16.4 | 16.6 | 16.9 | 17.1 | 17.4 | 17.6 | 17.8 | 18.1 | 18.3 | 18.6 |
| 139.7 | 55 | | 14.2 | 14.4 | 14.6 | 14.9 | 15.1 | 15.3 | 15.6 | 15.8 | 16.0 | 16.3 | 16.5 | 16.7 | 17.0 | 17.2 | 17.4 | 17.7 | 17.9 |
| 142.2 | 56 | | 13.7 | 13.9 | 14.1 | 14.3 | 14.6 | 14.8 | 15.0 | 15.2 | 15.5 | 15.7 | 15.9 | 16.1 | 16.4 | 16.6 | 16.8 | 17.0 | 17.3 |
| 144.8 | 57 | | 13.2 | 13.4 | 13.6 | 13.8 | 14.1 | 14.3 | 14.5 | 14.7 | 14.9 | 15.1 | 15.4 | 15.6 | 15.8 | 16.0 | 16.2 | 16.4 | 16.7 |
| 147.3 | 58 | | | | 13.2 | 13.4 | 13.6 | 13.8 | 14.0 | 14.2 | 14.4 | 14.6 | 14.8 | 15.0 | 15.3 | 15.5 | 15.7 | 15.9 | 16.1 |
| 149.9 | 59 | | | | | | 13.1 | 13.3 | 13.5 | 13.7 | 13.9 | 14.1 | 14.3 | 14.5 | 14.7 | 14.9 | 15.1 | 15.3 | 15.6 |
| 152.4 | 60 | | | | | | | | 13.1 | 13.3 | 13.5 | 13.7 | 13.9 | 14.1 | 14.3 | 14.5 | 14.6 | 14.8 | 15.0 |
| 154.9 | 61 | | | | | | | | | | 13.0 | 13.2 | 13.4 | 13.6 | 13.8 | 14.0 | 14.2 | 14.4 | 14.5 |
| 157.5 | 62 | | | | | | | | | | | | | 13.2 | 13.4 | 13.5 | 13.7 | 13.9 | 14.1 |
| 160.0 | 63 | | | | | | | | | | | | | | | 13.1 | 13.3 | 13.5 | 13.6 |
| 162.6 | 64 | | | | | | | | | | | | | | | | | 13.0 | 13.2 |

*Whenever a child's specific height or weight measurement is not listed, round to the closest number in the table.*

## CALCULATED BODY MASS INDEX   40.5 in.–60 in. AND 78 LB–94 LB

Weight

| Height (cm) | Height (in) | 78 / 35.4 | 79 / 35.8 | 80 / 36.3 | 81 / 36.7 | 82 / 37.2 | 83 / 37.6 | 84 / 38.1 | 85 / 38.6 | 86 / 39.0 | 87 / 39.5 | 88 / 39.9 | 89 / 40.4 | 90 / 40.8 | 91 / 41.3 | 92 / 41.7 | 93 / 42.2 | 94 / 42.6 |
|---|---|---|---|---|---|---|---|---|---|---|---|---|---|---|---|---|---|---|
| | | lb / kg | | | | | | | | | | | | | | | | |
| 101.6 | 40 | 34.3 | 34.7 | | | | | | | | | | | | | | | |
| 102.9 | 40.5 | 33.4 | 33.9 | 34.3 | 34.7 | | | | | | | | | | | | | |
| 104.1 | 41 | 32.6 | 33.0 | 33.5 | 33.9 | 34.3 | 34.7 | | | | | | | | | | | |
| 105.4 | 41.5 | 31.8 | 32.2 | 32.7 | 33.1 | 33.5 | 33.9 | 34.3 | 34.7 | | | | | | | | | |
| 106.7 | 42 | 31.1 | 31.5 | 31.9 | 32.3 | 32.7 | 33.1 | 33.5 | 33.9 | 34.3 | 34.7 | | | | | | | |
| 108.0 | 42.5 | 30.4 | 30.8 | 31.1 | 31.5 | 31.9 | 32.3 | 32.7 | 33.1 | 33.5 | 33.9 | 34.3 | 34.6 | | | | | |
| 109.2 | 43 | 29.7 | 30.0 | 30.4 | 30.8 | 31.2 | 31.6 | 31.9 | 32.3 | 32.7 | 33.1 | 33.5 | 33.8 | 34.2 | 34.6 | 35.0 | | |
| 110.5 | 43.5 | 29.0 | 29.4 | 29.7 | 30.1 | 30.5 | 30.8 | 31.2 | 31.6 | 32.0 | 32.3 | 32.7 | 33.1 | 33.4 | 33.8 | 34.2 | 34.6 | 34.9 |
| 111.8 | 44 | 28.3 | 28.7 | 29.1 | 29.4 | 29.8 | 30.1 | 30.5 | 30.9 | 31.2 | 31.6 | 32.0 | 32.3 | 32.7 | 33.0 | 33.4 | 33.8 | 34.1 |
| 113.0 | 44.5 | 27.7 | 28.0 | 28.4 | 28.8 | 29.1 | 29.5 | 29.8 | 30.2 | 30.5 | 30.9 | 31.2 | 31.6 | 32.0 | 32.3 | 32.7 | 33.0 | 33.4 |
| 114.3 | 45 | 27.1 | 27.4 | 27.8 | 28.1 | 28.5 | 28.8 | 29.2 | 29.5 | 29.9 | 30.2 | 30.6 | 30.9 | 31.2 | 31.6 | 31.9 | 32.3 | 32.6 |
| 115.6 | 45.5 | 26.5 | 26.8 | 27.2 | 27.5 | 27.8 | 28.2 | 28.5 | 28.9 | 29.2 | 29.5 | 29.9 | 30.2 | 30.6 | 30.9 | 31.2 | 31.6 | 31.9 |
| 116.8 | 46 | 25.9 | 26.2 | 26.6 | 26.9 | 27.2 | 27.6 | 27.9 | 28.2 | 28.6 | 28.9 | 29.2 | 29.6 | 29.9 | 30.2 | 30.6 | 30.9 | 31.2 |
| 118.1 | 46.5 | 25.4 | 25.7 | 26.0 | 26.3 | 26.7 | 27.0 | 27.3 | 27.6 | 28.0 | 28.3 | 28.6 | 28.9 | 29.3 | 29.6 | 29.9 | 30.2 | 30.6 |
| 119.4 | 47 | 24.8 | 25.1 | 25.5 | 25.8 | 26.1 | 26.4 | 26.7 | 27.1 | 27.4 | 27.7 | 28.0 | 28.3 | 28.6 | 29.0 | 29.3 | 29.6 | 29.9 |
| 120.7 | 47.5 | 24.3 | 24.6 | 24.9 | 25.2 | 25.6 | 25.9 | 26.2 | 26.5 | 26.8 | 27.1 | 27.4 | 27.7 | 28.0 | 28.4 | 28.7 | 29.0 | 29.3 |
| 121.9 | 48 | 23.8 | 24.1 | 24.4 | 24.7 | 25.0 | 25.3 | 25.6 | 25.9 | 26.2 | 26.5 | 26.9 | 27.2 | 27.5 | 27.8 | 28.1 | 28.4 | 28.7 |
| 124.5 | 49 | 22.8 | 23.1 | 23.4 | 23.7 | 24.0 | 24.3 | 24.6 | 24.9 | 25.2 | 25.5 | 25.8 | 26.1 | 26.4 | 26.6 | 26.9 | 27.2 | 27.5 |
| 127.0 | 50 | 21.9 | 22.2 | 22.5 | 22.8 | 23.1 | 23.3 | 23.6 | 23.9 | 24.2 | 24.5 | 24.7 | 25.0 | 25.3 | 25.6 | 25.9 | 26.2 | 26.4 |
| 129.5 | 51 | 21.1 | 21.4 | 21.6 | 21.9 | 22.2 | 22.4 | 22.7 | 23.0 | 23.2 | 23.5 | 23.8 | 24.1 | 24.3 | 24.6 | 24.9 | 25.1 | 25.4 |
| 132.1 | 52 | 20.3 | 20.5 | 20.8 | 21.1 | 21.3 | 21.6 | 21.8 | 22.1 | 22.4 | 22.6 | 22.9 | 23.1 | 23.4 | 23.7 | 23.9 | 24.2 | 24.4 |
| 134.6 | 53 | 19.5 | 19.8 | 20.0 | 20.3 | 20.5 | 20.8 | 21.0 | 21.3 | 21.5 | 21.8 | 22.0 | 22.3 | 22.5 | 22.8 | 23.0 | 23.3 | 23.5 |
| 137.2 | 54 | 18.8 | 19.0 | 19.3 | 19.5 | 19.8 | 20.0 | 20.3 | 20.5 | 20.7 | 21.0 | 21.2 | 21.5 | 21.7 | 21.9 | 22.2 | 22.4 | 22.7 |
| 139.7 | 55 | 18.1 | 18.4 | 18.6 | 18.8 | 19.1 | 19.3 | 19.5 | 19.8 | 20.0 | 20.2 | 20.5 | 20.7 | 20.9 | 21.2 | 21.4 | 21.6 | 21.8 |
| 142.2 | 56 | 17.5 | 17.7 | 17.9 | 18.2 | 18.4 | 18.6 | 18.8 | 19.1 | 19.3 | 19.5 | 19.7 | 20.0 | 20.2 | 20.4 | 20.6 | 20.8 | 21.1 |
| 144.8 | 57 | 16.9 | 17.1 | 17.3 | 17.5 | 17.7 | 18.0 | 18.2 | 18.4 | 18.6 | 18.8 | 19.0 | 19.3 | 19.5 | 19.7 | 19.9 | 20.1 | 20.3 |
| 147.3 | 58 | 16.3 | 16.5 | 16.7 | 16.9 | 17.1 | 17.3 | 17.6 | 17.8 | 18.0 | 18.2 | 18.4 | 18.6 | 18.8 | 19.0 | 19.2 | 19.4 | 19.6 |
| 149.9 | 59 | 15.8 | 16.0 | 16.2 | 16.4 | 16.6 | 16.8 | 17.0 | 17.2 | 17.4 | 17.6 | 17.8 | 18.0 | 18.2 | 18.4 | 18.6 | 18.8 | 19.0 |
| 152.4 | 60 | 15.2 | 15.4 | 15.6 | 15.8 | 16.0 | 16.2 | 16.4 | 16.6 | 16.8 | 17.0 | 17.2 | 17.4 | 17.6 | 17.8 | 18.0 | 18.2 | 18.4 |

*Whenever a child's specific height or weight measurement is not listed, round to the closest number in the table.*

## CALCULATED BODY MASS INDEX    61 in.–71 in. AND 78 LB–94 LB

|  |  | Weight | | | | | | | | | | | | | | | | |
|---|---|---|---|---|---|---|---|---|---|---|---|---|---|---|---|---|---|---|
| kg |  | 35.4 | 35.8 | 36.3 | 36.7 | 37.2 | 37.6 | 38.1 | 38.6 | 39.0 | 39.5 | 39.9 | 40.4 | 40.8 | 41.3 | 41.7 | 42.2 | 42.6 |
| lb |  | 78 | 79 | 80 | 81 | 82 | 83 | 84 | 85 | 86 | 87 | 88 | 89 | 90 | 91 | 92 | 93 | 94 |
| **Height** | | | | | | | | | | | | | | | | | | |
| cm | in | | | | | | | | | | | | | | | | | |
| 154.9 | 61 | 14.7 | 14.9 | 15.1 | 15.3 | 15.5 | 15.7 | 15.9 | 16.1 | 16.2 | 16.4 | 16.6 | 16.8 | 17.0 | 17.2 | 17.4 | 17.6 | 17.8 |
| 157.5 | 62 | 14.3 | 14.4 | 14.6 | 14.8 | 15.0 | 15.2 | 15.4 | 15.5 | 15.7 | 15.9 | 16.1 | 16.3 | 16.5 | 16.6 | 16.8 | 17.0 | 17.2 |
| 160.0 | 63 | 13.8 | 14.0 | 14.2 | 14.3 | 14.5 | 14.7 | 14.9 | 15.1 | 15.2 | 15.4 | 15.6 | 15.8 | 15.9 | 16.1 | 16.3 | 16.5 | 16.7 |
| 162.6 | 64 | 13.4 | 13.6 | 13.7 | 13.9 | 14.1 | 14.2 | 14.4 | 14.6 | 14.8 | 14.9 | 15.1 | 15.3 | 15.4 | 15.6 | 15.8 | 16.0 | 16.1 |
| 165.1 | 65 |  | 13.1 | 13.3 | 13.5 | 13.6 | 13.8 | 14.0 | 14.1 | 14.3 | 14.5 | 14.6 | 14.8 | 15.0 | 15.1 | 15.3 | 15.5 | 15.6 |
| 167.6 | 66 |  |  |  | 13.1 | 13.2 | 13.4 | 13.6 | 13.7 | 13.9 | 14.0 | 14.2 | 14.4 | 14.5 | 14.7 | 14.8 | 15.0 | 15.2 |
| 170.2 | 67 |  |  |  |  |  |  | 13.2 | 13.3 | 13.5 | 13.6 | 13.8 | 13.9 | 14.1 | 14.3 | 14.4 | 14.6 | 14.7 |
| 172.7 | 68 |  |  |  |  |  |  |  |  | 13.1 | 13.2 | 13.4 | 13.5 | 13.7 | 13.8 | 14.0 | 14.1 | 14.3 |
| 175.3 | 69 |  |  |  |  |  |  |  |  |  |  |  | 13.1 | 13.3 | 13.4 | 13.6 | 13.7 | 13.9 |
| 177.8 | 70 |  |  |  |  |  |  |  |  |  |  |  |  |  | 13.1 | 13.2 | 13.3 | 13.5 |
| 180.3 | 71 |  |  |  |  |  |  |  |  |  |  |  |  |  |  |  |  | 13.1 |

*Whenever a child's specific height or weight measurement is not listed, round to the closest number in the table.*

## CALCULATED BODY MASS INDEX 44 in.–68 in. AND 95 LB–112 LB

| Height | | Weight | | | | | | | | | | | | | | | | |
|---|---|---|---|---|---|---|---|---|---|---|---|---|---|---|---|---|---|---|
| cm | in (kg) | 43.1 | 43.5 | 44.0 | 44.5 | 44.9 | 45.4 | 45.8 | 46.3 | 46.7 | 47.2 | 47.6 | 48.1 | 48.5 | 49.0 | 49.4 | 49.9 | 50.8 |
| | (lb) | 95 | 96 | 97 | 98 | 99 | 100 | 101 | 102 | 103 | 104 | 105 | 106 | 107 | 108 | 109 | 110 | 112 |
| 111.8 | 44 | 34.5 | 34.9 | | | | | | | | | | | | | | | |
| 113.0 | 44.5 | 33.7 | 34.1 | 34.4 | 34.8 | | | | | | | | | | | | | |
| 114.3 | 45 | 33.0 | 33.3 | 33.7 | 34.0 | 34.4 | 34.7 | | | | | | | | | | | |
| 115.6 | 45.5 | 32.3 | 32.6 | 32.9 | 33.3 | 33.6 | 34.0 | 34.3 | 34.6 | 35.0 | | | | | | | | |
| 116.8 | 46 | 31.6 | 31.9 | 32.2 | 32.6 | 32.9 | 33.2 | 33.6 | 33.9 | 34.2 | 34.6 | 34.9 | | | | | | |
| 118.1 | 46.5 | 30.9 | 31.2 | 31.5 | 31.9 | 32.2 | 32.5 | 32.8 | 33.2 | 33.5 | 33.8 | 34.1 | 34.5 | 34.8 | | | | |
| 119.4 | 47 | 30.2 | 30.6 | 30.9 | 31.2 | 31.5 | 31.8 | 32.1 | 32.5 | 32.8 | 33.1 | 33.4 | 33.7 | 34.1 | 34.4 | 34.7 | | |
| 120.7 | 47.5 | 29.6 | 29.9 | 30.2 | 30.5 | 30.8 | 31.2 | 31.5 | 31.8 | 32.1 | 32.4 | 32.7 | 33.0 | 33.3 | 33.7 | 34.0 | 34.3 | 34.9 |
| 121.9 | 48 | 29.0 | 29.3 | 29.6 | 29.9 | 30.2 | 30.5 | 30.8 | 31.1 | 31.4 | 31.7 | 32.0 | 32.3 | 32.7 | 33.0 | 33.3 | 33.6 | 34.2 |
| 124.5 | 49 | 27.8 | 28.1 | 28.4 | 28.7 | 29.0 | 29.3 | 29.6 | 29.9 | 30.2 | 30.5 | 30.7 | 31.0 | 31.3 | 31.6 | 31.9 | 32.2 | 32.8 |
| 127.0 | 50 | 26.7 | 27.0 | 27.3 | 27.6 | 27.8 | 28.1 | 28.4 | 28.7 | 29.0 | 29.2 | 29.5 | 29.8 | 30.1 | 30.4 | 30.7 | 30.9 | 31.5 |
| 129.5 | 51 | 25.7 | 25.9 | 26.2 | 26.5 | 26.8 | 27.0 | 27.3 | 27.6 | 27.8 | 28.1 | 28.4 | 28.7 | 28.9 | 29.2 | 29.5 | 29.7 | 30.3 |
| 132.1 | 52 | 24.7 | 25.0 | 25.2 | 25.5 | 25.7 | 26.0 | 26.3 | 26.5 | 26.8 | 27.0 | 27.3 | 27.6 | 27.8 | 28.1 | 28.3 | 28.6 | 29.1 |
| 134.6 | 53 | 23.8 | 24.0 | 24.3 | 24.5 | 24.8 | 25.0 | 25.3 | 25.5 | 25.8 | 26.0 | 26.3 | 26.5 | 26.8 | 27.0 | 27.3 | 27.5 | 28.0 |
| 137.2 | 54 | 22.9 | 23.1 | 23.4 | 23.6 | 23.9 | 24.1 | 24.4 | 24.6 | 24.8 | 25.1 | 25.3 | 25.6 | 25.8 | 26.0 | 26.3 | 26.5 | 27.0 |
| 139.7 | 55 | 22.1 | 22.3 | 22.5 | 22.8 | 23.0 | 23.2 | 23.5 | 23.7 | 23.9 | 24.2 | 24.4 | 24.6 | 24.9 | 25.1 | 25.3 | 25.6 | 26.0 |
| 142.2 | 56 | 21.3 | 21.5 | 21.7 | 22.0 | 22.2 | 22.4 | 22.6 | 22.9 | 23.1 | 23.3 | 23.5 | 23.8 | 24.0 | 24.2 | 24.4 | 24.7 | 25.1 |
| 144.8 | 57 | 20.6 | 20.8 | 21.0 | 21.2 | 21.4 | 21.6 | 21.9 | 22.1 | 22.3 | 22.5 | 22.7 | 22.9 | 23.2 | 23.4 | 23.6 | 23.8 | 24.2 |
| 147.3 | 58 | 19.9 | 20.1 | 20.3 | 20.5 | 20.7 | 20.9 | 21.1 | 21.3 | 21.5 | 21.7 | 21.9 | 22.2 | 22.4 | 22.6 | 22.8 | 23.0 | 23.4 |
| 149.9 | 59 | 19.2 | 19.4 | 19.6 | 19.8 | 20.0 | 20.2 | 20.4 | 20.6 | 20.8 | 21.0 | 21.2 | 21.4 | 21.6 | 21.8 | 22.0 | 22.2 | 22.6 |
| 152.4 | 60 | 18.6 | 18.7 | 18.9 | 19.1 | 19.3 | 19.5 | 19.7 | 19.9 | 20.1 | 20.3 | 20.5 | 20.7 | 20.9 | 21.1 | 21.3 | 21.5 | 21.9 |
| 154.9 | 61 | 17.9 | 18.1 | 18.3 | 18.5 | 18.7 | 18.9 | 19.1 | 19.3 | 19.5 | 19.7 | 19.8 | 20.0 | 20.2 | 20.4 | 20.6 | 20.8 | 21.2 |
| 157.5 | 62 | 17.4 | 17.6 | 17.7 | 17.9 | 18.1 | 18.3 | 18.5 | 18.7 | 18.8 | 19.0 | 19.2 | 19.4 | 19.6 | 19.8 | 19.9 | 20.1 | 20.5 |
| 160.0 | 63 | 16.8 | 17.0 | 17.2 | 17.4 | 17.5 | 17.7 | 17.9 | 18.1 | 18.2 | 18.4 | 18.6 | 18.8 | 19.0 | 19.1 | 19.3 | 19.5 | 19.8 |
| 162.6 | 64 | 16.3 | 16.5 | 16.6 | 16.8 | 17.0 | 17.2 | 17.3 | 17.5 | 17.7 | 17.9 | 18.0 | 18.2 | 18.4 | 18.5 | 18.7 | 18.9 | 19.2 |
| 165.1 | 65 | 15.8 | 16.0 | 16.1 | 16.3 | 16.5 | 16.6 | 16.8 | 17.0 | 17.1 | 17.3 | 17.5 | 17.6 | 17.8 | 18.0 | 18.1 | 18.3 | 18.6 |
| 167.6 | 66 | 15.3 | 15.5 | 15.7 | 15.8 | 16.0 | 16.1 | 16.3 | 16.5 | 16.6 | 16.8 | 16.9 | 17.1 | 17.3 | 17.4 | 17.6 | 17.8 | 18.1 |
| 170.2 | 67 | 14.9 | 15.0 | 15.2 | 15.3 | 15.5 | 15.7 | 15.8 | 16.0 | 16.1 | 16.3 | 16.4 | 16.6 | 16.8 | 16.9 | 17.1 | 17.2 | 17.5 |
| 172.7 | 68 | 14.4 | 14.6 | 14.7 | 14.9 | 15.1 | 15.2 | 15.4 | 15.5 | 15.7 | 15.8 | 16.0 | 16.1 | 16.3 | 16.4 | 16.6 | 16.7 | 17.0 |

*Whenever a child's specific height or weight measurement is not listed, round to the closest number in the table.*

## CALCULATED BODY MASS INDEX    69 in.–77 in. AND 95 LB–112 LB

| Height | | Weight | | | | | | | | | | | | | | | | | |
|---|---|---|---|---|---|---|---|---|---|---|---|---|---|---|---|---|---|---|---|---|
| | | kg | 43.1 | 43.5 | 44.0 | 44.5 | 44.9 | 45.4 | 45.8 | 46.3 | 46.7 | 47.2 | 47.6 | 48.1 | 48.5 | 49.0 | 49.4 | 49.9 | 50.8 |
| | | lb | 95 | 96 | 97 | 98 | 99 | 100 | 101 | 102 | 103 | 104 | 105 | 106 | 107 | 108 | 109 | 110 | 112 |
| cm | in | | | | | | | | | | | | | | | | | | | |
| 175.3 | 69 | | 14.0 | 14.2 | 14.3 | 14.5 | 14.6 | 14.8 | 14.9 | 15.1 | 15.2 | 15.4 | 15.5 | 15.7 | 15.8 | 15.9 | 16.1 | 16.2 | 16.5 |
| 177.8 | 70 | | 13.6 | 13.8 | 13.9 | 14.1 | 14.2 | 14.3 | 14.5 | 14.6 | 14.8 | 14.9 | 15.1 | 15.2 | 15.4 | 15.5 | 15.6 | 15.8 | 16.1 |
| 180.3 | 71 | | 13.2 | 13.4 | 13.5 | 13.7 | 13.8 | 13.9 | 14.1 | 14.2 | 14.4 | 14.5 | 14.6 | 14.8 | 14.9 | 15.1 | 15.2 | 15.3 | 15.6 |
| 182.9 | 72 | | | 13.0 | 13.2 | 13.3 | 13.4 | 13.6 | 13.7 | 13.8 | 14.0 | 14.1 | 14.2 | 14.4 | 14.5 | 14.6 | 14.8 | 14.9 | 15.2 |
| 185.4 | 73 | | | | | | 13.1 | 13.2 | 13.3 | 13.5 | 13.6 | 13.7 | 13.9 | 14.0 | 14.1 | 14.2 | 14.4 | 14.5 | 14.8 |
| 188.0 | 74 | | | | | | | | | 13.1 | 13.2 | 13.4 | 13.5 | 13.6 | 13.7 | 13.9 | 14.0 | 14.1 | 14.4 |
| 190.5 | 75 | | | | | | | | | | | | 13.1 | 13.2 | 13.4 | 13.5 | 13.6 | 13.7 | 14.0 |
| 193.0 | 76 | | | | | | | | | | | | | | 13.0 | 13.1 | 13.3 | 13.4 | 13.6 |
| 195.6 | 77 | | | | | | | | | | | | | | | | | 13.0 | 13.3 |

*Whenever a child's specific height or weight measurement is not listed, round to the closest number in the table.*

## CALCULATED BODY MASS INDEX  48 in.–76 in. AND 114 LB–146 LB

| Height | | Weight | | | | | | | | | | | | | | | | |
| cm | in | kg 51.7 / lb 114 | 52.6 / 116 | 53.5 / 118 | 54.4 / 120 | 55.3 / 122 | 56.2 / 124 | 57.2 / 126 | 58.1 / 128 | 59.0 / 130 | 59.9 / 132 | 60.8 / 134 | 61.7 / 136 | 62.6 / 138 | 63.5 / 140 | 64.4 / 142 | 65.3 / 144 | 66.2 / 146 |
|---|---|---|---|---|---|---|---|---|---|---|---|---|---|---|---|---|---|---|
| 121.9 | 48 | 34.8 | | | | | | | | | | | | | | | | |
| 124.5 | 49 | 33.4 | 34.0 | 34.6 | | | | | | | | | | | | | | |
| 127.0 | 50 | 32.1 | 32.6 | 33.2 | 33.7 | 34.3 | 34.9 | | | | | | | | | | | |
| 129.5 | 51 | 30.8 | 31.4 | 31.9 | 32.4 | 33.0 | 33.5 | 34.1 | 34.6 | | | | | | | | | |
| 132.1 | 52 | 29.6 | 30.2 | 30.7 | 31.2 | 31.7 | 32.2 | 32.8 | 33.3 | 33.8 | 34.3 | 34.8 | | | | | | |
| 134.6 | 53 | 28.5 | 29.0 | 29.5 | 30.0 | 30.5 | 31.0 | 31.5 | 32.0 | 32.5 | 33.0 | 33.5 | 34.0 | 34.5 | | | | |
| 137.2 | 54 | 27.5 | 28.0 | 28.5 | 28.9 | 29.4 | 29.9 | 30.4 | 30.9 | 31.3 | 31.8 | 32.3 | 32.8 | 33.3 | 33.8 | 34.2 | 34.7 | |
| 139.7 | 55 | 26.5 | 27.0 | 27.4 | 27.9 | 28.4 | 28.8 | 29.3 | 29.7 | 30.2 | 30.7 | 31.1 | 31.6 | 32.1 | 32.5 | 33.0 | 33.5 | 33.9 |
| 142.2 | 56 | 25.6 | 26.0 | 26.5 | 26.9 | 27.4 | 27.8 | 28.2 | 28.7 | 29.1 | 29.6 | 30.0 | 30.5 | 30.9 | 31.4 | 31.8 | 32.3 | 32.7 |
| 144.8 | 57 | 24.7 | 25.1 | 25.5 | 26.0 | 26.4 | 26.8 | 27.3 | 27.7 | 28.1 | 28.6 | 29.0 | 29.4 | 29.9 | 30.3 | 30.7 | 31.2 | 31.6 |
| 147.3 | 58 | 23.8 | 24.2 | 24.7 | 25.1 | 25.5 | 25.9 | 26.3 | 26.8 | 27.2 | 27.6 | 28.0 | 28.4 | 28.8 | 29.3 | 29.7 | 30.1 | 30.5 |
| 149.9 | 59 | 23.0 | 23.4 | 23.8 | 24.2 | 24.6 | 25.0 | 25.4 | 25.9 | 26.3 | 26.7 | 27.1 | 27.5 | 27.9 | 28.3 | 28.7 | 29.1 | 29.5 |
| 152.4 | 60 | 22.3 | 22.7 | 23.0 | 23.4 | 23.8 | 24.2 | 24.6 | 25.0 | 25.4 | 25.8 | 26.2 | 26.6 | 27.0 | 27.3 | 27.7 | 28.1 | 28.5 |
| 154.9 | 61 | 21.5 | 21.9 | 22.3 | 22.7 | 23.1 | 23.4 | 23.8 | 24.2 | 24.6 | 24.9 | 25.3 | 25.7 | 26.1 | 26.5 | 26.8 | 27.2 | 27.6 |
| 157.5 | 62 | 20.9 | 21.2 | 21.6 | 21.9 | 22.3 | 22.7 | 23.0 | 23.4 | 23.8 | 24.1 | 24.5 | 24.9 | 25.2 | 25.6 | 26.0 | 26.3 | 26.7 |
| 160.0 | 63 | 20.2 | 20.5 | 20.9 | 21.3 | 21.6 | 22.0 | 22.3 | 22.7 | 23.0 | 23.4 | 23.7 | 24.1 | 24.4 | 24.8 | 25.2 | 25.5 | 25.9 |
| 162.6 | 64 | 19.6 | 19.9 | 20.3 | 20.6 | 20.9 | 21.3 | 21.6 | 22.0 | 22.3 | 22.7 | 23.0 | 23.3 | 23.7 | 24.0 | 24.4 | 24.7 | 25.1 |
| 165.1 | 65 | 19.0 | 19.3 | 19.6 | 20.0 | 20.3 | 20.6 | 21.0 | 21.3 | 21.6 | 22.0 | 22.3 | 22.6 | 23.0 | 23.3 | 23.6 | 24.0 | 24.3 |
| 167.6 | 66 | 18.4 | 18.7 | 19.0 | 19.4 | 19.7 | 20.0 | 20.3 | 20.7 | 21.0 | 21.3 | 21.6 | 22.0 | 22.3 | 22.6 | 22.9 | 23.2 | 23.6 |
| 170.2 | 67 | 17.9 | 18.2 | 18.5 | 18.8 | 19.1 | 19.4 | 19.7 | 20.0 | 20.4 | 20.7 | 21.0 | 21.3 | 21.6 | 21.9 | 22.2 | 22.6 | 22.9 |
| 172.7 | 68 | 17.3 | 17.6 | 17.9 | 18.2 | 18.5 | 18.9 | 19.2 | 19.5 | 19.8 | 20.1 | 20.4 | 20.7 | 21.0 | 21.3 | 21.6 | 21.9 | 22.2 |
| 175.3 | 69 | 16.8 | 17.1 | 17.4 | 17.7 | 18.0 | 18.3 | 18.6 | 18.9 | 19.2 | 19.5 | 19.8 | 20.1 | 20.4 | 20.7 | 21.0 | 21.3 | 21.6 |
| 177.8 | 70 | 16.4 | 16.6 | 16.9 | 17.2 | 17.5 | 17.8 | 18.1 | 18.4 | 18.7 | 18.9 | 19.2 | 19.5 | 19.8 | 20.1 | 20.4 | 20.7 | 20.9 |
| 180.3 | 71 | 15.9 | 16.2 | 16.5 | 16.7 | 17.0 | 17.3 | 17.6 | 17.9 | 18.1 | 18.4 | 18.7 | 19.0 | 19.2 | 19.5 | 19.8 | 20.1 | 20.4 |
| 182.9 | 72 | 15.5 | 15.7 | 16.0 | 16.3 | 16.5 | 16.8 | 17.1 | 17.4 | 17.6 | 17.9 | 18.2 | 18.4 | 18.7 | 19.0 | 19.3 | 19.5 | 19.8 |
| 185.4 | 73 | 15.0 | 15.3 | 15.6 | 15.8 | 16.1 | 16.4 | 16.6 | 16.9 | 17.2 | 17.4 | 17.7 | 17.9 | 18.2 | 18.5 | 18.7 | 19.0 | 19.3 |
| 188.0 | 74 | 14.6 | 14.9 | 15.2 | 15.4 | 15.7 | 15.9 | 16.2 | 16.4 | 16.7 | 16.9 | 17.2 | 17.5 | 17.7 | 18.0 | 18.2 | 18.5 | 18.7 |
| 190.5 | 75 | 14.2 | 14.5 | 14.7 | 15.0 | 15.2 | 15.5 | 15.7 | 16.0 | 16.2 | 16.5 | 16.7 | 17.0 | 17.2 | 17.5 | 17.7 | 18.0 | 18.2 |
| 193.0 | 76 | 13.9 | 14.1 | 14.4 | 14.6 | 14.7 | 15.1 | 15.3 | 15.6 | 15.8 | 16.1 | 16.3 | 16.6 | 16.8 | 17.0 | 17.3 | 17.5 | 17.8 |
| 195.6 | 77 | 13.5 | 13.8 | 14.0 | 14.2 | 14.5 | 14.7 | 14.9 | 15.2 | 15.4 | 15.7 | 15.9 | 16.1 | 16.4 | 16.6 | 16.8 | 17.1 | 17.3 |
| 198.1 | 78 | 13.2 | 13.4 | 13.6 | 13.9 | 14.1 | 14.3 | 14.6 | 14.8 | 15.0 | 15.3 | 15.5 | 15.7 | 15.9 | 16.2 | 16.4 | 16.6 | 16.9 |

*Whenever a child's specific height or weight measurement is not listed, round to the closest number in the table.*

## CALCULATED BODY MASS INDEX   55 in.–78 in. AND 148 LB–180 LB

| Height (cm) | (in) | 148 | 150 | 152 | 154 | 156 | 158 | 160 | 162 | 164 | 166 | 168 | 170 | 172 | 174 | 176 | 178 | 180 |
|---|---|---|---|---|---|---|---|---|---|---|---|---|---|---|---|---|---|---|
| **Weight (kg)** → | | 67.1 | 68.0 | 68.9 | 69.9 | 70.8 | 71.7 | 72.6 | 73.5 | 74.4 | 75.3 | 76.2 | 77.1 | 78.0 | 78.9 | 79.8 | 80.7 | 81.6 |
| 139.7 | 55 | 34.4 | 34.9 | | | | | | | | | | | | | | | |
| 142.2 | 56 | 33.2 | 33.6 | 34.1 | 34.5 | 35.0 | | | | | | | | | | | | |
| 144.8 | 57 | 32.0 | 32.5 | 32.9 | 33.3 | 33.8 | 34.2 | 34.6 | | | | | | | | | | |
| 147.3 | 58 | 30.9 | 31.3 | 31.8 | 32.2 | 32.6 | 33.0 | 33.4 | 33.9 | 34.3 | 34.7 | | | | | | | |
| 149.9 | 59 | 29.9 | 30.3 | 30.7 | 31.1 | 31.5 | 31.9 | 32.3 | 32.7 | 33.1 | 33.5 | 33.9 | 34.3 | 34.7 | | | | |
| 152.4 | 60 | 28.9 | 29.3 | 29.7 | 30.1 | 30.5 | 30.9 | 31.2 | 31.6 | 32.0 | 32.4 | 32.8 | 33.2 | 33.6 | 34.0 | 34.4 | 34.8 | |
| 154.9 | 61 | 28.0 | 28.3 | 28.7 | 29.1 | 29.5 | 29.9 | 30.2 | 30.6 | 31.0 | 31.4 | 31.7 | 32.1 | 32.5 | 32.9 | 33.3 | 33.6 | 34.0 |
| 157.5 | 62 | 27.1 | 27.4 | 27.8 | 28.2 | 28.5 | 28.9 | 29.3 | 29.6 | 30.0 | 30.4 | 30.7 | 31.1 | 31.5 | 31.8 | 32.2 | 32.6 | 32.9 |
| 160.0 | 63 | 26.2 | 26.6 | 26.9 | 27.3 | 27.6 | 28.0 | 28.3 | 28.7 | 29.1 | 29.4 | 29.8 | 30.1 | 30.5 | 30.8 | 31.2 | 31.5 | 31.9 |
| 162.6 | 64 | 25.4 | 25.7 | 26.1 | 26.4 | 26.8 | 27.1 | 27.5 | 27.8 | 28.2 | 28.5 | 28.8 | 29.2 | 29.5 | 29.9 | 30.2 | 30.6 | 30.9 |
| 165.1 | 65 | 24.6 | 25.0 | 25.3 | 25.6 | 26.0 | 26.3 | 26.6 | 27.0 | 27.3 | 27.6 | 28.0 | 28.3 | 28.6 | 29.0 | 29.3 | 29.6 | 30.0 |
| 167.6 | 66 | 23.9 | 24.2 | 24.5 | 24.9 | 25.2 | 25.5 | 25.8 | 26.1 | 26.5 | 26.8 | 27.1 | 27.4 | 27.8 | 28.1 | 28.4 | 28.7 | 29.1 |
| 170.2 | 67 | 23.2 | 23.5 | 23.8 | 24.1 | 24.4 | 24.7 | 25.1 | 25.4 | 25.7 | 26.0 | 26.3 | 26.6 | 26.9 | 27.3 | 27.6 | 27.9 | 28.2 |
| 172.7 | 68 | 22.5 | 22.8 | 23.1 | 23.4 | 23.7 | 24.0 | 24.3 | 24.6 | 24.9 | 25.2 | 25.5 | 25.8 | 26.2 | 26.5 | 26.8 | 27.1 | 27.4 |
| 175.3 | 69 | 21.9 | 22.2 | 22.4 | 22.7 | 23.0 | 23.3 | 23.6 | 23.9 | 24.2 | 24.5 | 24.8 | 25.1 | 25.4 | 25.7 | 26.0 | 26.3 | 26.6 |
| 177.8 | 70 | 21.2 | 21.5 | 21.8 | 22.1 | 22.4 | 22.7 | 23.0 | 23.2 | 23.5 | 23.8 | 24.1 | 24.4 | 24.7 | 25.0 | 25.3 | 25.5 | 25.8 |
| 180.3 | 71 | 20.6 | 20.9 | 21.2 | 21.5 | 21.8 | 22.0 | 22.3 | 22.6 | 22.9 | 23.1 | 23.4 | 23.7 | 24.0 | 24.3 | 24.5 | 24.8 | 25.1 |
| 182.9 | 72 | 20.1 | 20.3 | 20.6 | 20.9 | 21.2 | 21.4 | 21.7 | 22.0 | 22.2 | 22.5 | 22.8 | 23.1 | 23.3 | 23.6 | 23.9 | 24.1 | 24.4 |
| 185.4 | 73 | 19.5 | 19.8 | 20.1 | 20.3 | 20.6 | 20.8 | 21.1 | 21.4 | 21.6 | 21.9 | 22.2 | 22.4 | 22.7 | 23.0 | 23.2 | 23.5 | 23.7 |
| 188.0 | 74 | 19.0 | 19.3 | 19.5 | 19.8 | 20.0 | 20.3 | 20.5 | 20.8 | 21.1 | 21.3 | 21.6 | 21.8 | 22.1 | 22.3 | 22.6 | 22.9 | 23.1 |
| 190.5 | 75 | 18.5 | 18.7 | 19.0 | 19.2 | 19.5 | 19.7 | 20.0 | 20.2 | 20.5 | 20.7 | 21.0 | 21.2 | 21.5 | 21.7 | 22.0 | 22.2 | 22.5 |
| 193.0 | 76 | 18.0 | 18.3 | 18.5 | 18.7 | 19.0 | 19.2 | 19.5 | 19.7 | 20.0 | 20.2 | 20.4 | 20.7 | 20.9 | 21.2 | 21.4 | 21.7 | 21.9 |
| 195.6 | 77 | 17.6 | 17.8 | 18.0 | 18.3 | 18.5 | 18.7 | 19.0 | 19.2 | 19.4 | 19.7 | 19.9 | 20.2 | 20.4 | 20.6 | 20.9 | 21.1 | 21.3 |
| 198.1 | 78 | 17.1 | 17.3 | 17.6 | 17.8 | 18.0 | 18.3 | 18.5 | 18.7 | 19.0 | 19.2 | 19.4 | 19.6 | 19.9 | 20.1 | 20.3 | 20.6 | 20.8 |

*Whenever a child's specific height or weight measurement is not listed, round to the closest number in the table.*

## CALCULATED BODY MASS INDEX     61 in.–78 in. AND 182 LB–214 LB

| Height | | Weight | | | | | | | | | | | | | | | | |
|---|---|---|---|---|---|---|---|---|---|---|---|---|---|---|---|---|---|---|
| **cm** | **in** | kg 82.6 | 83.5 | 84.4 | 85.3 | 86.2 | 87.1 | 88.0 | 88.9 | 89.8 | 90.7 | 91.6 | 92.5 | 93.4 | 94.3 | 95.3 | 96.2 | 97.1 |
| | | lb 182 | 184 | 186 | 188 | 190 | 192 | 194 | 196 | 198 | 200 | 202 | 204 | 206 | 208 | 210 | 212 | 214 |
| 154.9 | 61 | 34.4 | 34.8 | | | | | | | | | | | | | | | |
| 157.5 | 62 | 33.3 | 33.7 | 34.0 | 34.4 | 34.8 | | | | | | | | | | | | |
| 160.0 | 63 | 32.2 | 32.6 | 32.9 | 33.3 | 33.7 | 34.0 | 34.4 | 34.7 | | | | | | | | | |
| 162.6 | 64 | 31.2 | 31.6 | 31.9 | 32.3 | 32.6 | 33.0 | 33.3 | 33.6 | 34.0 | 34.3 | 34.7 | | | | | | |
| 165.1 | 65 | 30.3 | 30.6 | 31.0 | 31.3 | 31.6 | 32.0 | 32.3 | 32.6 | 32.9 | 33.3 | 33.6 | 33.9 | 34.3 | 34.6 | 34.9 | | |
| 167.6 | 66 | 29.4 | 29.7 | 30.0 | 30.3 | 30.7 | 31.0 | 31.3 | 31.6 | 32.0 | 32.3 | 32.6 | 32.9 | 33.2 | 33.6 | 33.9 | 34.2 | 34.5 |
| 170.2 | 67 | 28.5 | 28.8 | 29.1 | 29.4 | 29.8 | 30.1 | 30.4 | 30.7 | 31.0 | 31.3 | 31.6 | 32.0 | 32.3 | 32.6 | 32.9 | 33.2 | 33.5 |
| 172.7 | 68 | 27.7 | 28.0 | 28.3 | 28.6 | 28.9 | 29.2 | 29.5 | 29.8 | 30.1 | 30.4 | 30.7 | 31.0 | 31.3 | 31.6 | 31.9 | 32.2 | 32.5 |
| 175.3 | 69 | 26.9 | 27.2 | 27.5 | 27.8 | 28.1 | 28.4 | 28.6 | 28.9 | 29.2 | 29.5 | 29.8 | 30.1 | 30.4 | 30.7 | 31.0 | 31.3 | 31.6 |
| 177.8 | 70 | 26.1 | 26.4 | 26.7 | 27.0 | 27.3 | 27.5 | 27.8 | 28.1 | 28.4 | 28.7 | 29.0 | 29.3 | 29.6 | 29.8 | 30.1 | 30.4 | 30.7 |
| 180.3 | 71 | 25.4 | 25.7 | 25.9 | 26.2 | 26.5 | 26.8 | 27.1 | 27.3 | 27.6 | 27.9 | 28.2 | 28.5 | 28.7 | 29.0 | 29.3 | 29.6 | 29.8 |
| 182.9 | 72 | 24.7 | 25.0 | 25.2 | 25.5 | 25.8 | 26.0 | 26.3 | 26.6 | 26.9 | 27.1 | 27.4 | 27.7 | 27.9 | 28.2 | 28.5 | 28.8 | 29.0 |
| 185.4 | 73 | 24.0 | 24.3 | 24.5 | 24.8 | 25.1 | 25.3 | 25.6 | 25.9 | 26.1 | 26.4 | 26.7 | 26.9 | 27.2 | 27.4 | 27.7 | 28.0 | 28.2 |
| 188.0 | 74 | 23.4 | 23.6 | 23.9 | 24.1 | 24.4 | 24.7 | 24.9 | 25.2 | 25.4 | 25.7 | 25.9 | 26.2 | 26.4 | 26.7 | 27.0 | 27.2 | 27.5 |
| 190.5 | 75 | 22.7 | 23.0 | 23.2 | 23.5 | 23.7 | 24.0 | 24.2 | 24.5 | 24.7 | 25.0 | 25.2 | 25.5 | 25.7 | 26.0 | 26.2 | 26.5 | 26.7 |
| 193.0 | 76 | 22.2 | 22.4 | 22.6 | 22.9 | 23.1 | 23.4 | 23.6 | 23.9 | 24.1 | 24.3 | 24.6 | 24.8 | 25.1 | 25.3 | 25.6 | 25.8 | 26.0 |
| 195.6 | 77 | 21.6 | 21.8 | 22.1 | 22.3 | 22.5 | 22.8 | 23.0 | 23.2 | 23.5 | 23.7 | 24.0 | 24.2 | 24.4 | 24.7 | 24.9 | 25.1 | 25.4 |
| 198.1 | 78 | 21.0 | 21.3 | 21.5 | 21.7 | 22.0 | 22.2 | 22.4 | 22.6 | 22.9 | 23.1 | 23.3 | 23.6 | 23.8 | 24.0 | 24.3 | 24.5 | 24.7 |

*Whenever a child's specific height or weight measurement is not listed, round to the closest number in the table.*

## CALCULATED BODY MASS INDEX   66 in.–78 in. AND 216 LB–250 LB

| Height cm | in | kg: 98.0 | 98.9 | 99.8 | 100.7 | 101.6 | 102.5 | 103.4 | 104.3 | 105.2 | 106.1 | 107.0 | 108.0 | 108.9 | 109.8 | 110.7 | 111.6 | 112.5 | 113.4 |
| | | lb: 216 | 218 | 220 | 222 | 224 | 226 | 228 | 230 | 232 | 234 | 236 | 238 | 240 | 242 | 244 | 246 | 248 | 250 |
|---|---|---|---|---|---|---|---|---|---|---|---|---|---|---|---|---|---|---|---|
| 167.6 | 66 | 34.9 | | | | | | | | | | | | | | | | | |
| 170.2 | 67 | 33.8 | 34.1 | 34.5 | 34.8 | | | | | | | | | | | | | | |
| 172.7 | 68 | 32.8 | 33.1 | 33.5 | 33.8 | 34.1 | 34.4 | 34.7 | 35.0 | | | | | | | | | | |
| 175.3 | 69 | 31.9 | 32.2 | 32.5 | 32.8 | 33.1 | 33.4 | 33.7 | 34.0 | 34.3 | 34.6 | 34.9 | | | | | | | |
| 177.8 | 70 | 31.0 | 31.3 | 31.6 | 31.9 | 32.1 | 32.4 | 32.7 | 33.0 | 33.3 | 33.6 | 33.9 | 34.1 | 34.4 | 34.7 | | | | |
| 180.3 | 71 | 30.1 | 30.4 | 30.7 | 31.0 | 31.2 | 31.5 | 31.8 | 32.1 | 32.4 | 32.6 | 32.9 | 33.2 | 33.5 | 33.8 | 34.0 | 34.3 | 34.6 | 34.9 |
| 182.9 | 72 | 29.3 | 29.6 | 29.8 | 30.1 | 30.4 | 30.7 | 30.9 | 31.2 | 31.5 | 31.7 | 32.0 | 32.3 | 32.5 | 32.8 | 33.1 | 33.4 | 33.6 | 33.9 |
| 185.4 | 73 | 28.5 | 28.8 | 29.0 | 29.3 | 29.6 | 29.8 | 30.1 | 30.3 | 30.6 | 30.9 | 31.1 | 31.4 | 31.7 | 31.9 | 32.2 | 32.5 | 32.7 | 33.0 |
| 188.0 | 74 | 27.7 | 28.0 | 28.2 | 28.5 | 28.8 | 29.0 | 29.3 | 29.5 | 29.8 | 30.0 | 30.3 | 30.6 | 30.8 | 31.1 | 31.3 | 31.6 | 31.8 | 32.1 |
| 190.5 | 75 | 27.0 | 27.2 | 27.5 | 27.7 | 28.0 | 28.2 | 28.5 | 28.7 | 29.0 | 29.2 | 29.5 | 29.7 | 30.0 | 30.2 | 30.5 | 30.7 | 31.0 | 31.2 |
| 193.0 | 76 | 26.3 | 26.5 | 26.8 | 27.0 | 27.3 | 27.5 | 27.8 | 28.0 | 28.2 | 28.5 | 28.7 | 29.0 | 29.2 | 29.5 | 29.7 | 29.9 | 30.2 | 30.4 |
| 195.6 | 77 | 25.6 | 25.9 | 26.1 | 26.3 | 26.6 | 26.8 | 27.0 | 27.3 | 27.5 | 27.7 | 28.0 | 28.2 | 28.5 | 28.7 | 28.9 | 29.2 | 29.4 | 29.6 |
| 198.1 | 78 | 25.0 | 25.2 | 25.4 | 25.7 | 25.9 | 26.1 | 26.3 | 26.6 | 26.8 | 27.0 | 27.3 | 27.5 | 27.7 | 28.0 | 28.2 | 28.4 | 28.7 | 28.9 |

*Whenever a child's specific height or weight measurement is not listed, round to the closest number in the table.*

# BIBLIOGRAPHY

Abraham, Jame, M.D., and Carmen Allegra, M.D. *Bethesda Handbook of Clinical Oncology.* New York: Lippincott Williams & Wilkins, 2001.

Ackerknecht, Erwin H., M.D. *A Short History of Medicine.* Rev. ed. Baltimore: Johns Hopkins University Press, 1982.

Adams, Robert, M.D., et al. "Prompt Differentiation of Addison's Disease from Anorexia Nervosa during Weight Loss and Vomiting." *Southern Medical Journal* 91, no. 2 (February 1998): 208–211.

Altman, Robert, and Michael J. Sarg. *The Cancer Dictionary.* Rev. ed. New York: Facts On File, 2000.

American Gastroenterological Association. "American Gastroenterological Association Medical Position Statement: Guidelines for the Evaluation of Food Allergies." *Gastroenterology* 120 (2001): 1,023–1,025.

Ammer, Christine. *The New A to Z of Women's Health.* 4th ed. New York: Facts On File, 2000.

Andersson, Roland E., M.D. et al. "Appendectomy and Protection against Ulcerative Colitis." *New England Journal of Medicine* 344, no. 11 (March 15, 2001): 808–814.

Andrews, Nancy C., M.D. "Disorders of Iron Metabolism." *New England Journal of Medicine* 341, no. 26 (December 23, 1999): 1,986–1,995.

Angulo, Paul, M.D. "Nonalcoholic Fatty Liver Disease." *New England Journal of Medicine* 346, no. 16 (April 18, 2002): 1,221–1,231.

Antman, Karen, M.D., and Yuan Chang, M.D. "Kaposi's Sarcoma." *New England Journal of Medicine* 342, no. 14 (April 6, 2000): 1,027–1,038.

Aparasu, Rajender R., and Jane R. Mort. "Inappropriate Prescribing for the Elderly: Beers Criteria-Based Review." *The Annals of Pharmacotherapy* 34 (2000): 338–346.

Avunduk, Canan. *Manual of Gastroenterology.* 3d ed. Philadelphia: Lippincott Williams & Wilkins, 2002.

Bacon, Bruce R., M.D., et al. "*HFE* Genotype in Patients with Hemochromotosis and Other Liver Diseases," *Annals of Internal Medicine* 130, no. 12 (June 15, 1999): 953–962.

Bagnardi, Vincenzo, et al. "Alcohol Consumption and the Risk of Cancer." *Alcohol Research & Health* 25, no. 4 (2001): 263–269.

Baris, Dalsu, M.D., and Sheilia Hoar Zahm. "Epidemiology of Lymphomas." *Current Opinion in Oncology* 12 (2000): 383–394.

Barlow, Sarah E., M.D., et al. "Treatment of Child and Adolescent Obesity: Reports from Pediatricians, Pediatric Nurse Practitioners, and Registered Dietitians." *Pediatrics* 110, no. 1 (July 2002): 229–235.

Barnes, Warner, and L. A. Fingerhut. "Injury and Poisoning Episodes and Conditions: National Health Interview Study: 1997." Vital Health Statistics 10, no. 202 (July 2000).

Bartlett, John G., M.D. "Antibiotic-Associated Diarrhea." *New England Journal of Medicine* 346, no. 5 (January 31, 2002): 334–339.

Becker, Anne E., M.D., et al. "Eating Disorders." *New England Journal of Medicine* 340, no. 14 (April 8, 1999): 1,092–1,098.

Belluzzi, Andrea, M.D., et al. "Effect of an Enteric-Coated Fish-Oil Preparation on Relapses in Crohn's Disease." *New England Journal of Medicine* 334, no. 24 (June 13, 1996): 1,557–1,560.

Belmont, John W., et al. "Congenital Sucrase-Isomaltose Deficiency Presenting with Failure to Thrive, Hypercalcemia, and Nephrocalcinosis." *BMC Pediatrics* 2 (April 2002).

Bensoussan, Alan, et al. "Treatment of Irritable Bowel Syndrome with Chinese Herbal Medicine: A Randomized Controlled Trial." *Journal of the American Medical Association* 280, no. 18 (November 11, 1998): 1,585–1,589.

Bernstein, Charles N., M.D., et al. "The Incidence of Fracture among Patients with Inflammatory Bowel Disease: A Population-Based Cohort Study." *Annals of Internal Medicine* 133, no. 10 (November 21, 2000): 795–799.

Bingham, Sheila, A., et al. "Dietary Fibre in Food and Protection against Colorectal Cancer in the European Prospective Investigation into Cancer and Nutrition (EPIC): An Observational Study." *Lancet* 361, no. 9368 (May 3, 2003): 1,496–1,501.

Black, M. M., et al. "A Randomized Clinical Trial of Home Intervention for Children with Failure to Thrive." *Pediatrics* 95, no. 6 (June 1, 1995): 807–814.

Blackwell, D. L., J. G. Collins, and R. Coles. "Summary Health Statistics for U.S. Adults: National Health Interview Survey, 1997." National Center for Health Statistics. *Vital Health Statistics* 10, no. 205 (2002).

Blanck, Heidi Michels, Laura Kettel Khan, and Mary K. Serdula, M.D. "Use of Nonprescription Weight Loss Products: Results from a Multistate Survey." *Journal of American Medical Association* 286, no. 8 (August 22/29, 2001): 930–935.

Bloomgarden, Zachary T., M.D. "New Insights in Obesity." *Diabetes Care* 25, no. 4 (April 2002): 789–795.

Bond, John H., M.D. "Polyp Guideline: Diagnosis, Treatment, and Surveillance for Patients with Colorectal Polyps." *American Journal of Gastroenterology* 95, no. 11 (November 2000): 3,053–3,063.

Brandi, Maria Luisa, et al. "Guidelines for Diagnosis and Therapy of MEN Type 1 and Type 2." *Journal of Clinical Endocrinology & Metabolism* 86, no. 12 (2001): 5,658–5,671.

Brock, Jane, M.D. "Process of Care and Outcomes for Elderly Patients Hospitalized with Peptic Ulcer Disease: Results from a Quality Improvement Project." *Journal of the American Medical Association* 286, no. 16 (October 24/31, 2001): 1,985–1,993.

Brolin, Robert E., M.D. "Bariatric Surgery and Long-Term Control of Morbid Obesity." *Journal of the American Medical Association* 288, no. 22 (December 11, 2002): 2,793–2,796.

Brown, Robert S., Jr., M.D., et al. "A Survey of Liver Transplantation from Living Adult Donors in the United States." *New England Journal of Medicine* 348, no. 9 (February 27, 2003): 818–825.

Brugge, William R., M.D., and Jacques Van Dam, M.D. "Pancreatic and Biliary Endoscopy." *New England Journal of Medicine* 341, no. 24 (December 9, 1999): 1,808–1,818.

Bulaj, Zaneta J., M.D., et al. "Disease-Related Conditions in Relatives of Patients with Hemochromatosis." *New England Journal of Medicine* 343, no. 21 (November 23, 2000): 1,529–1,535.

Bytzer, Peter, M.D., et al. "Prevalence of Gastrointestinal Symptoms Associated with Diabetes Mellitus: A Population-Based Survey of 15000 Adults." *Archives of Internal Medicine* 161 (September 10, 2001): 1,989–1,996.

Bytzer, Peter, M.D., and Nicholas J. Talley, M.D. "Dyspepsia." *Annals of Internal Medicine* 134, no. 9, part 2 (2001): 815–822.

Calle, Eugenia E., et al. "Overweight, Obesity, and Mortality from Cancer in a Prospectively Studied Cohort of U.S. Adults." *New England Journal of Medicine* 348, no. 17 (April 24, 2003): 1,625–1,638.

Calvert, Paula M., M.D., and Harold Frucht, M.D. "The Genetics of Colorectal Cancer." *Annals of Internal Medicine* 137, no. 7 (2002): 603–612.

Calvo, M. M., et al. "Role of Magnetic Resonance Cholangiopancreatography with Suspected Choledo-cholithiasis." *Mayo Clinic Proceedings* 77, no. 5 (May 2002): 422–428.

Cannon, Richard O., et al. "Imipramine in Patients with Chest Pain despite Normal Coronary Angiograms." *New England Journal of Medicine* 330, no. 20 (May 19, 1994): 1,411–1,417.

Cassell, Dana K., and David H. Gleaves. *Obesity and Eating Disorders.* 2d ed. New York: Facts On File, 2000.

Cavicchi, Maryan, M.D., et al. "Prevalence of Liver Disease and Contributing Factors in Patients Receiving Home Parenteral Nutrition for Permanent Intestinal Failure." *Annals of Internal Medicine* 132, no. 7 (2000): 525–532.

Centers for Disease Control and Prevention. "At a Glance: Colorectal Cancer: The Importance of Prevention and Early Detection, 2001." 2001.

Centers for Disease Control and Prevention. "Intussusception among Recipients of Rotavirus Vaccine—United States, 1998–1999." *Morbidity and Mortality Report* 48 (1999): 577–581.

Charatan, Fred. "New York Outbreak of *E. coli* Poisoning Affects 1000 and Kills Two." *British Medical Journal* 319 (October 2, 1999): 873.

Chen, Xian-Ming, M.D., et al. "Cryptosporidiosis." New England Journal of Medicine 346, no. 2 (May 30, 2002): 1,723–1,731.

Cherry, Donald K., and David A. Woodwell, Division of Health Care Statistics. "National Ambulatory Medical Care Survey: 2000 Summary." *Advance Data* no. 328 (June 5, 2002).

Chow, W. H., et al. "Gallstones, Cholecystectomy and Risk of Cancers of the Liver, Biliary Tract and Pancreas." *British Journal of Cancer* 79, no. 3/4 (1999): 640–644.

Clark, Robin E., Judith Freeman Clark, with Christine Adamec. *The Encyclopedia of Child Abuse.* 2d ed. New York: Facts On File, 2000.

Colgan, S. M., E. B. Faragher, and P. J. Whorwell. "Controlled Trial of Hypnotherapy in Relapse Prevention of Duodenal Ulceration." *Lancet* (June 11, 1988): 1,299–1,300.

Corcoran, Colleen, N.P., and Steven Grinspoon, M.D. "Treatments for Wasting in Patients with the Acquired Immunodeficiency Syndrome." *New England Journal of Medicine* 340, no. 22 (June 3, 1999): 1,740–1,750.

Cox, Cheryl A., and Stephen J. Bickston. "Right Upper Quadrant Pain: Gallbladder Disease and Its Complications." In *20 Common Problems in Gastroenterology.* New York: McGraw-Hill Medical Publishing Division, 2002.

Crump, John A., et al. "An Outbreak of *Escherichia coli* 0157:H7 Infections among Visitors to a Dairy Farm." *New England Journal of Medicine* 347, no. 8 (August 22, 2002): 555–560.

Cummings, David E., M.D., et al. "Plasma Ghrelin Levels after Diet-Induced Weight Loss or Gastric Bypass Surgery." *New England Journal of Medicine* 346, no. 21 (May 23, 2002): 1,623–1,630.

Dang, Chi V., M.D. "Runner's Anemia." *Journal of the American Medical Association* 286, no. 6 (August 8, 2001): 714–716.

Davis, Dirk R., M.D. "Esophageal Infections." *GI/Liver Secrets.* 2d ed. Philadelphia: Hanley & Belfus, 2001.

De Groen, Piet C., M.D., et al. "Biliary Tract Cancers." *New England Journal of Medicine* 341, no. 18 (October 28, 1999): 1,368–1,378.

Despres, Jen-Pierre, Isabelle Lemieux, and Denis Prud'homme. "Treatment of Obesity: Need to Focus on High Risk Abdominally Obese Patients." *British Medical Journal* 322 (March 24, 2001): 716–720.

Deutsch, John C., M.D. "Gastric Cancer." In *GI/Liver Secrets.* 2d ed. Philadelphia: Hanley & Belfus, 2001.

Devesa, Susan S., William J. Blot, and Joseph F. Fraumeni, Jr., M.D. "Changing Patterns in the Incidence of Esophageal and Gastric Carcinoma in the United States." *Cancer* 83, no. 10 (November 15, 1998): 2,049–2,053.

Diamant, Allison L., M.D., et al. "Lesbians' Sexual History with Men: Implications for Taking a Sexual History." *Archives of Internal Medicine* 159 (December 13/27, 1999): 2,730–2,736.

Dibs, Susan D., M.D., and M. Douglas Baker, M.D. "Anaphylaxis in Children: A 5-Year Experience." *Pediatrics* 99, no. 1: Available online. URL:http://pediatrics.aappublications.orgcgi/content/full/99/1/e7 Posted January 1997.

Dixon, John B., and Paul E. O'Brien, M.D. "Gastro-esophageal Reflux in Obesity: The Effect of Lap-Band Placement." *Obesity Surgery* 9 (1999): 527–531.

Dolin, Raphael, M.D. "Enterovirus 71—Emerging Infections and Emerging Questions." *New England Journal of Medicine* 341, no. 13 (September 23, 1999): 984–985.

Eberhardt, M. S., D. D. Ingram, D. M. Makuc, et al. National Center for Health Statistics, *Health, United States, 2001 with Urban and Rural Health Chartbook.* Hyattsville, Md.: 2001.

Edmundowicz, Steven A., ed. *20 Common Problems in Gastroenterology.* New York: McGraw-Hill, 2002.

El Mahdy, Christine. *Mummies, Myth and Magic in Ancient Egypt.* New York: Thames and Hudson, 1989.

El-Serag, Hashem B., M.D., et al. "Prevention of Complicated Ulcer Disease among Chronic Users of Nonsteroidal Anti-inflammatory Drugs: The Use of a Nomogram in Cost-effectiveness Analysis." *Archives of Internal Medicine* 162 (October 14, 2002): 2,105–2,110.

El-Serag, Hashem B., M.D., John M. Inadomi, M.D., and Kris V. Kowdley, M.D. "Screening for Hereditary Hemochromatosis in Siblings and Children of Affected Parents." *Annals of Internal Medicine* 132, no. 4 (February 15, 2000): 261–269.

El-Serag, Hashem B., M.D., and Andrew C. Mason, M.D. "Risk Factors for the Rising Rates of Primary Liver Cancer in the United States." *Archives of Internal Medicine* 160 (November 27, 2000): 3,227–3,230.

Elson, Charles O., M.D. "Genes, Microbes, and T Cells—New Therapeutic Targets in Crohn's Disease." *New England Journal of Medicine* 346, no. 8 (February 21, 2002): 614–616.

Ettinger, Mark P., M.D., et al. "Recombinant Variant of Ciliary Neurotrophic Factor for Weight Loss in Obese Adults: A Randomized, Dose-Ranging Study." *Journal of the American Medical Association* 289, no. 13 (April 9, 2003): 1,826–1,832.

Falk, Rodney H., M.D., Raymond L. Comenzo, M.D., and Martha Skinner, M.D. "The Systemic Amyloidoses." *New England Journal of Medicine* 337, no. 13 (September 25, 1997): 898–909.

Fallone, Carlo A., M.D., et al. "Association of *Helicobacter pylori* Genotype with Gastroesophageal Reflux Disease and Other Upper Gastrointestinal Diseases." *American Journal of Gastroenterology* 95, no. 3 (2000): 659–669.

Fan, S. T., et al. "Early Treatment of Acute Biliary Pancreatitis by Endoscopic Papillotomy." *New England Journal of Medicine* 328, no. 4 (January 28, 1993): 228–232.

Farci, Patrizia, et al. "Treatment of Chronic Hepatitis D with Interferon Alfa-2a." *New England Journal of Medicine* 330, no. 2 (January 13, 1994): 88–94.

Farrell, Richard J., M.D., and Ciaran P. Kelly, M.D. "Celiac Sprue." *New England Journal of Medicine* 346, no. 3 (January 17, 2002): 180–188.

Farrell, Philip M., M.D., et al. "Early Diagnosis of Cystic Fibrosis through Neonatal Screening Prevents Severe

Malnutrition and Improves Long-Term Growth." *Pediatrics* 107, no. 1 (January 2001): 1–13.

Ferzoco, L. B., M.D., V. Raptopoulos, M.D., and W. Silen, M.D. "Acute Diverticulitis." *New England Journal of Medicine* 338, no. 21 (May 21, 1998): 1,521–1,526.

Field, Alison E., et al. "Impact of Overweight on the Risk of Developing Common Chronic Diseases during a 10-Year Period." *Archives of Internal Medicine* 161 (July 9, 2001): 1,581–1,586.

Fisher, Richard S., M.D., and Henry P. Parkman, M.D. "Management of Nonulcer Dyspepsia." *New England Journal of Medicine* 339, no. 19 (November 5, 1998): 1,376–1,381.

Flegal, Katherine M., et al. "Prevalence and Trends in Obesity among U.S. Adults, 1999–2000." *Journal of the American Medical Association* 288, no. 14 (October 9, 2002): 1,723–1,727.

Folsch, Ulrich R., M.D., et al. "Early ERCP and Papillotomy Compared with Conservative Treatment for Acute Biliary Pancreatitis." *New England Journal of Medicine* 336, no. 4 (January 23, 1997): 237–242.

Folsom, Aaron R., M.D., et al. "Associations of General and Abdominal Obesity with Multiple Health Outcomes in Older Women." *Archives of Internal Medicine* 160 (July 24, 2000): 2,117–2,128.

Fontaine, Kevin R., et al. "Years of Life Lost Due to Obesity." *Journal of the American Medical Association* 289, no. 2 (January 8, 2003): 187–193.

Food Safety and Inspection Service. "Food Safety Facts: Basics for Handling Food Safely." United States Department of Agriculture, July 2002.

Foote, Mary Ann, Alan Colowick, M.D., and David A. Goodin, M.D. "Basics of Anatomy and Physiology: Red Blood Cells and Anemia." *AMWA Journal* 17, no. 2 (2002): 13–19.

Franz, Marion J. "The Answers to Weight Loss Is Easy—Doing It is Hard!" *Clinical Diabetes* 19, no. 2 (2001): 105–109.

Frisch, Morten, M.D., et al. "Sexually Transmitted Infection as a Cause of Anal Cancer." *New England Journal of Medicine* 337, no. 19 (November 6, 1997): 1,350–1,358.

Fuchs, Charles S., M.D., and Robert J. Mayer, M.D. "Gastric Cancer." *New England Journal of Medicine* 331 (July 6, 1995): 32–41.

Gadde, Kishore M., M.D., et al. "Zonisamide for Weight Loss in Obese Adults: A Randomized Controlled Trial." *Journal of the American Medical Association* 289, no. 14 (April 9, 2003): 1,820–1,825.

Gammon, Marilie, D., et al. "Tobacco, Alcohol, and Socioeconomic Status and Adenocarcinomas of the Esophagus and Gastric Cardia." *Journal of the National Cancer Institute* 89, no. 17 (September 3, 1997): 1,277–1,284.

Ghosh, Subrata, M.D., et al. "Natalizumab for Active Crohn's Disease." *New England Journal of Medicine* 348, no. 1 (January 2, 2003): 24–32.

Ghosh, Subrata, Alan Shand, and Anne Ferguson. "Ulcerative Colitis." *British Medical Journal* 320 (April 22, 2000): 1,119–1,123.

Gordis, Leon, M.D. *Epidemiology.* 2d ed. Philadelphia: W. B. Saunders Company, 2000.

Gordon, Benjamin Lee, M.D. *Medieval and Renaissance Medicine.* New York: Philosophical Library, 1959.

Goyal, Raj K., M.D., and Ikuo Hirano, M.D. "The Enteric Nervous System." *New England Journal of Medicine* 334, no. 17 (April 25, 1996): 1,106–1,115.

Graham, David Y., M.D. "Therapy of *Helicobacter pylori:* Current Status and Issues." *Gastroenterology* 188, no. 2 (2000): S2–S8.

Graham, David Y., M.D., et al. "Ulcer Prevention in Long-term Users of Nonsteroidal Anti-Inflammatory Drugs." *Archives of Internal Medicine* 162 (January 28, 2002): 169–175.

Gulley, James, and Chris H. Takimoto. "Pancreatic Cancer." In *Bethesda Handbook of Clinical Oncology.* New York: Lippincott Williams & Wilkins, 2001.

Hegde, Upendra, and Jean Grem. "Biliary Tract Cancer." In *Bethesda Handbook of Clinical Oncology.* New York: Lippincott Williams & Wilkins, 2001.

Hennessy, Thomas W., M.D., et al. "A National Outbreak of *Salmonella Enteritidis* Infections from Ice Cream." *New England Journal of Medicine* 334, no. 20 (May 16, 1996): 1,281–1,286.

Herrine, Steven K., M.D. "Approach to the Patient with Chronic Hepatitis C Virus Infection." *Annals of Internal Medicine* 136, no. 10 (May 21, 2002): 747–757.

Hirschmann, Jan V., M.D. "What Killed Mozart?" *Archives of Internal Medicine* 161 (June 11, 2001): 1,381–1,389.

Horwitz, Brenda J., M.D., and Robert S. Fisher, M.D. "The Irritable Bowel Syndrome." *New England Journal of Medicine* 344, no. 24 (June 14, 2001): 1,846–1,850.

Izaks, Gerbrand J., M.D., Rudi G. J. Westerndrop, M.D., and Dick L. Knook. "The Definition of Anemia in Older Persons." *Journal of the American Medical Association* 281, no. 18 (May 12, 1999): 1,714–1,717.

Jacobsen, Bjarne K., et al. "Increase in Weight in All Birth Cohorts in a General Population: The Tromso Study, 1974–1994." *Archives of Internal Medicine* 161 (February 12, 2001): 466–472.

Jailwala, Jeegr, M.D., Thomas F. Imperiale, M.D., and Kurt Kroenke, M.D. "Pharmacologic Treatment of the Irritable Bowel Syndrome: A Systematic Review of Randomized, Controlled Trials." *Annals of Internal Medicine* 133, no. 2 (2000): 136–147.

Jasmer, Robert M., M.D., Payam Nahid, M.D., and Philip C. Hopewell, M.D. "Latent Tuberculosis Infection." *New England Journal of Medicine* 347, no. 23 (December 5, 2002): 1,860–1,866.

Jennette, J. Charles, M.D., and Ronald J. Falk, M.D. "Small-Vessel Vasculitis." *New England Journal of Medicine* 337, no. 21 (November 20, 1997): 1,512–1,523.

Joint World Health Organization and Food and Agriculture Organization of the United Nations. "Diet, Nutrition and the Prevention of Chronic Diseases. Report of a Joint WHO/FAO Expert Consultation." *WHO Technical Report Series* 916, Geneva, Switzerland, 2003.

Kandel, Joseph, M.D., and Christine Adamec. *The Encyclopedia of Senior Health and Well-Being.* New York: Facts On File, 2003.

Kaplan, Marshall M., M.D. "Primary Biliary Cirrhosis." *New England Journal of Medicine* 335, no. 21 (November 21, 1996): 1,570–1,580.

———. "Toward Better Treatment of Primary Sclerosing Cholangitis." *New England Journal of Medicine* 336, no. 10 (March 6, 1997): 719–721.

Keene, William E., et al. "A Swimming-Associated Outbreak of Hemorrhagic Colitis Caused by Escherichia coli 0157:H7 and Shigella Sonnei." *New England Journal of Medicine* 331, no. 9 (September 1, 1994): 579–584.

Kenchaiah, Satish, M.D., et al. "Obesity and the Risk of Heart Failure." *New England Journal of Medicine* 347, no. 5 (August 1, 2002): 305–313.

Kenyon, Thomas, A., M.D. "Immigration and Tuberculosis Among Children on the United States–Mexico Border, County of San Diego, California." *Pediatrics* 104, no. 1 (July 1999): e8.

Key, Timothy J., et al. "The Effect of Diet on Risk of Cancer." *Lancet* 360, no. 9336 (September 14, 2002): 861–868.

Khaitan, Leena, M.D., and Michael D. Holzman, M.D. "Laparoscopic Advances in General Surgery." *Journal of the American Medical Association* 287, no. 12 (March 27, 2002): 1,502–1,505.

Khan, Kamran, M.D., et al. "Global Drug-Resistance Patterns and the Management of Latent Tuberculosis Infection in Immigrants to the United States." *New England Journal of Medicine* 347, no. 23 (December 5, 2002): 1,850–1,859.

Khan, Laura Kettel, et al. "Use of Prescription Weight Loss Pills among U.S. Adults in 1996–1998." *Annals of Internal Medicine* 134, no. 4 (2001): 282–286.

Kim, George P., and Chris H. Takimoto. "Gastric Cancer." In *Bethesda Handbook of Clinical Oncology.* New York: Lippincott Williams & Wilkins, 2001.

Kim, George P., Chris H. Takimoto, and Carmen Allegra. "Colorectal Cancer." In *Bethesda Handbook of Clinical Oncology.* Philadelphia: Lippincott, Williams & Wilkins, 2001.

Kjaegard, Lise L., M.D., et al. "Artificial and Bioartificial Support Systems for Acute and Acute-on-Chronic Liver Failure." *Journal of the American Medical Association* 289, no. 2 (January 8, 2003): 217–222.

Knowles, Michael R., M.D., and Peter R. Durie, M.D. "What Is Cystic Fibrosis?" *New England Journal of Medicine* 347, no. 6 (August 8, 2002): 439–442.

Knox, Tamsin A., M.D., and Lori B. Olans, M.D. "Liver Disease in Pregnancy." *New England Journal of Medicine* 335, no. 8 (August 22, 1996): 569–576.

Kotler, Donald P., M.D. "Cachexia." *Annals of Internal Medicine* 133, no. 8 (2000): 622–634.

Kumar, Shaji, M.D., Michael G. Sarr, M.D., and Patrick S. Kamath, M.D. "Mesenteric Venous Thrombosis." *New England Journal of Medicine* 345, no. 23 (December 6, 2001): 1,683–1,688.

Laine, Loren, and Walter L. Peterson. "Bleeding Peptic Ulcer." *New England Journal of Medicine* 331, no. 11 (September 15, 1994): 717–727.

Lanas, A. I., et al. "Risk Factors Associated with Refractory Peptic Ulcers." *Gastroenterology* 109, no. 4 (1995): 1,124–1,133.

Lange, Paul H., M.D., and Christine Adamec. *Prostate Cancer for Dummies.* New York: Wiley Publishing, 2003.

Langman, Michael J., M.D. "Adverse Upper Gastrointestinal Effects of Rofecoxib Compared with NSAIDs." *Journal of the American Medical Association* 282, no. 20 (November 24, 1999): 1,929–1,933.

Langner, Elke, Stefan Greifenberg, and Joeg Gruenwald. "Ginger: History and Use." *Advances in Therapy* 15, no. 1 (January/February 1998): 25–44.

Lawrence, Steven P., M.D. "Evaluation of Focal Liver Masses." In *GI/Liver Secrets.* 2d ed. Philadelphia: Hanley & Belfus, 2001.

Lee, Thomas H., M.D., and Lee Goldman, M.D. "Evaluation of the Patient with Acute Chest Pain." *New England Journal of Medicine* 342, no. 16 (April 20, 2000): 1,187–1,195.

Leitzmann, Michael F., M.D., et al. "Recreational Physical Activity and the Risk of Cholecystectomy in Women." *New England Journal of Medicine* 341, no. 11 (September 9, 1999): 777–784.

Leung, Donald Y. M., M.D., et al. "Effect of Anti-IgE Therapy in Patients with Peanut Allergy." *New England Journal of Medicine* 348, no. 11 (March 13, 2003): 986–993.

Levenstein, Susan, et al. "Stress and Peptic Ulcer Disease." *Journal of the American Medical Association* 281, no. 1 (January 6, 1999): 10–11.

Lewey, Scott M., and Peter R. McNally. "Endoscopic Cancer Screening and Surveillance." In *GI/Liver Secrets*. 2d ed. Philadelphia: Hanley & Belfus, 2001.

Lieber, Charles S., M.D. "Alcohol and Hepatitis C." *Alcohol Research & Health* 25, no. 4 (2001): 245–254.

Lieberman, David A., et al. "Patterns of Endoscopy Use in the United States." *Gastroenterology* 118, no. 3 (2000): 619–624.

Lieberman, David A., M.D., et al. "Use of Colonoscopy to Screen Asymptomatic Adults for Colorectal Cancer. *New England Journal of Medicine* 343, no. 3 (July 20, 2000): 162–168.

List, James F., M.D., and Joel F. Habener, M.D. "Defective Melanocortin 4 Receptors in Hyperphagia and Morbid Obesity." *New England Journal of Medicine* 348, no. 12 (March 20, 2003): 1,160–1,163.

MacKenzie, William R., et al. "A Massive Outbreak in Milwaukee of *Cryptosporidium* Infection Transmitted through the Public Water Supply." *New England Journal of Medicine* 331, no. 3 (July 21, 1994): 161–167.

Maisels, M. Jeffrey, and Elizabeth Kring. "Length of Stay, Jaundice, and Hospital Readmission." *Pediatrics* 101, no. 6 (June 1998): 995–998.

Mayne, Susan T., et al. "Nutrient Intake and Risk of Subtypes of Esophageal and Gastric Cancer." *Cancer Epidemiology, Biomarkers & Prevention* 10 (October 2001): 1,055–1,062.

McCarthy, Nicole, and Jean Grem. "Esophageal Cancer." In *Bethesda Handbook of Clinical Oncology*. New York: Lippincott Williams & Wilkins, 2001.

McGlynn, Katherine A., et al. "International Trends and Patterns of Primary Liver Cancer." *International Journal of Cancer* 94 (2001): 290–296.

McNally, Peter R. *GI/Liver Secrets*. 2d ed. Philadelphia: Hanley & Belfus, 2001.

McTigue, Kathleen M., M.D., et al. "The Natural History of the Development of Obesity in a Cohort of Young U.S. Adults between 1981 and 1998." *Annals of Internal Medicine* 136, no. 12 (June 2002): 857–864.

Mehler, Philip S., M.D. "Diagnosis and Care of Patients with Anorexia Nervosa in Primary Care Settings." *Annals of Internal Medicine* 134, no. 11 (June 2001): 1,048–1,059.

Mesiya, Sikander A., M.D., and Anil Minocha, M.D. "Gastrointestinal Disease in Diabetes Mellitus." *Southern Medical Journal* (Winter 1998/1999): 33–38.

Meyer, Joette M., et al. "Risk Factors for *Helicobacter pylori* Resistance in the United States: The Surveillance of *H. pylori* Antimicrobial Resistance Partnership (SHARP) Study, 1993–1998." *Annals of Internal Medicine* 136, no. 1 (2002): 13–24.

Miniño, Arialdi, M., et al. "Deaths: Final Data for 2000." *National Vital Statistics Report* 50, no. 15 (September 15, 2002).

Minocha, Anil, M.D., et al. "Alterations in Upper Gastrointestinal Motility in *Helicobacter pylori*-positive Nonulcer Dyspepsia." *American Journal of Gastroenterology* 89, no. 10, (1994): 1,797–1,800.

Minocha, Anil, M.D., and Srinivasan, Radhika, M.D. "Conscious Sedation: Pearls and Perils." *Digestive Diseases and Sciences* 43, no. 8 (August 1998): 1,835–1,844.

Minocha, Anil, M.D. *The Gastroenterology Resident Pocket Survival Guide*. McLean, Va.: International Medical Publishing, 1999.

Minocha, Anil, M.D., et al. "*Helicobacter pylori* Is Associated with Alterations in Intestinal Gas Profile among Patients with Nonulcer Dyspepsia." *Digestive Diseases and Sciences* 39, no. 8 (August 1994): 1,613–1,617.

Minocha, Anil, M.D., and Christine Adamec. *How to Stop Heartburn: Simple Ways to Heal Heartburn and Acid Reflux*. New York: John Wiley & Sons, 2001.

Minocha, Anil, M.D., C. A. Racakowski, M.D., and Robert J. Richards, M.D. "Is a History of Tonsillectomy Associated with a Decreased Risk of *Helicobacter pylori* Infection?" *Journal of Clinical Gastroenterology* 25, no. 4 (1997): 580–582.

Minocha, Anil, M.D., and David Carroll. *Natural Stomach Care*. New York: Penguin Putnam, 2003.

Minocha, Anil, M.D. "Noncardiac Chest Pain: Where Does It Start?" *Postgraduate Medicine* 100, no. 6 (December 1996): 107–114.

Minocha, Anil, M.D., and Abraham S. Joseph, M.D. "Pathophysiology and Management of Noncardiac Pain." *KMA Journal* 93, no. 5 (May 1995): 196–201.

Minocha, Anil, M.D., and David S. Greenbaum, M.D. "Pill-Esophagitis Caused by Nonsteroidal Antiinflammatory Drugs." *American Journal of Gastroenterology* 86, no. 8 (1991): 1,086–1,089.

Minocha, Anil, M.D., et al. "Prevalence of Previous Appendectomy among Patients Needing Gastrointestinal Endoscopy." *Southern Medical Journal* 92, no. 1 (January 1999): 41–43.

Minocha, A., and C. A. Raczkowski. "Role of Appendectomy and Tonsillectomy in Pathogenesis of Ulcerative Colitis." *Digestive Disease Sciences* 42 (1997): 1,567–1,569.

Montague, Carl T., and Stephen O'Rahilly. "The Perils of Portliness: Causes and Consequences of Visceral Adiposity." *Diabetes* 49 (June 2000): 883–888.

Morris Brown, Linda, and Susan S. Devesa. "Epidemiologic Trends in Esophageal and Gastric Cancer in the United States." *Surgical Oncology Clinics of North America* 11 (2002): 235–256.

Morris Brown, Linda, Susan S. Devesa, and Joseph F. Fraumeni, M.D. "Epidemiology of Esophageal Cancer." In *Atlas of Clinical Oncology: Cancer of the Upper Gastrointestinal Tract.* London: B. C. Decker, 2002.

Murray, Karen F., M.D., and Kris V. Kowdley, M.D. "Neonatal Hemochromatosis." *Pediatrics* 108, no. 4 (October 2001): 960–964.

National Cancer Institute. "What You Need to Know about Cancer of the Pancreas." NIH Publication no. 01-1560, February 8, 2002.

National Center for Chronic Disease Prevention and Health Promotion. "The Burden of Chronic Diseases and Their Risk Factors: National and State Perspectives." Centers for Disease Control and Prevention, 2002.

National Cholesterol Education Program. "Third Report of the National Cholesterol Education Program (NCEP) Expert Panel on Detection, Evaluation, and Treatment of High Blood Cholesterol in Adults (Adult Treatment Panel III)." NIH Publication no. 02-5215, September 2002.

National Institute of Allergy and Infectious Diseases. "Fact Sheet: Foodborne Diseases." National Institutes of Health, April 2002.

National Institute of Allergy and Infectious Diseases. "Deciphering Pathogens: Blueprints for New Medical Tools." National Institutes of Health, NIH Publication no. 02-4987, September 2002.

National Institute of Allergy and Infectious Diseases. "Microbes: In Sickness and in Health." National Institutes of Health, NIH Publication no. 01-4914, September 2001.

National Institute of Allergy and Infectious Diseases. "NIAID Global Health Research Plan for HIV/AIDS, Malaria, and Tuberculosis." Undated.

National Institute of Diabetes and Digestive and Kidney Diseases. "Conquering Diabetes: Highlights of Program Efforts, Research Advances and Opportunities." U.S. Department of Health and Human Services, NIH Publication no. 02-5137, September 2002.

National Task Force on the Prevention and Treatment of Obesity. "Overweight, Obesity, and Health Risk." *Archives of Internal Medicine* 160 (April 10, 2000): 898–904.

Newman, Julliana. "Radiographic and Endoscopic Evaluation of the Upper GI Tract." *Radiologic Technology* 69, no. 3 (January/February 1998): 213–227.

Newman, Lee S., et al. "Sarcoidosis." *New England Journal of Medicine* 336, no. 17 (April 24, 1997): 1,224–1,234.

Noll, Richard. *The Encyclopedia of Schizophrenia and Other Psychotic Disorders.* 2d ed. New York: Facts On File, 2001.

O'Leary, Paula F. G., M.D., M.R.C.P.I., M.R.C. Path., and Fergus Shanahan, M.D., F.R.C.P. (UK). "Food Allergies," *Current Gastroenterology Reports* 4 (2002): 373–382.

Olivieri, Nancy F., M.D. "The ß-Thalssemias." *New England Journal of Medicine* 341, no. 2 (July 8, 1999): 99–109.

Ostapowicz G., et al. "Results of a Prospective Study of Acute Liver Failure at 17 Tertiary Care Centers in the United States." *Annals of Internal Medicine* 137 (December 2002): 947–954.

Pallis, Athanasios G., Ioannis G. Vlchonikolis, and Ioannis A. Mouzas. "Assessing Health-Related Quality of Life in Patients with Inflammatory Bowel Disease in Crete, Greece." *BMC Gastroenterology* 2, no. 1 (January 10, 2002). Available on-line. URL: www.biomedcentral.com/ 1471-230X/2/1.

Pandit, Manjula K., M.D., et al. "Drug-induced Disorders of Glucose Tolerance." *Annals of Internal Medicine* 118, no. 7 (April 1, 1993): 529–539.

Parashar, Umesh D., et al. "Trends in Intussusception-Associated Hospitalizations and Deaths among US Infants." *Pediatrics* 106, no. 6 (December 2000): 1,413–1,421.

Parker, Alex, et al. "A Gene Conferring Susceptibility to Type 2 Diabetes in Conjunction with Obesity is Located on Chromosome 18p11," *Diabetes* 50 (March 2001): 675–680.

Pearlman, Brian L., M.D. "The New Cholesterol Guidelines: Applying Them in Clinical Practice." *Postgraduate Medicine* 11, no. 2 (August 2002): 13–26.

Petit, William, Jr., M.D., and Christine Adamec. *The Encyclopedia of Diabetes.* New York: Facts On File, 2002.

Petrakis, John, M.D., et al. "Enhancement of Gastric Emptying of Solids by Erythromycin in Patients with Roux-en-Y Gastrojejunostomy." *Archives of Surgery* 133, no. 7 (July 1998): 709–714.

Pfenninger, John L. "Common Anorectal Conditions. Part III. Lesions." *American Family Physician,* July 1, 2001.

Podolsky, Daniel K., M.D. "Inflammatory Bowel Disease." *New England Journal of Medicine* 347, no. 6 (August 8, 2002): 417–429.

Ponec, Robert J., M.D., Michael D. Saunders, M.D., and Michael B. Kimmey, M.D. "Neostigmine for the Treatment of Acute Colonic Pseudo-Obstruction." *New England Journal of Medicine* 341, no. 3 (July 15, 1999): 137–141.

Ponsky, Lee E., et al. "Contemporary 'Urobiologic' Intervention in the Pancreaticobiliary Tree." *Urology* 57, no. 1 (2001): 21–25.

Prasad, K. R., and J. P. A. Lodge. "Transplantation of the Liver and Pancreas." *British Medical Journal* 322 (April 7, 2001): 845–847.

Pratt, Daniel S., M.D., and Marshall M. Kaplan, M.D. "Evaluation of Abnormal Liver-Enzyme Results in Asymptomatic Patients." *New England Journal of Medicine* 342, no. 17 (April 27, 2000): 1,266–1,271.

Quick, Clive R. G., et al. "Appendicitis." In *Essential Surgery: Problems, Diagnosis and Management.* 3d ed. Edinburgh, Scotland: Churchill Livingstone, 2001.

Rabbani, G. H., M.D. "The Search for a Better Oral Rehydration Solution for Cholera." *New England Journal of Medicine* 342, no. 5 (February 3, 2000): 345–347.

Räihä, Ismo, M.D., et al. "Lifestyle, Stress, and Genes in Peptic Ulcer Disease: A Nationwide Twin Cohort Study." *Archives of Internal Medicine* 158 (April 13, 1998): 698–704.

Rao, Patrick M., M.D., et al. "Effect of Computer Tomography of the Appendix on Treatment of Patients and Use of Hospital Resources." *New England Journal of Medicine* 338, no. 3 (January 15, 1998): 141–146.

Raoult, Didier, M.D., et al. "Cultivation of the Bacillus of Whipple's Disease." *New England Journal of Medicine* 342, no. 9 (March 2, 2000): 620–625.

Rayner, Christopher K. "Relationships of Upper Gastrointestinal Motor and Sensory Function with Glycemic Control." *Diabetes Care* 24, no. 2 (February 2001): 371–381.

Rockey, Don C., M.D. "Occult Gastrointestinal Bleeding." *New England Journal of Medicine* 341, no. 1 (July 1, 1999): 38–46.

Ruskone-Fourmestraux, A., et al. "Multiple Lymphomatous Polyposis of the Gastrointestinal Tract: Prospective Clinicopathologic Study of 31 Cases." *Gastroenterology* 112, no. 1 (January 1997): 7–16.

Ryan, David P., M.D., Carolyn C. Compton, M.D., and Robert J. Mayer, M.D. "Carcinoma of the Anal Canal." *New England Journal of the Medicine* 342, no. 11 (March 16, 2000): 792–800.

Ryan, David P., M.D., and Kevin C. Kain, M.D. "Health Advice and Immunizations for Travelers." *New England Journal of Medicine* 342, no. 23 (June 8, 2000): 1,716–1,725.

Ryan, Edward T., M.D., Mary E. Wison, M.D., and Kevin C. Kain, M.D. "Illness after International Travel." *New England Journal of Medicine* 347, no. 7 (August 15, 2002): 505–516.

Safdar, Nasia, M.D., and Dennis G. Maki, M.D. "The Commonality of Risk Factors for Nosocomial Colonization and Infection with Antimicrobial-Resistant *Staphylococcus aureus*, Enterococcus, Gram-Negative Bacilli, *Clostridium difficile*, and *Candida*." *Annals of Internal Medicine* 136 (2002): 834–844.

Sakane, Tsuyoshi, M.D., et al. "Behçet's Disease." *New England Journal of Medicine* 341, no. 17 (October 21, 1999): 1,284–1,291.

Salam, Gohar A. "Lipoma Excision." *American Family Physician* 65 (March 1, 2002): 901–904, 905.

Salbe, Arline D., et al. "Assessing Risk Factors for Obesity between Childhood and Adolescence. I. Birth Weight, Childhood Adiposity, Parental Obesity, Insulin, and Leptin." *Pediatrics* 110, no. 2 (August 2002): 299–306.

Salbe, Arline D., et al. "Assessing Risk Factors for Obesity between Childhood and Adolescence. II. Energy Metabolism and Physical Activity." *Pediatrics* 110, no. 2 (August 2002): 307–314.

Sampliner, Richard E., M.D. "Barrett's esophagus." In *GI/Liver Secrets.* 2d ed. Philadelphia: PA: Hanley & Belfus, 2001.

Sandler, Adrian D., M.D., et al. "Lack of Benefit of a Single Dose of Synthetic Human Secretin in the Treatment of Autism and Pervasive Development Disorder." *New England Journal of Medicine* 341, no. 24 (December 9, 1999): 1,801–1,806.

Satin, Morton. *Food Alert! The Ultimate Sourcebook for Food Safety.* New York: Facts On File, 1999.

Schaaf, H. Simon, M.Med., et al. "Evaluation of Young Children in Contact with Adult Multidrug-Resistant Pulmonary Tuberculosis: A 30-Month Follow-up." *Pediatrics* 109, no. 5 (May 2002): 765–771.

Schoenborn, Charlotte A., Patricia F. Adams, and Patricia M. Barnes. "Body Weight Status of Adults: United States, 1997–1998." *Advance Data from Vital and Health Statistics* no. 330 (September 6, 2002).

Schoenborn, Charlotte A., Patricia M. Barnes, and Division of Health Interview Statistics. "Leisure-Time Physical Activity among Adults: United States, 1997–98." *Advance Data from Vital and Health Statistics* no. 325 (April 7, 2002).

Schoenborn, Charlotte A., Jackline A. Vickerie, Patricia M. Barnes, and Division of Health Interview Statistics. "Cigarette Smoking Behavior of Adults: United States, 1997–1998." *Advance Data from Vital and Health Statistics* no. 331 (February 7, 2003).

Sciamanna, Christopher N., M.D., et al. "Who Reports Receiving Advice to Lose Weight? Results from a Multistate Survey." *Archives of Internal Medicine* 160 (August 14/28, 2000): 2,334–2,339.

Shaheen, Nicholas, M.D., and David F. Ransohoff, M.D. "Gastroesophageal Reflux, Barrett Esophagus, and Esophageal Cancer: Clinical Applications." *Journal of the American Medical Association* 287, no. 15 (April 17, 2002): 1,982–1,996.

Showstack, Jonathan, et al. "Resource Utilization in Liver Transplantation: Effects of Patient Characteristics and

Clinical Practice." *Journal of the American Medical Association* 281, no. 15 (April 21, 1999): 1,381–1,386.

Sicherer, Scott H., M.D., and Jerry A. Winkelstein, M.D. "Primary Immunodeficiency Diseases in Adults." *Journal of the American Medical Association* 279, no. 1 (January 7, 1998): 58–61.

Slonim, Alfred E., M.D., et al. "A Preliminary Study of Growth Hormone Therapy for Crohn's Disease." *New England Journal of Medicine* 342, no. 22 (June 1, 2000): 1,633–1,637.

Small, Peter M., M.D., and Paula I. Fujiwara, M.D. "Management of Tuberculosis in the United States." *The New England Journal of Medicine* 345, no. 3 (July 19, 2001): 189–200.

Srinivasan, Radhika, M.D., and Anil Minocha, M.D. "When to Suspect Lactose Intolerance." *Postgraduate Medicine* 104, no. 3 (September 1998): 109–123.

Starzl, Thomas E. "The Contribution of Transplantation to Gastroenterologic Knowledge." In *The Growth of Gastroenterologic Knowledge During the Twentieth Century.* Philadelphia: Lea & Ferbiger, 1994.

Staud, Roland, M.D., and Christine Adamec. *Fibromyalgia for Dummies.* New York: John Wiley & Sons, 2002.

Steinberg, William, and Scott Tenner. "Acute Pancreatitis." *New England Journal of Medicine* 330, no. 17 (April 28, 1994): 1,198–1,210.

Stern, Robert C., M.D. "The Diagnosis of Cystic Fibrosis." *New England Journal of Medicine* 3336, no. 7 (February 13, 1997): 487–491.

Stewart, Paul M., et al. "Cortisol Metabolism in Human Obesity: Impaired Cortisone [arrow] Cortisol Conversion in Subjects with Central Adiposity." *Journal of Clinical Endocrinology & Metabolism* 84, no. 3 (1999): 1,022–1,027.

Story, Mary T. "Management of Child and Adolescent Obesity: Attitudes, Barriers, Skills, and Training Needs among Health Care Professionals." *Pediatrics* 110, no. 1 (July 2002): 210–214.

St. Peter, Shawn D., M.D., Maher A. Abbas, M.D., and Keith A. Kelly, M.D. "The Spectrum of Pneumatosis Intestinalis." *Archives of Surgery* 138, no. 1 (January 200?): 68–75.

Stuart, Jon Spechler, M.D. "Barrett's Esophagus." *New England Journal of Medicine* 346, no. 11 (March 14, 2002): 836–842.

Suerbaum, Sebastian, M.D., and Michetti, Pierre, M.D. "*Helicobacter pylori* Infection." *New England Journal of Medicine* 347, no. 15 (October 10, 2002): 1,175–1,186.

Swagerty, Daniel L., Jr., M.D., M.P.H., Anne D. Walling, M.D., and Robert M. Klein. "Lactose Intolerance." *American Family Physician* 65, no. 9 (May 1, 2002): 1,845–1,850.

Swartz, Morton N., M.D. "Whipple's Disease—Past, Present, and Future." *New England Journal of Medicine* 342, no. 9 (March 2, 2000): 648–650.

Syngal, Sapna, et al. "Long-Term Weight Patterns and Risk for Cholecystectomy in Women." *Annals of Internal Medicine* 130, no. 6 (March 16, 1999): 471–477.

Tauxe, Robert V., and James M. Hughes. "International Investigation of Outbreaks of Foodborne Disease." *British Medical Journal* 313 (November 2, 1996): 1,093–1,094.

Tibbles, Patrick M., M.D., and John S. Edelsberg, M.D. "Hyerbaric-Oxygen Therapy." *New England Journal of Medicine* 334, no. 25 (June 20, 1996): 1,642–1,648.

Tierney, Lawrence M., Jr., M.D., Stephen J. McPhee, M.D., and Maxine A. Papadakis, M.D., eds. *Current Medical Diagnosis and Treatment 2002.* New York: Lange Medical Books, 2002.

Toh, Ban-Hock, Ian R. van Direl, and Paul A. Gleeson. "Pernicious Anemia." *New England Journal of Medicine* 447, no. 20 (November 13, 1997): 1,441–1,448.

Toribara, Neil, M.D. "Colorectal Cancer." In *GI Liver Secrets.* 2d ed. Philadelphia: Hanley & Belfus, 2001.

Trudgill, Nigel J., et al. "Familial Clustering of Reflux Symptoms." *American Journal of Gastroenterology* 94, no. 5 (1999): 1,172–1,178.

Uemura, Naomi, M.D., et al. "*Helicobacter Pylori* Infection and the Development of Gastric Cancer." *New England Journal of Medicine* 345, no. 11 (September 13, 2001): 784–789.

United States Department of Agriculture. "Foodborne Illness: What Consumers Need to Know." Undated.

United States Department of Agriculture's Meat and Poultry Hotline. "Molds on Food: Are They Dangerous?" April 2002.

Vaira, Dino, M.D., et al. "The Stool Antigen Test for Detection of *Helicobacter pylori* after Eradication Therapy." *Annals of Internal Medicine* 136, no. 4 (February 19, 2002): 280–287.

Van Dam, Jacques, M.D., and William R. Brugge, M.D. "Endoscopy of the Upper Gastrointestinal Tract." *New England Journal of Medicine* 341, no. 23 (December 2, 1999): 1,738–1,748.

Vinik, Aaron, M.D., et al. "Gastrointestinal, Genitourinary, and Neurovascular Disturbances in Diabetes." *Diabetes Reviews* 7, no. 4 (1996): 346–366.

Wannamethee, S. Goya, and A. Gerald Shaper. "Weight Change and Duration of Overweight and Obesity in the Incidence of Type 2 Diabetes." *Diabetes Care* 22, no. 8 (August 1999): 1,266–1,272.

Weil, Evette, et al. "Obesity among Adults with Disabling Conditions." *Journal of the American Medical*

*Association* 288, no. 10 (September 11, 2002): 1,265–1,268.

Weinberg, David S., and Christine Laine. "Colorectal Cancer Screening." In *20 Common Problems in Gastroenterology.* New York: McGraw-Hill Medical Publishing Division, 2002.

Whitaker, Robert C., M.D., et al. "Predicting Obesity in Young Adulthood from Childhood and Parental Obesity." *New England Journal of Medicine* 337, no. 13 (September 25, 1997): 869–873.

White, David G., et al. "The Isolation of Antibiotic-Resistant *Salmonella* from Retail Ground Meats." *New England Journal of Medicine* 345, no. 16 (October 18, 2001): 1,147–1,154.

Whitehead, William E., and Marvin M. Schuster, M.D. "Behavioral Approaches to the Treatment of Gastrointestinal Motility Disorders." *Medical Clinics of North America* 65, no. 5 (November 1981): 1,397–1,410.

Whitley, Richard J., M.D., et al. "Guidelines for the Treatment of Cytomegalovirus Diseases in Patients with AIDS in the Era of Potent Antiretroviral Therapy: Recommendations of an International Panel." *Archives of Internal Medicine* 158 (May 11, 1998): 957–969.

Wilschanski, Michael, et al. "Clinical and Genetic Risk Factors for Cystic Fibrosis-related Liver Disease." *Pediatrics* 103, no. 1 (January 1999): 52–57.

Wing, Rena R., et al. "Behavioral Science Research in Diabetes: Lifestyle Changes Related to Obesity, Eating Behavior, and Physical Activity." *Diabetes Care* 24, no. 1 (January 2001): 117–123.

Wirth, Alfred, M.D., and Jutta Krause. "Long-Term Weight Loss with Sibutramine: A Randomized Controlled Trial." *Journal of the American Medical Association* 286, no. 11 (September 19, 2001): 1,331–1,339.

Wolosin, James D., M.D., and Steven V. Edelman. "Diabetes and the Gastrointestinal Tract." *Clinical Diabetes* 18, no. 4 (Fall 2000): 148–151.

World Health Organization. *Diet, Food Supply and Obesity in the Pacific.* Geneva, Switzerland, 2003.

World Health Organization. "Diet, Nutrition and the Prevention of Chronic Diseases." WHO Technical Report Series 916, Geneva, Switzerland, 2003.

World Health Organization. *The World Health Report 2002: Reducing Risks, Promoting Healthy Life.* Geneva, Switzerland, 2002.

Wright, Charlotte M., et al. "Effect of Community Based Management in Failure to Thrive: Randomised Controlled Trial." *British Medical Journal* 317 (1998): 571–574.

Wood, Bradford J., and Razavi Pouneh. "Virtual Endoscopy: A Promising New Technology." *American Family Physician* 66, no. 66 (July 1, 2002): 107–112.

Wynbrandt, James, and Mark D. Ludman. "Gilbert disease." In *The Encyclopedia of Genetic Disorders and Birth Defects.* 2d ed. New York: Facts On File, 2000.

Yang, Hwai-I, et al. "Hepatitis B e Antigen and the Risk of Hepatocellular Carcinoma." *New England Journal of Medicine* 347, no. 3 (July 18, 2002): 168–174.

Yanovski, Susan Z., M.D., and Jack A. Yanovski, M.D. "Obesity." *New England Journal of Medicine* 346, no. 8 (February 21, 2002): 591–602.

Zebrack, Brad J., et al. "Psychological Outcomes in Long-Term Survivors of Childhood Leukemia, Hodgkin's Disease, and Non-Hodgkin's Lymphoma: A Report from the Childhood Cancer Survivor Study." *Pediatrics* 110, no. 1 (July 2002): 42–52.

# INDEX